Foreword

The success of this Review series to date has been a tribute to Dr Kaufman's undoubted skill as an editor in his selection and treatment of such a range of important current topics of paramount interest to the anaesthetist and in acquiring such a panel of excellent contributors.

The sheer bulk of published literature can deter if not defeat even the best intentioned seeker after knowledge, particularly in arriving at a balanced and critical judgement of what is and what is not of real importance to the maintenance of the highest standards of practice. In this respect, up-to-date and authoritative reviews of this kind can be of great value to clinicians who wish to be well informed. Readability is also an important matter since even the greatest truths can be obscured by poor presentation.

This volume maintains the high standard of its two predecessors in that it presents in a splendidly readable form a distillation of current knowledge on a wide range of anaesthetic and related matters. It is a model of its kind and it is to be hoped that its predictable success will encourage Dr Kaufman to continue his labours on behalf of his grateful colleagues.

1985   D.C.

Anaesthesia: Review 3

Anaesthesia:
Review 3

Edited by

Leon Kaufman

MD, FFARCS

Consultant Anaesthetist, University College Hospital, London;
Consultant Anaesthetist, St Mark's Hospital, London;
Honorary Senior Lecturer, University College London School of Medicine

Foreword by
Donald Campbell

MB, ChB, FFARCS, FRCP (Glasg)

Professor of Anaesthesia, University of Glasgow;
Honorary Consultant Anaesthetist, Glasgow Royal Infirmary

CHURCHILL LIVINGSTONE
EDINBURGH LONDON MELBOURNE AND NEW YORK 1985

CHURCHILL LIVINGSTONE
Medical Division of Longman Group Limited

Distributed in the United States of America by Churchill
Livingstone Inc., 1560 Broadway, New York, N.Y. 10036,
and by associated companies, branches and representatives
throughout the world.

First published 1985

ISBN 0 443 03202 5
ISSN 0263-1512

British Library Cataloguing in Publication Data
Anaesthesia.—Review 3.
  1. Anesthesia—Periodicals
  617'.96'05   RD78.3

Printed in Great Britain by
Butler & Tanner Ltd, Frome and London

Preface

The plethora of literature appertaining to anaesthesia has prompted the early appearance of Review 3 despite pleas of some critics for a longer interval between publication. The reviewers have been generous in their comments and constructive in their criticism, but recent published reviews have appeared too late to influence the presentation of this volume. As before there is a distinct emphasis on the medical problems confronting the anaesthetist. There are chapters on drugs and disease as they affect the course of anaesthesia, the assessment of patients with cardiac disease for non-cardiac operations, the assessment of patients with liver disease, and a chapter on myopathies. An anaesthetist and a pharmacologist consider different aspects of endorphins and although the relevance of opioid receptors may still be speculative the subject and terminology cannot be dismissed lightly.

There is also an historical review of the muscle relaxants culminating in the development of short acting drugs including one which is destroyed by non-enzymatic means. Some repetition is inevitable but the emphasis differs as is seen in the chapters on obstetric anaesthesia and analgesia. The problems associated with blood transfusion are extensively reviewed with comments on the introduction of modified haemoglobin solutions and the introduction of synthetic substitutes: an update has had to be appended to this section.

There is a study of the assessment of normal brain function during general anaesthesia while a chapter on neurosurgery which originally appeared in Review 1 has been extensively revised. The introduction of isoflurane has prompted chapters on inhalational agents and gaseous exchange during general anaesthesia. The management of inhalational burns is followed by a review of modern concepts of resuscitation. A short appendix revises some of the material found in Review 2.

I am grateful for the expertise and enthusiasm shown by my colleagues and their secretaries in the prompt preparation of their contributions. The co-ordination of the whole volume was made possible by the constant commitment of our secretary, Miss S. Wiggins while Mr T. Wells provided advice and assistance on the programming of the DEC computers.

1985   L.K.

Contributors

Rodney F. Armstrong MB, BS, FFARCS
Consultant, Departments of Anaesthesia and Intensive Care, University College Hospital, London

M. A. Branthwaite MD, FRCP, FFARCS
Consultant Physician and Anaesthetist, Brompton Hospital, London

John Efthimiou BSc, MRCP
North East Thames Regional Research Fellow and Honorary Clinical Lecturer, Department of Medicine, University College Hospital, The Rayne Institute, London

Stanley Feldman BSc, MB, BS, FFARCS
Consultant Anaesthetist, Magill Department of Anaesthesia, Westminster Hospital, London

A. H. Goldstone MA (Oxon), FRCP, FRCPE, MRCPath
Consultant Haematologist, University College Hospital, London; and Honorary Senior Lecturer in Haematology, University College Hospital Medical School, London

Ronald Greenbaum MB, ChB, DObst RCOG, FFARCS
Consultant Anaesthetist, University College Hospital, London; and Clinical Teacher, University College London

Christopher Heneghan BA, BM, BCh, FFARCS
Consultant Anaesthetist, Division of Anaesthesia, Clinical Research Centre, Harrow, Middlesex; and Honorary Consultant Anaesthetist, Department of Anaesthetics, Northwick Park Hospital, Harrow, Middlesex

C. W. Howell MB, FFARCS
Consultant Anaesthetist, King's College Hospital, London

G. Stewart Ingram MB, BS, FFARCS
Consultant Anaesthetist, The National Hospital for Nervous Diseases, Queen Square, and University College Hospital, London; and Honorary Senior Lecturer, University of London

J. Gareth Jones MD, FRCP, FFARCS
MRC Scientific Staff and Honorary Consultant Anaesthetist, Northwick Park Hospital, Harrow, Middlesex

Christopher C. Jordan BSc, PhD
Senior Research Leader, Department of Neuropharmacology, Glaxo Group Research Ltd, Ware, Hertfordshire

Leon Kaufman MD, FFARCS
Consultant Anaesthetist, University College Hospital, London, and St Mark's Hospital, London; and Honorary Senior Lecturer, University College London School of Medicine

Colin A. Pinnock MB, BS, FFARCS
Lecturer and Honorary Senior Registrar, University Department of Anaesthesia, Leicester

A. P. Rubin MB, BChir, FFARCS
Consultant Anaesthetist, Charing Cross Hospital, London

Charles R. J. Singer BSc, MB, ChB, MRCP (UK)
Lecturer in Haematology, University College London; and Honorary Senior Registrar, University College Hospital, London

Heather F. Slowey MB, BS, FFARCS
Lecturer, University of Wales College of Medicine, Cardiff

Christine Thornton BSc, MSc
Senior Research Officer, Division of Anaesthesia, Clinical Research Centre, Harrow, Middlesex

M. D. Vickers MB, BS, FFARCS
Professor of Anaesthetics, University of Wales College of Medicine, Cardiff

David White MB, BS, FFARCS
Consultant Anaesthetist, Northwick Park Hospital, Harrow, Middlesex, and Division of Anaesthesia, Clinical Research Centre, Harrow, Middlesex

Contents

Medicine for anaesthetists

RESPIRATORY FUNCTION IN COLITIS

The extraintestinal manifestations of inflammatory bowel disease such as skin rashes and joint inflammation are well known. Recently, cases have been reported which support a link between diseases such as ulcerative colitis and Crohn's disease and pulmonary dysfunction.

The pulmonary changes are not those of sulphasalazine-induced pulmonary disease, which presents as dyspnoea (usually within a few months of initiating therapy) and is typified by cough, sputum and fever and is associated with allergy to aspirin or sulphonamides (Editorial 1974). In the sulphasalazine-induced condition the chest radiograph may show infiltration and impaired pulmonary function. The disease resolves on cessation of therapy and recrudesces if sulphasalazine is restarted.

Pulmonary disease apparently unassociated with sulphasalazine has been reported in non-smokers with inflammatory bowel disease. Patients have presented with dyspnoea and/or a chronic productive cough which may occur in the quiescent stage of bowel disease, postcolectomy or even preceding bowel symptoms. Chest radiography has characteristically shown interstitial infiltration and changes compatible with bronchiectasis (Higenbottam *et al* 1980, Butland *et al* 1981).

Heatley *et al* (1982) examined pulmonary function in 102 patients with ulcerative colitis and Crohn's disease and found abnormality in 50% with a reduced lung transfer factor in 25%. There was no apparent correlation with the site of the bowel disease, its activity, the drug therapy or with circulating autoimmune complexes. Pulmonary function appears to be restrictive, with mild hypoxaemia and hypocapnia. The progress of the disease can be slowed by non-steroidal, anti-inflammatory agents and steroids but the condition appears to be progressive and may accelerate if therapy is withdrawn.

Patwardhan *et al* (1983) have recently reported three cases of pleuropericarditis complicating inflammatory bowel disease with no obvious underlying cause.

The clinical picture and family history of inflammatory bowel disease suggest an autoimmune aetiology.

INSULINS

In the early days of insulin therapy, technology was directed to the production of purer and more stable forms of insulin, achieved by crystallisation with zinc. The duration of action was then extended by combination with protamine or globin and by increasing the size of the crystal. Subsequently, work turned to the production of purified insulin giving increased potency and reduced immunogenicity. Despite a high incidence of insulin antibodies in patients receiving regular insulin, non-specific local or systemic allergic reactions have been rare using conventional insulins and have occurred even with the highly purified and synthetic human insulins.

The terms, purified, highly purified and monocomponent refer to the reduction in the insulin-like contaminants (mainly proinsulin) which cause local and allergic reactions. Human insulin (emp) produced by chemical manipulation of animal insulin (enzymatically modified porcine) is now available commercially and that produced by recombinant DNA technology (chain recombinant DNA bacteria, denoted-crb) may be marked in the near future.

Table 1.1 correlates the various types of insulin available, according to the old classification.

Table 1.1 Available insulins classified according to duration of action

Insulin type	Initial time (hours)	Peak time (hours)	Duration (hours)	Species
Rapid acting				
Soluble	½–1	2–3	5–8	Beef
Actrapid	½–1	2–4	6–8	Porcine
Human Actrapid (emp)	½–1	2–4	6–8	'Human'
Semilente	1–2	4–8	12–16	Beef
Semitard	1½–2	5–9	15–22	Porcine
Intermediate acting				
Globin	2–4	6–10	14–20	Beef
NPH	2–4	8–12	18–26	Beef
Lente	2–4	8–16	18–28	Beef
Lentard	2–6	7–15	18–24	Bovine/porcine
Montard	3–6	7–15	18–22	Porcine
Human Monotard (emp)	3–6	7–15	18–22	'Human'
Human Protophane (emp)	2–4	4–12	15–24	'Human'
Long acting				
PZI	6–8	14–24	24–36 +	Bovine
Ultralente	6–8	16–24	24–36 +	Bovine
Ultratard	4–8	10–30	32–36 +	Bovine
Mixed (biphasic)				
Rapitard	1–2	4–12	18–22	Porcine + bovine

BLOOD TRANSMISSIBLE DISEASES

Transfusion of blood is virtually an everyday part of the work of anaesthetists, who are all very well aware of the possible risks of transfusion, yet problems are rare. Indeed, infection after blood transfusion is extremely uncommon. In Western countries, transmissible diseases such as malaria and Chaga's disease can virtually be discounted, whereas bacterial infection or reactions to bacterial toxins are kept to a minimum using strict collection and storage techniques.

The diseases of clinical importance today are the viral infections — hepatitis A, hepatitis B, non-A, non-B hepatitis and cytomegalovirus (CMV) — and the bacterial infection, syphilis. Acquired immune deficiency syndrome (AIDS) may need to be added to the list as there has recently been a report of blood-borne transmission (Curran 1984). Most of our information on this topic comes from the USA where the population is larger, the techniques of collection of donors were less fastidious, and consequently there have been a greater number of clinical problems. The DHSS has recently requested male homosexuals not to donate blood.

The regional transfusion centres in the UK currently screen donor blood for hepatitis B surface antigen (HB$_s$Ag) and syphilis. Looking to the future, some centres are starting to screen for CMV prior to releasing blood to recipients at risk (renal transplant patients, for example). Bacterial screening is limited to fresh products such as platelets and white cell-poor blood, while random checks are carried out on unused whole blood.

Prior to the isolation of identifiable antigenic material, the terms hepatitis A and hepatitis B were used to describe the clinical features of infective and serum hepatitis (incubation periods 15–50 days and 50–180 days, respectively). The identification of hepatitis B surface antigen (HB$_s$Ag) and hepatitis A antigen (HAAg), coupled with animal research revealed that the viruses can be transmitted both orally and parenterally. In addition, a clinical picture similar to hepatitis B can be induced by transfusing blood not containing either of these antigens; the condition is termed non-A non-B hepatitis and is said to account for 80–90% of cases of post-transfusion hepatitis, after the exclusion of HB$_s$Ag donors.

Hepatitis A

This is a very rare cause of post-transfusion hepatitis, the oral/faecal route being the usual mode of transmission. The illness is most likely to occur if a donor gives blood during the in-cubation period, as the serum has been shown to be infective only for two to three weeks prior to the onset of jaundice and for a few days afterwards. The chronic carrier state has not been demonstrated. The illness is relatively mild and does not progress to chronic disease. The transmissable agent can be identified as typical particles in a stool specimen under electron microscopy or by using specific antibodies (Dienstag 1981). Hepatitis A antigen is found in 50% of the adult population, indicating widespread subclinical infections. Should a blood donor develop jaundice, the recipient may be treated with immune human serum gamma-globulin, which will confer long acting passive immunity.

Hepatitis B

Australia antigen HB$_s$Ag appears to be part of the outer coat of the larger 'Dane particle' which is probably the complete virus. A core antigen has also been identified and is termed HB$_c$Ag (hepatitis core antigen).

Screening of donor blood and the abolition of paid volunteers in the USA has reduced type B post-transfusion hepatitis considerably but not reduced the overall incidence of post-transfusion hepatitis, most of which must therefore be attributed to the existence of non-A non-B virus. The failure to abolish hepatitis B altogether is thought to be due to the presence of anti-Hb$_s$Ag antibodies in 40% of seropositive donors which can render the antigen un-detectable by routine laboratory testing.

In acutely infected patients, HB$_s$Ag can be found before the onset of clinical illness and is more likely to persist in patients who have no jaundice; patients with chronic active hepatitis often give no history of illness. The antibody anti-HB$_c$ is found during the acute stage whereas anti-HB$_s$ is not found until late in convalescence. The incidence of HB$_s$Ag carriers is quoted as $0·1$–$0·2$% in the USA with 10–25% of adults having anti-HB$_s$. Subtypes of HB$_s$Ag have been identified and combinations of up to three antigens are found in the subtypes. Most subtypes contain a common antigen a and either d or y and w or r (the commonest are adw, adr and ayw); these vary between regions, w being found in America, Europe and Africa. Antigens d and y are found in acute hepatitis and d is found in chronic hepatitis. The carrier state 'y' type is common in drug abusers and renal dialysis units. These subtypes are particularly useful markers in epidemiological studies.

The outcome of hepatitis B infection is determined by cell-mediated immunity in the host and those at greater risk are the immunosuppressed and immunodeficient. Treatment of exposed persons in the past has been limited to passive or active-passive immunisation with immuno-globulin preparations; however, active immunisation with hepatitis B vaccine is being evaluated in clinical trials (Continho et al 1983).

Non-A non-B hepatitis

Prior to the recognition of this disease, the agents thought to produce post-transfusion hepatitis other than Australia antigen were hepatitis A, CMV, toxoplasmosis and Ebstein Barr virus. However, clinical studies eliminated these infectious agents, and the term non-A non-B hepatitis was introduced. The clinical features, described by Dienstag in 1983, are similar to those of hepatitis B, but the incubation period (two weeks to four months) is shorter, the acute illness is less severe and chronic hepatitis occurs more frequently.

Patients are usually asymptomatic and anicteric (about 20% are jaundiced). Liver amino-transferases are the indicator of the disease. Twenty-five to 60% of the cases will have recurrent or persistently high transminases for more than 6 months. The patients are often asymptomatic but liver biopsy usually reveals chronic active hepatitis which presumably resolves in most cases; 10–20% proceed to cirrhosis. Transmission by other routes appears possible and a carrier state probably exists.

To date there are no serological methods of detection available for blood bank screening and prevention is limited to avoidance of use of commercial blood donors.

ACQUIRED IMMUNE DEFICIENCY SYNDROME

This new disease has rapidly achieved notoriety since 1979. It is characterised by an irreversible and profound acquired deficiency of cell mediated immune responses while normal humoral immunity is preserved. The mortality is high and predictions of as much as 70% mortality have been made from the original 300 cases reported.

The patients present specifically with Pneumocystis carinii pneumonia or Kaposis sarcoma, neither of which are usually found in healthy persons. Typically, non-specific problems such as fever, loss of weight, lymphadenopathy and diarrhoea may be present and other opportunist infections may have occurred. Patients are typically male adult homo-sexuals or drug abusers, though cases have occurred in haemophiliacs and even in infants.

The aetiology of this disease is not clear. It is obviously a communicable disease and a specific virus has been claimed to have been isolated in both France and the USA. It may be the result of multifactorial insults to the body including drugs and infection. Waterson (1983) deals with the problem to date.

The argument for possible transmission of this disease by blood and blood products was put strongly by Curran (1984) and adds to the possible risks of blood transfusion. Even so the incidence of infection following blood transfusion appears to be very low. However, until the introduction of human serum for vaccination in the 1920s and the widespread use of blood products, hepatitis B virus also had little opportunity to cause serious infection problems in man. Thus there may be more microbial agents, particularly those with a long incubation period, causing illnesses awaiting recognition.

ENFLURANE HEPATITIS

The establishment of a suitable animal model (Cousins et al 1979) and prospective clinical trials, have provided a definite link between halothane anaesthesia and associated liver damage. Halothane hepatitis is a rare condition. Its precise incidence is not known as clinical methods of determination of hepatic dysfunction are non-specific. Its aetiology, however, appears to be due to two, possibly interacting, mechanisms; toxicity due to halothane metabolism and an immune hypersensitivity response.

In an editorial (1980) Cousins reviewed the current knowledge of the subject. He concluded that reactive intermediates (such as 'free radicles'), may cause direct cellular damage. The presence of reactive metabolites has been indicated by the recovery of volatile reductive metabolites such as tri- and di-fluoroethane (CTF and CDF). These metabolites have been measured in man during halothane anaesthesia even using high inspired oxygen concentrations. It is presumed that they are formed in the relatively poorly oxygenated areas of the liver. The author also concluded that an immune mechanism may be implicated, as small numbers of patients have responded immunologically to a halothane challenge. However, cases of halothane hepatotoxicity have been reported after a single exposure. Cousins suggests that the identification of volatile reductive metabolites also implies binding of reactive intermediates to protein and lipid, which would facilitate an allergic response.

The identification of halothane-induced hepatic injury in the clinical situation, however, relies on relatively non-specific indicators, such as fever, jaundice and eosinophilia, associated with elevated transaminases, when the commoner causes of postoperative jaundice have been excluded. The relatively rare coincidence of anaesthesia being administered during the incubation phase of hepatitis A is difficult to exclude and may account for a few cases.

Enflurane is less readily metabolised and does not appear to have a reductive pathway. Lewis et al (1983) reviewed 24 cases of enflurane-associated hepatic injury, having excluded the usual causes of postoperative hepatic injury, such as drug induced cholestatic jaundice, post-transfusion viral hepatitis, hypoxaemia and shock. The authors concluded that the findings supported the occurrence of enflurane-associated hepatitis and that a fatal outcome is possible. The authors suggest that there is a lower incidence of the disease than that associated with halothane, but that otherwise the illness demonstrates the characteristics of halothane induced hepatitis. This condition could be attributable to an immune mechanism; the low incidence put forward by the authors would support this theory.

ETOMIDATE INFUSION FOR SEDATION

Sedation of patients requiring long-term ventilation continues to pose problems. There is a requirement for an agent which is non-cumulative, has negligible effect on cardiovascular performance and is non-toxic. Etomidate appeared to offer these attributes and was advocated for use in intensive care.

Any new drug must undergo rigorous animal testing and limited clinical trials to exclude possible adverse reactions, prior to its general release. Nevertheless, it is recognised that surveillance by individual medical practitioners must continue after the release of a new 'safe' drug, as side effects may only be revealed when large numbers of patients under varying conditions are exposed to the drug.

The promotion of the use of etomidate as a continuous infusion for sedation of patients in intensive care was suspended in 1983 by the Committee on Safety of Medicines 1983 following a report by Ledingham and Watt (1983) of an increased mortality rate amongst patients with multiple injuries, nursed in an intensive care unit. Direct adrenocortical suppression was the suspected underlying mechanism.

This suspicion has been strengthened in a report by Fellows *et al* (1983), of a prospective study of pituitary-adrenocortical function in six multiple injured patients admitted to their intensive care unit. The authors found evidence of direct adrenocortical suppression (as determined by response to short tetracosactrin tests, plasma adrenocorticotrophic hormone and plasma cortisol concentrations), in the patients who had received etomidate by infusion. They also found that normal adrenocortical function returned on withdrawal of the drug. Cardiovascular stability did not appear to depend on adrenocortical function. More recently Fragen *et al* (1983), and Sebel *et al* (1983) have given evidence of adrenocortical suppression associated with single doses of etomidate.

The search for a universally suitable drug for long-term sedation continues: the severely ill and unstable intensive care patient requiring a multiplicity of drugs is a poor subject for the identification of possible adverse drug reactions or interactions. Nevertheless, these reports do emphasise the need for case review and enquiry into any unexplained complications.

THE HISTAMINE RECEPTOR ANTAGONISTS

Recently, the use of type 2 (H_2)receptor antagonists (referred to in *Anaesthesia Review 2* 1983), has been advocated to reduce both the volume and acidity of gastric secretions in patients at risk of aspiration, particularly for obstetric patients in labour and presenting for Caesarean section (Johnstone *et al* 1982a, 1982b). A recent report by Manchikanti *et al* (1984) suggests that paediatric patients undergoing elective surgery may have low gastric pH and high gastric volumes. They found cimetidine to be effective and superior to glycopyrrolate in reducing gastric pH and volume.

The initial experimental work involved cimetidine. However, ranitidine offers advantages, lacking central nervous system effects, microsomal enzyme inhibition, antiandrogenic and renal tubule effects and having a longer duration of inhibition of gastric secretion. McAuley *et al* (1983) have investigated the use of oral ranitidine in patients presenting for elective Caesarean section. They found that a dose of 150 mg gave a pH greater than $2 \cdot 5$ in 79 out of 80 patients for 2–6 hours after administration. The volume of gastric aspirate was significantly less than in a group given magnesium trisilicate. Subsequently, McAuley *et al* (1984) have demonstrated oral ranitidine to be less effective in association with administration of opiate analgesics, and in the previously unfasted patient in labour. A preliminary trial of ranitidine 50 mg intravenously demonstrated that, despite crossing the placenta, there was no adverse effect on the neonate, neurobehavioural assessment, feeding, gastric aspirate pH and culture.

More generally, histamine release due to drug administration during anaesthesia may elicit clinical signs ranging from tachycardia and urticaria to hypotension, bronchospasm and cardiac arrest. A symposium in Munich in 1982 examined the significance of histamine and antihistamines in clinical reactions. Thornton & Lorenz (1983) reported a sizeable list of drugs used by anaesthetists which are known to release histamine (Table 1.2). The use of H_1 and H_2 histamine antagonists as premedicants might seem appropriate to reduce reactions due to histamine release following drug administration or surgery; indeed the combined use of both types of antagonists has a greater effect than that of either given alone. However, histamine release itself is not considered a threat to life and therefore the routine prophylactic use of these drugs cannot be advocated. Treatment should be directed to supportive measures and avoidance of provoking factors.

Table 1.2 Anaesthetic drugs known to release histamine

Propanidid	Chlorpheniramine
Althesin	Cimetidine
Thiopentone	Ranitidine
Methohexitone	
Flunitrazepam	Polygeline
Lormetazepam	Oxypolygelatin
	Human albumin
Suxamethonium	
Tubocurarine	Mepivacaine
Alcuronium	Morphine
Pancuronium	Aprotinin
	Bone cement (Palacos)

REFERENCES

Butland R J, Cole P, Citron K M, Turner-Warwick M 1981 Chronic bronchial suppuration and inflammatory bowel disease. *Quarterly Journal of Medicine* **50(197)**: 63–75

Continho R A, Leslie N, Albrecht-Van Lent P, Reerink-Brongers E E, Stoutjesdijk L, Dees P *et al* 1983 Efficiency of heat inactivated hepatitis vaccine in male homosexuals: outcome of a placebo controlled double-blind trial. *British Medical Journal* **286**: 1305–1306

Cousins M J 1980 Halothane hepatitis: What's new? *Drugs* **19**: 1–6

Cousins M J, Sharp J H, Gourlay G K, *et al* 1979 Hepatotoxicity and halothane metabolism in an animal model with application for human toxicity. *Anaesthesia and Intensive Care* **7**: 9–24

Curran J W, Lawrence D N, Jaffe H, Kaplan J E, Zyla L D, Chamberland M *et al* 1984 Acquired immunodeficiency syndrome (AIDS) associated with transfusions. *New England Journal of Medicine* **310**: 69–75

Dienstag J L 1983 Non-A, non-B hepatitis. Experimental transmission. Putative virus agents and markers and prevention. *Review Gastroemterology* **85**: 743–768

Dienstag J L 1981 Hepatitis A virus: virologic, clinical and epidemiological studies. *Human Pathology* **12**: 1097–1106

Editorial 1974 Sulphasalazine-induced lung disease. *Lancet* **ii**: 504–505

Fellows I W, Bastow M D, Byrne A J, Allison S P 1983 Adrenocortical suppression in multiply injured patients: complication of etomidate treatment. *British Medical Journal* **287**: 1837

Fragen R J, Shanks C A, Molteni A 1983 Effect on plasma cortisol concentrations of a single induction dose of etomidate or thiopentone. *Lancet* **ii**: 625–626

Heatley R V, Thomas P, Prokipchuk E J, Gauldie J, Sieniewicz D J, Bienenstock J 1982 Pulmonary function abnormalities in patients with inflammatory bowel disease. *Quarterly Journal of Medicine New Series L1* **203**: 241–260

Higenbottam T, Cochrane G M, Clark T J, Turner D, Millis R, Seymour W 1980 Bronchial disease in ulcerative colitis. *Thorax* **35**: 581–585

Johnstone J R, McCaughey W, Moore J, Dundee J W 1982a Cimetidine as an oral antacid before elective Caesarean section. *Anaesthesia* **37**: 26–32

Johnstone J R, McCaughey W, Moore J, Dundee J W 1982b A field trial of cimetidine as the sole oral antacid in obstetric anaesthesia. *Anaesthesia* **37**: 33–38

Ledingham J McA, Watt I 1983 Influence of sedation on mortality in critically ill multiple trauma patients. *Lancet* **1**: 1270

Lewis J H, Zimmerman H J, Ishak K G, Mullick F G 1983 Enflurane hepatotoxicity. A clinicopathologic study of 24 cases. *Annals of Internal Medicine* **98**: 984–992

Manchikanti L, Hawkins J M, McCracken J E, Roush J R 1984 Effects of preanaesthetic glycopyrrolate and cimetidine on gastric fluid acidity and volume in children. *European Journal of Anaesthesiology* **1**: 123–132

McAuley D M, Moore J, McCaughey W, Donnelly B D, Dundee J W 1983 Ranitidine as an antacid before elective Caesarean section. *Anaesthesia* **38**: 108–114

McAuley D M, Moore J, Dundee J W, McCaughey W 1984 Oral ranitidine in labour. *Anaesthesia* **39**: 433–438

Patwardhan R V, Heilpern R J, Brewster A C, Darrah J J 1983 Pleuropericarditis: an extraintestinal complication of inflammatory bowel disease. *Archives of Internal Medicine* **143**: 94–96

Sebel P S, Verghese C, Makin H L J 1983 Effect on plasma cortisol concentrations of a single induction dose of etomidate or thiopentone. *Lancer* **ii**: 625

Thornton J A, Lorenz W 1983 Histamine and antihistamines in anaesthesia and surgery. *Anaesthesia* **38**: 373–379

Waterson A P 1983 Acquired immune deficiency syndrome. *British Medical Journal* **286**: 743–746

Assessment of cardiac risks and complications for patients requiring non-cardiac surgery

Patients with a healthy heart, intact cardiovascular reflexes and a normal circulating blood volume are well equipped to withstand the stresses of general anaesthesia and surgery. Adverse cardiovascular events do occur in such subjects but idiosyncratic reactions to drugs, errors of technique or the inadvertent use of drug combinations which predispose to disorders of cardiac rhythm are usually invoked to explain them. The same is not true for those with cardiac disease and so there is a need to identify patients at risk, predict the nature and magnitude of likely complications and alter management accordingly.

Risk factors associated with known cardiac disease
The most widely quoted study of cardiac complications associated with anaesthesia and non-cardiac surgery was published in 1977 by Goldman *et al.* The series consisted of 1001 patients over 40 years of age and, by an analysis of the incidence of cardiac complications associated with the 9 factors listed in Table 2.1, 4 categories of risk were defined. Patients in category IV (score more than 26/53) were considered suitable only for life-saving surgery. The most adverse features were myocardial infarction within the preceding 6 months, physical signs of heart failure (elevation of the jugular venous pressure, the presence of a third heart sound), rhythm other than sinus, or more than 5 ventricular ectopic beats per minute. This scoring system is particularly valuable in identifying high-risk patients, but it may be an underestimate for some class I patients, for example those requiring abdominal aortic surgery (Jeffrey *et al* 1982).

The significance of ischaemic heart disease
The importance of cardiovascular disease in general and ischaemic heart disease in particular received renewed emphasis in 1982 from the publication of a survey of mortality associated with anaesthesia (Lunn & Mushin 1982). Cardiovascular disease was given as the cause of death for 84 of 153 patients who died within 6 days of surgery (in whom autopsy was carried out) and was present preoperatively in 38 of 58 patients whose deaths were totally attributed to anaesthesia. Most studies assess the combined risk of anaesthesia and surgery and ischaemic heart disease always figures prominently. Thus Kaplan and Dunbar (1979) reported a series of 8238 patients requiring non-cardiac surgery which included 873 who suffered from ischaemic heart disease, diagnosed on the basis of angina pectoris, ischaemic e.c.g. changes or previous myocardial infarction. Perioperative cardiovascular complications occurred in 72 of these 873 patients, 10% proving fatal. Similarly in a prospective study of 12 654 procedures, von Knorring (1981) identified 214 patients with ischaemic heart disease as judged by an abnormal e.c.g. or a history of previous infarction. Perioperative infarction

Table 2.1 Multifactorial risk index

History	
Age over 70	5 points
Infarct within 6/12	10
Signs	
Third Heart sound &/or	
Raised JVP	11
Aortic stenosis	3
E.c.g.	
Rhythm other than sinus	7
More than 5 VES/min	7
General	
Respiratory failure, hypokalaemia, acidosis, renal failure, liver dysfunction, immobility	3
Operation	
Abdominal, thoracic or aortic	3
Emergency surgery	4
Total possible	53
Group I	0-5 points
Group II	6-12
Group III	13-25
Group IV	over 26 points

From Goldman *et al* 1977

JVP: jugular venous pressure; VES: ventricular extrasystoles

was sought by serial e.c.g. monitoring and was detected in 12 patients (0·1%) who had no preoperative history of heart disease and a normal e.c.g. whereas 38 of the 214 patients (18%) with ischaemic heart disease suffered an infarct within the first 3 days.

These figures draw attention to two important points. The first is the greatly increased risk associated with proven ischaemic heart disease, and second is that there is a small but definite risk of infarction in those who have neither symptoms nor signs on routine examination. Thus it is likely that a proportion of patients with significant ischaemic heart disease (that is sufficient to cause impairment of left ventricular function) will be missed at the time of preoperative assessment. A high index of suspicion is the best tool for identifying these subjects, and it is a simple matter to add questions about risk factors to the preoperative history. These include a personal or family history of diabetes, hypertension or ischaemic heart disease, as well as characteristics such as obesity, smoking and an inactive lifestyle. The magnitude of risk is such that the chances of developing ischaemic heart disease are doubled by regular smoking, quadrupled in those with hypertension who smoke, and increased by a factor of eight in those with hypertension, hyperlipidaemia and who also smoke. Questions about smoking are usually followed by those about alcohol intake. Alcohol taken regularly tends to raise the systemic blood pressure but, at least with modest intake, the lipid profile is altered to favour the high density lipoproteins which are associated with a lower incidence of atheroma. Measurements of the serum cholestorel and lipid profile are not part of the battery of 'routine' investigations requested preoperatively in the UK and, in the average surgical service, such information is unlikely to be available. Occasionally symptoms other than angina pectoris provide a useful warning of vascular disease. Thus the first indication of ischaemic heart disease is sometimes a complaint of excessive fatigue, inappropriate dyspnoea or dizziness on exertion, while cerebrovascular disease should be suspected if there is a history of visual disturbances or giddiness after abrupt postural changes or movement of the head.

Confirming the diagnosis of ischaemic heart disease

It is important to appreciate that a normal e.c.g. does not exclude the presence of significant ischaemic heart disease and that the resting trace is normal in up to two-thirds of patients with angina pectoris but no previous infarct. The exercise e.c.g. is more helpful because 75% of patients with angina develop ST-segment depression during the test. A refinement of the exercise e.c.g. has been advocated as a means of identifying the severity of ischaemic heart disease, ST-segment depression during exercise being related to the increment in heart rate (Elamin et al 1982). Nuclear imaging or angiography are more specific but are rarely appropriate in the context of non-cardiac surgery, whereas echocardiography can be considered more often. Using this non-invasive technique, left ventricular function can be assessed, and the state of the mitral and aortic valves examined. The movement of the ventricular wall and septum can be studied, so identifying dyskinetic areas which are present in a proportion of patients with ischaemic heart disease at rest, and which occur in a higher proportion during exercise. This functional assessment is often of more value to the anaesthetist than knowledge of the precise anatomy of the coronary arteries.

The role of previous myocardial infarction

Many studies carried out over more than two decades have confirmed that this is the single most important determinant of risk of further infarction during or after surgery (Portal 1982). The largest series, consisting of nearly 33 000 patients operated on at the Mayo Clinic between 1967 and 1968, was reported by Tarhan and colleagues in 1972. The incidence of myocardial infarction within the first postoperative week was $0 \cdot 13\%$ in those without a history of previous infarction, and averaged $6 \cdot 6\%$ in those who had had a previous infarct. The importance of the interval between previous infarction and subsequent anaesthesia and surgery has been apparent in all series and was demonstrated again by Steen et al in 1978. The overall incidence of reinfarction was similar to previous reports ($6 \cdot 1\%$) but rose from $4 \cdot 1\%$ when surgery was delayed more than 6 months after the infarct, to 11% in those operated on at between 3 and 6 months, and to 27% if surgery occurred within 3 months. Thus there is widespread agreement about the significance of a previous infarct and the importance of the interval between the infarct and subsequent surgery. Similarly most authors report that the mortality of reinfarction associated with surgery is high, usually between 50 and 70%, although in von Knorring's series (1981) the mortality was only just over 33%. A number of other risk factors have been suggested in one or more of these reports. Most consistent is the adverse effect of hypotension, defined as a reduction of 30% or more in systolic blood pressure lasting at least 10 minutes. Preoperative hypertension, surgery lasting longer than 3 hours, emergency operations and elective upper abdominal and non-cardiac thoracic surgery have been identified in some series as possible risk factors, whereas there has been no association with the nature of the anaesthetic (including at least one study of spinal anaesthesia), nor even with the presence preoperatively of anginal pain.

Armed with this information, it is appropriate to enquire how these adverse factors can be overcome. Rao and El-Etr in 1981 reported a series of 97 patients requiring non-cardiac surgery who had suffered a myocardial infarct within the previous 6 months. When operation was delayed until 3–6 months after the infarct, the incidence of reinfarction was $3 \cdot 4\%$ with no mortality, and even in those operated on within 3 months, the incidence of reinfarction was only $7 \cdot 8\%$ with a mortality of $5 \cdot 3\%$. These impressive figures emphasise that meticulous attention to cardiovascular monitoring and management can greatly minimise risk, the principles followed by these authors being outlined in Table 2.2. It must also be appreciated however that this quality of care cannot be confined to the operative period alone because the incidence of perioperative infarction is highest on the 3rd postoperative day, a time when many patients have returned to a general ward.

Table 2.2 Principles of management advocated by Rao & El-Etr

MONITOR E.C.G. LEAD V5 AS WELL AS BP, HR & PAWP
MAINTAIN HAEMATOCRIT AT MORE THAN 30%
PROMPT TREATMENT OF ANY HAEMODYNAMIC CHANGE

From Rao TLK & El-Etr HA 1981

BP: systemic blood pressure; HR: heart rate; PAWP: pulmonary arterial wedge pressure

A factor rarely considered when the role of previous infarction has been evaluated, is the extent and severity of myocardial damage and the likelihood of further ischaemic episodes. The availability of coronary arterial surgery and the controversy over the prophylactic role of drug treatment after myocardial infarction have led to attempts to identify patients whose infarct has placed them at greater than average risk. Currently there is growing interest in the findings of limited exercise tests, carried out in those without evidence of cardiac failure before discharge from hospital after an episode of infarction (Epstein *et al* 1982, Jennings *et al* 1984). The development of ST-segment depression, anginal pain or indices of impaired ventricular function such as exercise induced hypotension or a reduced ejection fraction identify patients who are at risk of further infarction or death within a year. Studies such as these may permit greater precision in identifying risk for patients requiring anaesthesia and surgery after a previous infarct. Another factor which must be considered today is the influence of coronorary arterial bypass grafting. Mahar *et al* (1978) reported 220 procedures on 148 patients who had previously undergone coronary arterial surgery, and there were no instances of myocardial infarction. Although coronary bypass surgery may diminish risk associated with subsequent non-cardiac surgery, it is only likely to be carried out in the UK when it is indicated in its own right, and not solely as a means of enhancing the safety of other procedures.

The significance of hypertension

Hypertension is primarily a disorder of vascular tone but many of its complications involve the heart and so its role as a determinant of cardiovascular risk associated with anaesthesia must be considered too. Most authors have reported an increased incidence of adverse cardiovascular complications in patients with moderate or severe hypertension (diastolic blood pressure greater than 100 mmHg) subjected to anaesthesia and surgery, although Goldman (1983) does not regard hypertension as an independent risk factor.

Three characteristics of the cardiovascular system of the hypertensive patient are important during anaesthesia. The *first* is an exaggerated haemodynamic response to stimuli which affect vascular tone. Thus the pressor response to laryngoscopy and intubation, and to surgical stimulation is far greater than normal; conversely the hypotensive effect of conventional doses of intravenous anaesthetic induction agents is also accentuated. *Second* is the development of left ventricular hypertrophy as a result of sustained systemic hypertension. The hypertrophied ventricle is non-compliant so that small changes in diastolic volume are associated with large changes in intraventricular pressure. This means that a marked fall in output will result when there is only modest hypovolaemia and, conversely, the ventricular end-diastolic and hence left atrial pressures can rise rapidly in response to a small increment of volume. Similarly the non-compliant left ventricle is intolerant of tachycardia, which reduces the time for diastolic filling and for coronary flow, and is often compromised if sinus rhythm is lost because the filling boost of atrial systole disappears. *Finally* there is an increased incidence of both cerebrovascular and ischaemic heart disease, and of impaired renal function in patients with hypertension. Superimposed on this background are the effects of drug treatment and the influence of pre-existing abnormalities of blood volume. Many hypotensive agents diminish the cardiovascular reaction to stimuli such as pain or hypovolaemia, but those which deplete the catecholamine stores at sympathetic nerve terminals enhance sensitivity to alpha-adrenergic agonists. Patients with sustained, untreated hypertension are likely to have a reduced blood volume and hypovolaemia can occur preoperatively as a consequence of treatment, when biochemical disturbances are sometimes also present.

Adverse cardiac or cerebral complications can follow either hyper- or hypotension. Myocardial damage is more common and, in both cases, the injury is mediated by ischaemia although the mechanisms causing the ischaemia differ in the two cases. Hypertension increases the demand on the left ventricle and so myocardial oxygen uptake must increase. The head of pressure available to perfuse the coronary circulation is increased when the diastolic blood pressure is raised but the duration of coronary flow is likely to fall as the systemic pressure rises. If myocardial function is already poor, the response to an increase in afterload is dilatation of the ventricle and an increase in ventricular end-diastolic pressure. This also impedes flow in the vulnerable subendocardial coronary vessels and so coronary perfusion falls when myocardial oxygen demands are increased. Areas of myocardial ischaemia result and e.c.g. evidence of ischaemia often persists long after the hypertensive episode has passed.

Systemic hypotension reduces the demand on the left ventricle but also reduces the head of pressure available to perfuse the coronary circulation. This is particularly liable to result in ischaemia when there is obstruction to flow in the main coronary vessels. Here too there is a paradox because if ventricular function is poor, the reduction in afterload will increase cardiac output and diminish the intraventricular diastolic pressure so that coronary perfusion is improved. This is the rationale for the use of vasodilator drugs in heart failure. Thus the hypertensive patient with an impaired myocardium is most likely to benefit and least likely to suffer if hypotension occurs as a result of a reduction in systemic resistance. Conversely, the hypertensive patient with a good left ventricle but proximal vessel disease is at greater risk of myocardial damage if the systemic pressure falls. Both types of patient are at risk if hypotension occurs as a result of hypovolaemia or myocardial depression. One final hazard is that areas of ischaemic myocardium are more depressed by anaesthetic agents than is normal heart muscle and so the combination of anaesthesia and enhanced ischaemia is particularly adverse.

With this analysis in mind, the risk factors for individual patients can be assessed by a series of questions. Is the hypertension mild, moderate or severe with diastolic pressures above 90, 100 and 110 mmHg respectively? There is little to suggest that mild, asymptomatic and untreated hypertension adds significantly to the risk associated with anaesthesia and surgery. Moderate or severe hypertension warrant more concern and both should be treated, or considered for treatment preoperatively. The cause and duration are also worth noting because hypertension which is secondary to renal or endocrine disease is often severe but carries a reasonably good prognosis if the cause is amenable to correction and the diagnosis is made early. Essential hypertension is much more common and attention should be given to whether it is controlled, whether the control is effective and what drug regime is used. It is preferable to defer elective surgery if severe hypertension is uncontrolled or control is poor.

Evidence of cardiac, renal or carebrovascular disease should be sought preoperatively and it is prudent to assume that the left ventricle is impaired if there is radiological or electro-cardiographic evidence of left ventricular hypertrophy, even in patients without a history of exertional dyspnoea or anginal pain. A better assessment of left ventricular function is possible if echocardiography is available. The presence of hypovolaemia should be considered, either as a consequence of hypertension, drug treatment to control the blood pressure, or intercurrent disease. Postural hypotension is common in hypovolaemic subjects but must be distinguished from the postural fall in blood pressure intended with some hypotensive medication.

Disorders of cardiac rhythm

Ectopic beats occur and are experienced by healthy patients, the incidence increasing with excesses of alcohol, caffeine, or nicotine, particularly in those who go for long periods without food. The advent of ambulatory e.c.g. monitoring has permitted analysis of the frequency and significance of these disturbances of rhythm, and they can be regarded as benign in subjects less than 40 years of age with no other evidence of cardiac disease.

Conversely however, the presence of more than five ventricular extrasystoles per minute, detected at any time before surgery, is a high-risk factor, contributing seven points to the Goldman risk index (Goldman *et al* 1977). Particular attention should be given to those with ventricular extrasystoles in whom coronary arterial disease is known to be present because the incidence of sudden death is magnified several-fold, independent of any added risk factor associated with surgery or anaesthesia.

Defects of conduction are often a source of anxiety, but the presence of symptoms related to the bradycardia, and the severity of the associated cardiac disease are of greater importance than the nature of the electrophysiological disturbance. Patients with congenital heart block as an isolated anomaly do not require preoperative pacing, whereas those with acquired, usually symptomatic, complete heart block, or Mobitz type II block with wide QRS complexes, warrant at least temporary pacing. The incidence of cardiac complications during anaesthesia and surgery in those with bifascicular block does not warrant the insertion of a pacemaker prophylactically (Bellocci *et al* 1980).

Risk factors associated with valvular or congenital heart disease

Serious valvular heart disease is amenable to surgical correction in all but exceptional circum-stances and so is now less common in patients presenting for non-cardiac surgery. The pattern of valvular disease has also changed so that significant mitral stenosis occurs in-frequently now in the UK, whereas mitral incompetence secondary to ischaemic heart disease, and aortic stenosis associated with atheroma are seen more often. Patients with prosthetic heart valves also present for non-cardiac surgery and here it is the use of anti-coagulants and the need for antibiotic prophylaxis which take precedence over the haemo-dynamic consequences. The valve lesion associated with the greatest risk is aortic stenosis, which is often accompanied by ischaemic heart disease in elderly patients. Effort-induced syncope is a particularly adverse feature because it indicates that the left ventricle cannot generate an increased output when necessary. Anginal pain, dyspnoea on exertion and any alteration of cardiac rhythm are also unfavourable features. Acute hypotension, sometimes fatal, is likely to occur as a result of systemic vasodilatation, hypovolaemia or any myocardial depression. Left ventricular failure, pulmonary oedema and rhythm disturbances, particu-larly conduction defects, are also common. Mitral incompetence presents fewer hazards, although here too it is relatively easy to precipitate pulmonary oedema by injudicious transfusion.

Patients with acyanotic congenital heart disease usually withstand anaesthesia and surgery without incident, although those with coarctation of the aorta are at some risk of intra-operative hypertension and cerebral or subarachnoid haemorrhage. Cyanotic heart disease is obviously less benign but, here too, youthful subjects at least are often well-compensated in haemodynamic terms and acclimatised to a low arterial oxygen tension. Specific risk factors apply in some circumstances, for example, severe pulmonary hypertension, infundibular hypertrophy or systemic embolism. These are best considered individually by consulting texts devoted to the care of such patients during cardiac surgery where the hazards associated with each condition are discussed in detail.

Pericardial disease, hypertrophic or congestive cardiomyopathy, and thromboembolic or primary pulmonary hypertension are unlikely to be encountered often. Here too an under-standing of the pathophysiology of each condition provides the best protection against un-toward cardiovascular complications, a reminder that there is much truth in the aphorism 'forewarned is forearmed'.

REFERENCES

Bellocci F, Santarelli P, Di Gennaro M, Ansalone G, Fenici R 1980 The risk of cardiac complications in surgical patients with bifascicular block: a clinical and electrophysiologic study in 98 patients. *Chest* **77:** 343–348

Elamin M S, Boyle R, Kardash M M *et al* 1982 Accurate detection of coronary heart disease by new exercise test. *British Heart Journal* **48:** 311–320

Epstein S E, Palmeri S T, Patterson R E 1982 Evaluation of patients after acute myocardial infarction: indications for cardiac catheterization and surgical intervention. *New England Journal of Medicine* **307:** 1487–1492

Goldman L, Caldera D L, Nussbaum S R *et al* 1977 Multifactorial index of cardiac risk in non-cardiac surgical procedures. *New England Journal of Medicine* **297:** 845–850

Goldman L 1983 Cardiac risks and complications of non-cardiac surgery. *Annals of Internal Medicine* **98:** 504–513

Jeffrey C C, Kunsman J, Cullen D L, Brewster D C 1982 The usefulness of the Goldman cardiac risk index. *Anesthesiology* **57:** suppl. A443

Jennings K, Reid D S, Hawkins T, Julian D J 1948 Role of exercise testing early after myocardial infarction in identifying candidates for coronary surgery. *British Medical Journal* **288:** 185–187

Kaplan J A, Dunbar R W 1979 Anesthesia for noncardiac surgery in patients with cardiac disease. In: Kaplan J A (ed) *Cardiac anesthesia*, Grune & Stratton, New York, ch 11, p 377

Lunn J N, Mushin W W 1982 Mortality associated with anaesthesia. *Nuffield Provincial Hospitals Trust London*, Tables 4.10, 6.4, p 61, 80

Mahar L J, Steen P A, Tinker J H, Vliestra R E, Smith H C, Pluth J R 1978 Perioperative myocardial infarction in patients with coronary artery disease with and without aortocoronary bypass grafts. *Journal of Thoracic and Cardiovascular Surgery* **76:** 533–537

Portal R W 1982 Elective surgery after myocardial infarction. *British Medical Journal* **284:** 843–844

Rao TLK, El-Etr H A 1981 Myocardial reinfarction following anesthesia in patients with recent infarction. *Anesthesia and Analgesia* **60:** 271–272 (abstract)

Steen P A, Tinker J H, Tarhan S 1978 Myocardial reinfarction after anesthesia and surgery. *Journal of the American Medical Association* **239:** 2566–2570

Tarhan S, Moffitt E A, Taylor W F, Giuliani E R 1972 Myocardial infarction after general anesthesia. *Journal of the American Medical Association* **220:** 1451–1454

von Knorring J 1981 Postoperative myocardial infarction: a prospective study in a risk group of surgical patients. *Surgery* **90:** 55–60

Myopathies and recent theories on myasthenia gravis

INTRODUCTION

Since the 1950s our knowledge of the number and diversity of muscle diseases has increased rapidly. This has largely been due to the development of sensitive electromyographic and histochemical techniques, supported by many advances in the field of muscle biochemistry. The field is so large, however, that only an introduction and guide to the relevant literature can be given here.

Muscle diseases may be expressed in many different ways, the most obvious of which is weakness. A child may fail to achieve the motor milestones such as sitting and walking, whereas an adult may not be able to rise from a chair or climb stairs. Such patients (e.g. with muscular dystrophies) are weak even when at rest, in contrast to a second group who are of normal strength at rest but in whom only a small amount of exercise leads to premature or excessive fatigue (e.g. in myasthenia gravis and muscle mitochondrial disorders). A third category are patients who are not necessarily weak or easily fatigued but have some disturbance of function such as myotonia, severe cramps or episodic weakness. This review attempts to summarise (1) the classification of myopathies, (2) the clinical and pathological features of some of the more widely recognised types of myopathies, and (3) recent theories on the pathogenesis of myasthenia gravis.

CLASSIFICATION OF MYOPATHIES

The myopathies include a large variety of diseases, many of which are exceedingly rare and as a result of which their classification is difficult. They can be classified on the basis of pathological appearances or, more readily, on the clinical presentations. In Table 3.1 I have

Table 3.1 Classification of myopathies

Genetically determined myopathies	**Drug-induced myopathies**
Pure muscular dystrophies	
Congenital myopathies	**Endocrine/metabolic myopathies**
Myotonic disorders	
Glycogen storage diseases	**Myopathies associated with malignant disease**
Familial periodic paralysis	
Myopathy of malignant hyperpyrexia	Carcinomatous myopathy
Familial myoglobinuria	Myasthenic-myopathic syndrome
Inflammatory myopathies	
Polymyositis/dermatomyositis	**Miscellaneous myopathies e.g.**
Granulomatous myositis	Alcoholic myopathy
Giant cell myositis	Nutritional myopathy
Infective myositis	Amyloid myopathy

tried to provide a simple working classification consisting of those disorders which seem to be separate entities on genetic, clinical and pathological grounds. The classification of myopathies has been extensively reviewed by Walton (1981).

MUSCULAR DYSTROPHIES

These are hereditary diseases characterised by painless degeneration and atrophy of skeletal muscle which becomes replaced with fat and fibrous tissues. The various dystrophies (Table 3.2) can usually be distinguished clinically by their progress, the muscles affected and the pattern of inheritance. In most dystrophies light microscopy reveals the presence of internal cell nuclei (as opposed to peripheral nuclei seen in normal fibres), with a wide variation in fibre size.

Table 3.2 Pure muscular dystrophies

X-linked muscular dystrophies
Severe (Duchenne)
Benign (Becker)
Scapuloperoneal

Autosomal recessive muscular dystrophies
Limb-girdle (scapulohumeral)
Childhood muscular dystrophy
Congenital muscular dystrophy

Autosomal dominant muscular dystrophies
Facioscapulohumeral (Landouzy-Dejerine)
Scapuloperoneal
Distal (infantile/adult forms)
Late onset proximal
Ocular/oculopharyngeal

Duchenne's muscular dystrophy (pseudohypertrophic type)

In 1868 Duchenne first described what is the most serious, though not the most common type of muscular dystrophy. This disorder typically manifests as progressive muscle weakness and atrophy in males between 2 and 5 years of age. The calf muscles often appear hypertrophied and the patient may walk with a waddling gait. Most patients deteriorate steadily and are unable to walk by about the age of 10 years (Walton 1978). Involvement of cardiac muscle is invariable, though not clinically detectable in the early stages (Walton 1978, Hunsaker et al 1982). Death usually occurs within 10 to 15 years of clinical onset.

Myopathies which affect limb muscles may also affect the respiratory muscles and respiratory disability is well recognised in muscular dystrophy (McCormack & Spalter 1966, Buchsbaum et al 1968, Burke et al 1971, Hapke et al 1972). Typical abnormalities of lung function in patients with respiratory muscle weakness include a reduced vital capacity (VC) with a restrictive ventilatory defect, reduced total lung capacity, raised residual volume and reduced maximal inspiratory and expiratory mouth pressures (Moxham 1982). Hypercapnia is said to be likely to occur when respiratory muscle strength is less than 30% of normal (in an uncomplicated myopathy), or when the VC is less than 50% of the predicted value (Braun et al 1983). In subjects without infection, hypercapnia is an extremely bad prognostic sign (Inkley et al 1974). The presence of scoliosis may further restrict ventilation and weak abdominal muscles may result in an ineffective cough. Respiratory failure and pulmonary infection contribute significantly to death in about 80% of patients with Duchenne muscular dystrophy (Gilroy *et al* 1963, Inkley *et al* 1974). Regular breathing exercises, the prevention of scoliosis, instruction of the patient and family in the use of postural drainage during respiratory infections, together with appropriate antibiotic therapy may all help in delaying the development of respiratory failure, and seems to be the only useful approach to prophylaxis.

Recent reviews on the management of Duchenne muscular dystrophy include those of Siegel (1978) and Dubowitz (1980).

The serum creatine kinase (CK) level is often markedly elevated, parallelling the magnitude of muscle necrosis as well as reflecting increased permeability of the muscle membrane (Pennington 1980). CK levels are often used for the diagnosis of putative carriers of Duchenne muscular dystrophy. In the last few years the non-invasive technique of nuclear magnetic resonance (NMR) has been used to study chemical changes in intact muscles, and unusual phosphodiesters have been found in dystrophic muscle (Chalovich *et al* 1979). It is now becoming possible to use topical NMR to study human muscle constituents in situ, and this may facilitate the investigation of the chemical composition and metabolism of both normal and diseased muscle (Edwards *et al* 1982).

The fundamental abnormalities in muscular dystrophies are not yet known, although a membrane defect, primary or co-existing, is often detectable (Rowland 1980). Most researchers agree that in Duchenne muscular dystrophy there is a selective change in sarcolemmal permeability which allows release of some enzymes and an increase in intracellular calcium. Recently it has been demonstrated that the platelets of patients with Duchenne muscular dystrophy also show altered membrane permeability accompanied by elevated intracellular calcium levels, suggesting a more widespread membrane defect (Yarom *et al* 1983).

Anaesthetic problems

The implications of increased muscle membrane permeability and decreased cardiac and pulmonary reserve in patients with muscular dystrophy must be considered prior to anaesthesia. Anaesthesia may be hazardous in these patients (Boba 1970, Yamashita *et al* 1976) and should be administered by an experienced anaesthetist, even for minor procedures. Malignant hyperpyrexia is said to be more common in patients with muscle disease (King *et al* 1972, Denborough *et al* 1973, Gronert 1980, Oka *et al* 1982). Indeed the diagnosis of Duchenne muscular dystrophy has occasionally been established after the development of malignant hyperpyrexia in those patients in whom these conditions have coexisted.

Becker muscular dystrophy

This is a less severe form of dystrophy, also with a sex-linked mode of inheritance, which appears in the teens (Moser *et al* 1966). Cardiac involvement is usually absent and contractures and skeletal deformities occur late. Some patients, though severely disabled, may survive to a normal age (Walton 1978).

Limb girdle (scapulohumeral) muscular dystrophy

This is usually transmitted as an autosomal recessive trait and has a more benign course than the previous two. Sufferers may survive late into adult life, but often have considerable disability due to profound limb girdle weakness. The clinical picture is very similar to that of the Kugelberg-Welander syndrome (spinal muscular atrophy) with which it was often confused in the past (Smith & Patel 1965, Walton 1978).

Facioscapulohumeral muscular dystrophy

This is inherited as an autosomal dominant trait, but there is a wide variation in gene expression within a family. Weakness predominately affects the face and upper limb girdle, but later in the disease the lower limbs may be affected. Most patients have a normal life span (Walton 1954).

MYOTONIC DISORDERS

Myotonic dystrophy (Steinert's disease)

This is the most common type of myopathy to be seen in adults in general clinical practice. It is dominantly inherited, but gene penetration varies considerably. It is a multisystem disorder in which myotonia (i.e. continuing muscle contraction after cessation of voluntary effort or stimulation) and distal muscular atrophy may be accompanied by cataracts, frontal baldness, gonadal atrophy, cardiomyopathy, respiratory muscle weakness, endocrine anomalies and dementia. The patients usually survive well into adult life, although severe forms may appear in childhood. Cardiac involvement, including conduction defects, arrhythmias and mitral valve prolapse, is common (Motta et al 1979) and rarely may lead to sudden death (Spillane 1951, Fisch & Evans 1954). Respiratory muscle weakness with alveolar hypoventilation is also common but its degree is often unsuspected clinically (Serisier et al 1982), and bronchopneumonia may be the commonest cause of death (Black & Ravin 1974, Walton 1978).

Anaesthetic problems

Anaesthesia is often complicated in these patients and this is thought to be due to impaired ventilation and ineffective coughing, as a result of respiratory and abdominal muscle weakness (Kaufman 1960, Gillam et al 1964), as well as to reduced cardiac reserve due to the presence of cardiomyopathy. The sternomastoid muscle, an important accessory muscle of inspiration, is often atrophied in this disease and this further reduces the respiratory reserve. The laryngeal muscles may also be atrophied and intubation therefore performed without the use of muscle relaxants.

Myotonia congenita (Thomsen's disease)

This is inherited as an autosomal trait and manifests at birth or in early childhood. Myotonia is generalised, but there is usually no involvement of other organs, and life expectancy is not reduced.

Paramyotonia

This condition is characterised by myotonia which appears only on exposure to the cold.

Although there are no cures for myotonic disorders, myotonia may be relieved by treatment with quinine, phenytoin or prednisolone.

CONGENITAL MYOPATHIES

Apart from the dystrophies there are a few so called congenital myopathies, which are usually manifest at birth with hypotonic muscles and later in life slowness in learning to walk, with diffuse, but mainly proximal muscle weakness. Included in this group are central core disease, nemaline myopathy, myotubular myopathy and idiopathic myopathies (Walton

1981). Diseases due to abnormalities of mitochondrial structure or chemistry are also often included in this category (Dubowitz 1978).

DISORDERS OF ENERGY METABOLISM

There are a number of genetically determined defects of muscle energy metabolism. These include defects in the glycolytic pathway (glycogen storage diseases) and mitochondrial enzymes of both pyruvate and fatty acid metabolism (DiMauro & Eastwood 1977). In general patients with metabolic defects are of normal or of near normal strength when rested, but limited in their exercise endurance.

Glycogen storage diseases

A number of glycolytic disorders may affect muscles. The cause of weakness in these disorders is not clear, but it is probably the result of mechanical damage to the contractile machinery resulting from accumulation of abnormal glycogen. They are inherited as autosomal recessive traits.

Type 2 (Pompe's disease)

This is due to a deficiency of acid maltase which usually presents at birth with severe muscle hypotonia and ventilatory failure. The disease is usually fatal in early life although there are now reports of adult patients presenting with similar problems, including proximal muscle weakness (DiMauro et al 1978). Ventilatory failure may be the presenting problem in the adult form of acid maltase deficiency (Keunen et al 1984), which is unlike most other neuromuscular diseases in which ventilatory failure is a late or terminal feature. This suggests there may be selective involvement of the respiratory muscles in this condition. Serum CK levels are generally increased but the diagnosis is best established by estimations of acid maltase activity in leucocytes and muscle. Muscle biopsy reveals a vacuolar myopathy with positive histochemical staining for glycogen. As yet there is no effective enzyme substitution therapy for acid maltase deficiency. However, it has been suggested that respiratory muscle training may improve pulmonary function in these patients (Martin et al 1983).

Type 3 (Cori-Forbes disease)

This is due to deficiency of a debranching enzyme leading to accumulation of structurally abnormal glycogen in the muscle. The clinical symptoms are diverse ranging from severe muscle weakness in childhood to an asymptomatic form in the adult.

Type 5 (McArdle's disease)

This is due to myophosphorylase deficiency. Patients usually have normal strength at rest but pain is experienced in the muscles during exercise (McArdle 1951). If exercise is continued at a high level, myoglobin may be released into the circulation with the consequent risk of renal damage (Bank et al 1972). Myophosphorylase deficiency may also give rise to progressive weakness rather than exercise intolerance (Engel et al 1963) and rarely may even result in rapidly progressive weakness with ventilatory failure (DiMauro & Hartlage 1978).

Type 7 (Tarui's disease)

This is due to a deficiency of phosphofructokinase (PFK), the clinical symptoms of which are very similar to those of McArdle's disease (Tarui's *et al* 1965). However, this defect is also seen in the red blood cells, giving rise to haemolytic anaemia, often detectable by a raised reticulocyte count (Layzer 1977).

DISORDERS OF FAT METABOLISM

These have only recently been described and include deficiencies of muscle carnitine and carnitine palmitoyltransferase. They present with weakness, exercise intolerance, muscle stiffness and pain which is sometimes accompanied by myoglobinuria (DiMauro *et al* 1980). Where there is evidence of carnitine deficiency, treatment with oral carnitine may improve exercise tolerance (Angelini *et al* 1976).

FAMILIAL PERIODIC PARALYSIS

Familial periodic paralysis is characterised by periodic attacks of weakness and is of considerable interest to anaesthetists.

Hypokalaemic periodic paralysis

This is an autosomal dominant condition, sometimes associated with thyrotoxicosis, in which attacks of flacid paralysis characteristically occur in association with a fall in plasma potassium concentration (Gordon *et al* 1970). The attacks of weakness first occur in the second decade of life and may last up to 24 hours. Attacks often occur after a carbohydrate meal or during a period of rest following exercise. The hypokalaemia is thought to be due to a shift of K^+ from the extracellular space into muscle. The ensuing hyperpolarisation of the cell membrane causes cardiac dysrhythmias and resistance to acetylcholine at the neuro-muscular junction. These patients may exhibit a myasthenic-like sensitivity to non-depolarising muscle relaxants during an acute episode of the disease. Potassium supple-mentation, restriction of sodium intake and avoidance of carbohydrates and heavy exercise all help the patient to avoid attacks of paralysis. Acetazolamide, a carbonic anhydrase inhibitor, has also proved valuable in the treatment of this condition.

Hyperkalaemic periodic paralysis

This too is an autosomal dominant condition, in which the attacks of paralysis are usually much shorter in duration than the hypokalaemic type, lasting on average 30 to 40 minutes, and may be precipitated immediately by exercise. In the attacks the plasma K^+ concentration usually rises and some patients develop myotonia (Layzer *et al* 1967). The hyperkalaemia is thought to be due to K^+ moving out of muscle, and possibly other tissues, into the plasma. During an attack the patient will be resistant to non-depolarising relaxants.

High carbohydrate intake, glucose and insulin all help to minimise attacks. Acetazolamide is very effective in the long term management (McArdle 1962), and may act by preventing K^+ flux across the muscle membrane, as well as by promoting K^+ excretion.

MALIGNANT HYPERPYREXIA

Malignant hyperpyrexia is a rare but serious disorder, first described in 1960 (Denborough & Lovell 1960), which presents considerable problems to anaesthetists. Apparently healthy individuals undergoing routine surgery develop alarming and often fatal hyperpyrexia.

Usually after anaesthesia is induced, muscle stiffness develops which is accompanied by a rapid rise in body temperature, increase in plasma K^+ and lactate levels and subsequent development of cardiac failure. Myoglobinuria and renal damage are additional problems. Unless the signs are recognised early during anaesthesia and treatment begun promptly, the prognosis is poor, death resulting in about 50% of cases. Many anaesthetic agents are known to induce malignant hyperpyrexia but the most frequently implicated are halothane, methoxyflurane, enflurane, cyclopropane, trichlorethylene and the muscle relaxant succinylcholine (Newson 1972, Gallant 1983). It has been suggested that nitrous oxide and some local anaesthetics may also induce this condition (Katz & Krick 1976, Klimaneck et al 1976, Wadhwa 1977), although this is certainly controversial in the case of nitrous oxide (Gallant 1983).

Malignant hyperpyrexia is inherited as autosomal dominant condition with reduced penetrance. Its incidence has been variously reported as 1 : 20 000 (Britt & Kalow 1970) or 1 : 200 000 (Ellis & Halsall 1980) persons subjected to anaesthesia, although this discrepancy in incidence may be due to differing anaesthetic techniques in Canada and the United Kingdom. Some muscle diseases, e.g. muscular dystrophy, central core disease and myotonic disorders, are said to be associated with or predisposed to malignant hyperpyrexia (Gronert 1980, Oka et al 1982). Elevated serum CK levels have been used to diagnose patients susceptible to malignant hyperpyrexia (Gallant 1983), but this is not a sufficiently reliable test, as 60% of patients with otherwise proven susceptibility have a normal CK level (Tan et al 1978).

The diagnosis of susceptible individuals can be made with reasonable confidence by use of an in vitro muscle preparation, which, when compared with normal human muscle, shows a greater propensity to contracture in the presence of caffeine (Moulds & Denborough 1974, Kallow et al 1977). An alternative diagnostic technique may be to measure the proportion of the active form of phosphorylase in muscle, as this seems to be increased in susceptible subjects (Willner et al 1980).

Hyperpyrexic attacks are not an inevitable consequence of halothane anaesthesia and it has been estimated that the probability of pyrexia developing in susceptible subjects is about 44% (Halsall et al 1979). This type of observation has led to the suggestion that there may be unidentified stress factors, which render the subjects more susceptible to the ill effects of halothane (Wingard 1974). A disease similar to human malignant hyperpyrexia has been described in pigs (Gallant 1983). These animals are particularly sensitive to stress and develop muscle rigidity, acidosis, hyperkalaemia and die of heart failure if kept in a stressful environment. Like humans, susceptible pigs are sensitive to halothane and depolarising muscle relaxants and so this porcine disease has become useful in furthering our understanding of malignant hyperpyrexia in humans. The major defect of muscle in malignant hyperpyrexia is thought to be in the control of intracellular calcium levels and the mechanisms involved in the regulation of excitation-contraction coupling (Britt 1979).

The only effective treatment for malignant hyperpyrexia is dantrolene, a peripheral muscle relaxant, which is thought to act by interfering with the mechanisms responsible for calcium release (Aldrete 1981). The management of susceptible patients requires avoidance of known precipitating agents and stress, as well as careful monitoring of body temperature. If hyperpyrexia develops, intravenous dantrolene should be administered and strenuous efforts made to cool the body and limit the rise in plasma lactate and K^+ levels. Prophylactic oral dantrolene for 48 hours prior to surgery, has been recommended in susceptible patients (Aldrete 1981).

INFLAMMATORY MYOPATHIES

Polymyositis and dermatomyositis are the most common types of acute muscle disease and may be subdivided into four groups:

1. Polymyositis (simple)
2. Dermatomyositis (simple)
3. Polymyositis/dermatomyositis associated with malignancy
4. Polymyositis/dermatomyositis associated with collagen vascular disease (e.g. rheumatoid arthritis, scleroderma, systemic lupus erythematosis).

These disorders are characterised by proximal muscle weakness with wasting, muscle tenderness and pain. The muscle weakness often leads to immobilisation with difficulty holding up the head, dysphagia, and if the respiratory muscles are involved there is the risk of life threatening ventilatory failure. Rarely myoglobinuria and renal failure may occur (Kreitzer et al 1978). Cutaneous manifestations include widespread erythema, a characteristic heliotrope erythema around the eyes and periorbital oedema. The erythrocyte sedimentation rate and serum CK level are often raised and the EMG demonstrates a myopathic pattern. Muscle biopsy usually demonstrates widespread necrosis with macrophage infiltration and marked variation of fibre size.

Polymyositis is almost certainly the result of an autoimmune reaction against muscle, which is probably cell mediated in origin. Several studies have shown that lymphocytes from patients with polymyositis are cytotoxic towards muscle cells grown in culture (Johnson et al 1972). The factors responsible for initiating the autoimmune response are not known but probably include virus infections, drugs and neoplasia.

The primary treatment is with high doses of corticosteroids and/or immunosuppressive drugs. Corticosteroids, however, may themselves cause muscle wasting and it is therefore important to balance the beneficial and harmful effects of treatment very carefully (Edward et al 1979).

DRUG-INDUCED MYOPATHIES

There are a number of myopathies which are thought to result from drug administration (Table 3.3). These have been well reviewed by Lane and Mastaglia (1978).

Table 3.3 Drug-induced muscle disorders

Disorder	Drug implicated
Acute/suabacute painful proximal myopathy	Clofibrate, aminocaproic acid, emetine, heroin, alcohol, vincristine, cimetidine, lithium
Acute rhabdomyolysis	Heroin, amphetamine, phencyclidine, alcohol
Subacute/chronic painless proximal myopathy	Corticosteroids, chloroquine, heroin, alcohol, perphexiline
Myasthenic syndromes	D-penicillamine, aminoglycosides, polymixins, tetracyclines, phenytoin, propranolol, chloropromazine, procainamide
Polymyositis/dermatomyositis	20, 25-Diazacholesterol, propranolol, suxamethonium
Malignant hyperpyrexia	Halothane, suxamethonium, enflurane cycloproprane, chloroform, methoxyflurane, diethyl-ether, ketamine, psychotropics

Adapted from Lane & Mastaglia 1978.

ENDOCRINE AND METABOLIC MYOPATHIES

These present the anaesthetist with the problems of the underlying disease process, together with the problems of a patient with generalised muscle weakness. The most well known disorders in this group are well reviewed by Walton (1981) and include:

1. Thyrotoxicosis:
   a. limb girdle myopathy
   b. myasthenia gravis
   c. periodic paralysis
2. Myxoedema:
   a. limb girdle myopathy
   b. Debré-Semelaigne syndrome (cretinism)
   c. Hoffman's syndrome (adults)
3. Hypopituitarism
4. Acromegaly
5. Cushing's disease
6. Addison's disease
7. Conn's syndrome (primary aldosteronism)
8. Hyperparathyroidism
9. Osteomalacia
10. Chronic renal failure

RECENT THEORIES ON THE PATHOGENESIS OF MYASTHENIA GRAVIS

There are a number of different types of myasthenia gravis, all of which can contribute to our understanding of the underlying pathogenesis of the disease (Compston *et al* 1980).

Generalised myasthenia

Three clinical varieties are recognised:

1. Generalised myasthenia may be associated with a thymoma, when there is no clear HLA (human leucocyte antigen) association. Patients have a high titre of antibodies to acetylcholine receptors (ACR), and usually also have high titres of antibodies to skeletal muscle.

2. Generalised myasthenia may be associated with thymitis in patients under the age of 40, and in this group there is an association with HLA-B8 or DR W3 (D locus related) or both. These patients may have other associated autoimmune diseases but do not usually possess antibodies to striated muscle. Such patients do well after thymectomy.

3. Generalised myasthenia may be associated with thymitis in patients over the age of 40. These patients have a high incidence of HLA-A3 and B7 or DR W2 or both. They have the lowest titres of antibodies to ACRs in patients with generalised myasthenia.

Ocular myasthenia

In this variety the weakness is confined clinically to the extraocular muscles. These patients have the lowest ACR antibody titres.

Neonatal myasthenia

This disorder occurs in babies born to myasthenic mothers and is due to the transplacental passage of ACR antibodies. The condition may be fatal unless treated with anticholinesterase drugs. It tends to persist for 1–6 weeks and muscle strength improves as the ACR antibody levels fall.

Penicillamine-induced myasthenia

Penicillamine-induced myasthenia results from the development of ACR antibodies in association with abnormal muscle fatigue. It usually occurs some months after treatment with penicillamine and like other autoimmune diseases induced by penicillamine, occurs in susceptible individuals. Thus, patients with rheumatoid arthritis are much more likely to develop myasthenia gravis when treated with penicillamine than patients suffering from Wilson's disease (Vincent et al 1978). The disorder usually remits after stopping the drug.

Congenital myasthenia

This comprises a group of rare disorders, some of which have a genetic origin. In some patients the defect is presynaptic. An absence of anticholinesterase at the motor end plate has also been described. ACR antibodies are not present.

PATHOGENESIS

In 1960 the high incidence of autoimmune phenomena in patients with myasthenia gravis led Simpson to formulate his hypothesis that the disease was due to antibodies to the motor end-plate (Simpson 1960). In the same year circulating antibodies to striated muscle, which cross-reacted with thymic myoid cells, were reported in some myasthenic patients (Strauss et al 1960). Only about one-third of myasthenic patients have such antibodies and these are usually patients with thymomas. Such antibodies also occur in association with thymoma without myasthenia and do not play any part in the pathogenesis of muscular weakness.

Evidence suggesting involvement of ACR antibodies

Further progress in our understanding of the pathogenesis of myasthenia gravis resulted from the discovery of α-bungarotoxin (α-BT), a snake venom protein which binds specifically and irreversibly to ACRs (Chang & Lee 1963). In 1974 Almon et al discovered a factor present in the globulin fraction of the sera of patients with myasthenia which blocked binding of α-BT to rat ACRs. Since then several other methods have shown humeral interference with ACRs.

Antibodies to ACRs have been found in about 90% of myasthenic patients. Although, the antibody titre does not correspond with the severity of the disease, patients with thymomas tend to have high titres, and those with predominantly ocular symptoms have the lowest mean titres. Within each individual there is usually a rise in antibody titre with increasing disease severity and vice versa.

Several lines of evidence suggest that ACR antibodies are the cause of the muscle weakness. Injection of α-BT into animals has shown that a decrease in functioning ACRs gives rise to myasthenic symptoms. Mice injected repeatedly with immunoglobulin prepared from myasthenic sera become weak, with a decreased number of ACRs as shown by α-BT binding (Toyka et al 1975). The third component of complement (C3), is necessary for this phenomenon to occur. Removal of ACR antibodies by plasma exchange increases muscular strength in most of the myasthenic patients so treated, and the return of weakness correlates with the reappearance of the ACR antibodies (Newsom-Davis et al 1978). Neonatal myasthenia is associated with the presence of ACR antibodies transferred via the placenta to the baby. Furthermore the infant appears to improve as the antibody level falls.

Mechanisms by which ACR antibodies may produce muscular weakness

There are probably three main mechanisms by which ACR antibodies interfere with neuromuscular transmission:

1. Complement-mediated lysis
2. Modulation of acetylcholine receptors
3. Direct block

Complement-mediated lysis

Immunoglogin-G and C3 (together with a little C9) have been demonstrated on the postsynaptic membrane where their distribution correspond to that of the ACRs. This is consistent with complement-mediated lysis of the postsynaptic membrane, leading to loss of ACRs.

Modulation of acetylcholine receptors

ACRs are constantly being degraded and synthesised. The average ACR in a normal individual has a life of about 7 days, while in a myasthenic individual this is reduced to about 1 day. The rate of degradation appears to be increased after cross-linking of ACRs by antibody (Drachman *et al* 1978).

Direct block

Antibodies against the acetylcholine binding site could directly inhibit ACR function. Such antibodies do exist in myasthenic patients, but they usually form only a small proportion of the total ACR antibody present (Shibuya *et al* 1978).

Reasons for poor correlation between ACR antibody levels and disease severity

The poor correlation between ACR antibody levels and disease severity remains to be explained. About 5% of patients with generalised myasthenia have no detectable ACR antibody. Antibody heterogeneity may be partly responsible for this (Vincent & Newsom-Davis 1980). In an individual patient there are probably several types of ACR antibody, some of which are more effective in blocking or destroying the ACR than others. Antibodies directed against the acetylcholine binding site of the ACR would, in theory, cause a profound decrease in neuromuscular transmission but these are not detected by the routine radioimmunoassay methods employed. The rate of resynthesis of ACRs after their destruction also varies between individuals, and this could also determine the severity of muscular weakness.

Role of the thymus

The normal role of the thymus is the education of the T-lymphocytes, which are not antibody producing cells, but subserve a variety of functions, such as helper cells, suppressor cells and cytotoxic T-cells. B-cells are rare in the normal thymus. That the thymus plays a part in myasthenia gravis is suggested by the histological appearances of the gland and the effect of thymectomy on the course of the disease. Between 10 and 15% of myasthenic patients have a thymoma, and over two-thirds of the remainder show thymitis (Castelman & Norris 1949), which is an infiltration of the thymic medulla with lymphocytes forming follicles with germinal centres, in which B-cells are found. Thymectomy results in remission or improvement in 60–80% of patients, though the delay before improvement varies considerably and may be several years (Papatestas *et al* 1976).

Recently it has been shown that the thymus is an active site of production of antibodies to ACRs in most patients with thymitis (Scadding *et al* 1981), suggesting that the thymus may be the site of autosensitisation to the ACR. Irradiated thymic cells, which are viable but incapable of antibody synthesis augment the production of antibodies to ACRs by autologous peripheral blood lymphocytes. This suggests that the thymus is a site of some helper factor, possibly an antigen presenting cell bearing ACRs, which enhances ACR antibody synthesis (Newsom-Davis *et al* 1980). ACRs have been found on muscle-like cells cultured from mouse and rat thymuses (Kao & Drachman 1977). It seems possible, therefore, that the thymus might also be the source of the original ACRs to which tolerance is broken, possibly as a result of viral infection.

In summary, myasthenia gravis is an autoimmune disorder in which autoantibodies directed against the acetylcholine receptor reduce the number of functioning receptor sites, resulting in impaired neuromuscular transmission. Treatment with plasma exchange reveals that serum ACR antibodies usually have an inverse relationship with muscle strength. The ACR antibody is heterogeneous and can lead to loss of muscle ACRs by several mechanisms. ACR antibody is produced by the thymus in small amounts and it is clear that the thymus plays an important part in the pathogenesis of this disease. Analysis of clinical, immunological and HLA characteristics in myasthenia gravis suggest that more than one mechanism may underlie the breakdown in tolerance to ACRs, leading to the production of ACR antibodies.

REFERENCES

Aldrete J A 1981 Advances in the diagnosis and treatment of malignant hyperpyrexia. *Acta Anaesthesiologica Scandinavica* **25:** 477–483

Almon R R, Andrew C G, Appel S H 1974 Serum globulin in myasthenia gravis: inhibition of alpha-bungarotoxin binding to acetylocholine receptors. *Science* **186:** 55–57

Angelini C, Lucke S, Canparutti S 1976 Carnitine deficiency of skeletal muscle: report of a treated case. *Neurology* **26:** 633–637

Bank W J, DiMauro S, Rowland L P 1972 Renal failure in McArdle's disease. *New England Journal of Medicine* **287:** 1102

Braun N M T, Arora N S, Rochester D F 1 983 Respiratory muscle and pulmonary function in polymyositis and other proximal myopathies. *Thorax* **38:** 616–623

Britt B A 1979 Etiology and pathophysiology of malignant hyperthermia. *Federation Proceedings* **38:** 44–48

Britt B A, Kalow W 1970 Malignant hyperthermia: etiology unknown. *Canadian Anaesthetists' Society Journal* **17:** 316–330

Buchsbaum H W *et al* 1968 Chronic alveolar hypoventilation due to muscular dystrophy. *Neurology (Minneapolis)* **18:** 319–324

Burke S S, Grove N M, Houser C R, Hohn D M 1971 Respiratory aspects of pseudohypertrophic muscular dystrophy. *American Journal of Diseases of Children* **121:** 230–234

Castleman B, Norris E H 1949 The pathology of the thymus in myasthenia gravis. A study of 35 cases. *Medicine* **28:** 27–58

Chalovich J M, Burt C T, Danon M J, Glonek T, Barany M 1979 Phosphodiesters in muscular dystrophies. *Annals of the New York Academy of Sciences* **317:** 649–669

Chang C C, Lee C Y 1963 Isolation of neurotoxins from the venom of *Bungarus multicinctus* and their modes of neuromuscular blocking action. *Archives Internationale de Pharmacodynamie et de Therapie* **144:** 241–257

Compston D A, Vincent A, Newsom-Davis H, Batchelor J R 1980 Clinical, pathological HLA antigen and immunological evidence for disease heterogeneity in myasthenia gravis. *Brain* **103:** 579–601

Denborough M A, Dennett X, Anderson R Mc D 1973 Central core disease and malignant hyperpyrexia. *British Medical Journal* **1:** 272–273

Denborough M A, Lovell R R H 1960 Anaesthetic deaths in a family. *Lancet* **ii:** 45

DiMauro S, Eastwood A B 1977 Disorders of glycogen and lipid metabolism. *Advances in Neurology* **17:** 123–142

DiMauro S, Stern L Z, Mehler M, Nagle R B, Payne C 1978 Adult-onset maltase deficiency: a postmortem study. *Muscle and Nerve* **1:** 27–36

Drachman D B, Angus C W, Adams R N, Michelson J D, Hoffman G J 1978 Myasthenic antibodies cross-link acetylcholine receptors to accelerate degradation. *New England Journal of Medicine* **298:** 1116–1122

Dubowitz V (ed) 1978 Muscle disorders in childhood. *Saunders, Philadelphia P A*

Dubowitz V, Heckmatt J 1980 Management of muscular dystrophy. *British Medical Bulletin* **36:** 139–144

Duchenne G B 1868 Recherche sur la paralysie musculaire pseudohypertrophique ou paralysie myo-sclerosique. *Archives Generale Medicine* **2:** 200–209

DiMauro S, Hartlage P L 1978 Fatal infantile form of muscle phosphorylase deficiency. *Neurology* **28:** 1124–1129

Edwards R H T, Wiles C M, Round J M, Jackson M J, Young A 1979 Muscle breakdown and repair in polymyositis: a case study. *Muscle and Nerve* **2:** 223–228

Ellis F R, Halsall P J 1980 Malignant hyperpyrexia. *British Journal of Hospital Medicine* **24:** 318–327

Engel W K, Eyerman I L, Williams H L 1963 Late onset type of skeletal muscle phosphorylase deficiency. A new familial variety with completely and partially affected subjects. *New England Journal of Medicine* **268:** 135–137

Fisch C, Evans P V 1954 The heart in dystrophia myotonica. *New England Journal of Medicine* **251:** 527–531

Gallant E M 1983 Malignant hyperthemia: responses of skeletal muscles to general anaesthetics. *Mayo Clinic Proceedings* **58:** 758–763

Gillam P M S, Heaf P J D, Kaufman L, Lucas B G B 1964 Respiration in dystrophia myotonica. *Thorax* **19:** 112–120

Gilroy J, Cahalan J L, Berman R, Newman M 1963 Cardiac and pulmonary complications in Duchenne's progressive muscular dystrophy. *Circulation* **27:** 484–489

Gordon A M, Green J R, Lagunoff D 1970 Studies on a patient with hypokalaemic familial periodic paralysis. *American Journal of Medicine* **48:** 185–195

Gronert G A 1980 Malignant hyperthermia. *Anesthesiology* **53:** 395–423

Halsall P J, Ellis F R 1979 A screening test for the malignant hyperpyrexia phenotype using suxamethonium-induced contracture of muscle treated with caffeine and its inhibition by dantrolene. *British Journal of Anaesthesia* **51:** 753–756

Hapke E J, Meed J C, Jacobs J 1972 Pulmonary function in progressive muscular dystrophy. *Chest* **61:** 41–47

Havard C W H, Scadding G K 1983 Myasthenia gravis: pathogenesis and current concepts in management. *Drugs* **26:** 174–184

Hunsaker R H, Fulkerson P K, Barry F J, Lewis R P, Leier C V, Unverferth D V 1982 Cardiac function in Duchenne's muscular dystrophy. *American Journal of Medicine* **73:** 235–238

Inkley S R, Oldenburg F C, Vignos P J 1974 Pulmonary function in Duchenne muscular dystrophy related to stage of disease. *American Journal of Medicine* **56:** 297–306

Johnson R L, Fink C W, Ziff M 1972 Lymphotoxin formation by lymphocytes and muscle in polymyositis. *Journal of Clinical Investigation* **51:** 2435–2449

Kalow W, Britt B A, Richter A 1977 The caffeine test of isolated human muscle in relation to malignant hyperthermia. *Canadian Anaesthetists' Society Journal* **24:** 678–694

Kao I, Drachman D B 1977 Thymic muscle cells bear accetylcholine receptors possible relation to myasthenia gravis. *Science* **195:** 74–75

Kaufman L 1960 Anaesthesia in dystrophia myotonica. A review of the hazards of anaesthesia. *Proceedings of the Royal Society of Medicine* **53:** 183–187

Keunen R W M, Lambregts P C L A, Op de Coul A A W, Joosten E M G 1984. Respiratory failure as initial symptom of acid maltase deficiency. *Journal of Neurology, Neurosurgery and Psychiatry* **47:** 549–552

King J O, Denborough M A, Zapf P W 1972 Inheritance of malignant hyperpyrexia. *Lancet* **i:** 365–370

Kreitzer S M, Ehrenpreis M, Miguel E, Petrasek J 1978 Acute myoglobinuric renal failure in polymyositis. *New York State Journal of Medicine* **2:** 295–297

Lane J M, Mastaglia F L 1978 Drug induced myopathies in man. *Lancet* **ii:** 562–565

Layzer, R B 1977 Glycolysis and glycogen. In: Rowland L P (ed) *Pathogenesis of human muscular dystrophies.* Excerpta Medica, Amsterdam, p 395–403

Layzer R B, Lovelace R E, Rowland L P 1967 Hyperkalaemic periodic paralysis. *Archives of Neurology, Chicago* **16:** 455–472

Martin R J, Sufit R L, Ringel S T, Hudgel D W, Hill P L 1938 Respiratory improvement by muscle training in adult onset acid and maltase deficiency. *Muscle and Nerve* **6:** 201–203

McArdle B 1951 Myopathy due to a defect in muscle glycogen breakdown. *Clinical Science* **10:** 13–25

McArdle B 1962 Adynamic episodica hereditaria and its treatment. *Brain* **85:** 121–148

MacComas A J 1977 Neuromuscular function and disorders. Butterworths, London.

McCormak, W M, Spalter H F 1966 Muscular dystrophy, alveolar hypoventilation and papilloedema. *Journal of the American Medical Association* **197:** 957–959

Miller E D, Sanders C B, Rowlinson J C, Berry F A, Sussman M D, Epstein R M 1978 Anaesthesia-induced rhabdomyolysis in a patient with Duchenne's muscular dystrophy. *Anesthesiology* **48:** 146–148

Moser H von, Weismann U, Richterich R, Rossi E 1966 Progressiv muskeldystropie Haufigkeit, Klinik und Genetik der Duchenne-Form. *Schweizerische Medizinische Wochenschrift* **94**: 1610–1621

Motta J et al 1979 Cardiac abnormalities in myotonic dystrophy electrophysiologic and histopathologic studies. *American Journal of Medicine* **67**: 467–473

Moulds R F W, Denborough M A 1974 A study of the action of caffeine, halothane, potassium chloride and procaine on normal human skeletal muscle. *Clinical Experimental Pharmacology and Physiology* **1**: 197–209

Moxham J 1982 Function and fatigue of respiratory muscles. In: Sarner M (ed) *Advanced medicine*. Pitman, London, p 127–137

Newsom-Davis J, Pinching A J, Vincent A, Wilson S G 1978 Function of circulating antibody to acetylcholine receptor in myasthenia gravis: investigated by plasma exchange.

Newson A J 1972 Malignant hyperthermia: three case reports. *New Zealand Medical Journal* **75**: 138–143

Oka S et al 1982 Malignant hyperpyrexia and Duchenne muscular dystrophy: a case report. *Canadian Anaesthetists' Society Journal* **29**: 627–629

Papatestas A E, Genkins G, Horowitz S H, Kornfeld P 1976 Thymectomy in myasthenia gravis: pathologic, clinical and electrophysiologic correlations. *Annals of the New York Academy of Science* **274**: 555–573

Pennington R J T 1980 Clinical biochemistry of muscular dystrophy. *British Medical Bulletin* **36**: 123–126

Scadding G K, Vincent A, Newsom-Davis J, Henry K 1981 Acetylcholine receptor antibody: synthesis by thymic lumphocytes: correlation with thymic histology. *Neurology* **31**: 935–943

Seay A R, Ziter F A, Thomson J A 1978 Cardiac arrest during induction of anaesthesia in Duchenne muscular dystrophy. *Journal of Paediatrics* **93**: 88–90

Shibuya N, Mori K, Nakazawa Y 1978 Serum factor blocks neuromuscular transmission in myasthenia gravis. *Neurology* **28**: 804–811

Siegel I M 1978 The management of muscular dystrophy: a clinical review. *Muscle and Nerve* **1**: 453–460

Simpson J A 1960 Myasthenia gravis. A new hypothesis. *Scottish Medical Journal* **5**: 419–436

Smith J B, Patel A 1965 The Wohlfart-Kugelberg-Welander disease, review of the literature and report of a case. *Neurology* **15**: 469–473

Spillane J D 1951 The heart in dystrophia myotonica. *British Heart Journal* **13**: 343–349

Strauss A J L, Seegal B C, Hsu K C, Burkholder P M, Nastuk W L, Osserman K E 1960 Immunofluorescence demonstration of a muscle binding complement-fixing serum globulin fraction in myasthenia gravis. *Proceedings of the Society of Experimental Biology* **105**: 184–191

Tan S, Aldrete J A, Solomons C C 1978 Correlation of serum creatine phosphokinase and pyrophosphate during surgery in patients with malignant hyperthermia susceptibility. In: Aldrete J A, Britt B A (eds) *Malignant hyperthermia*. Grune & Stratton, New York, p 389–400

Tarui S et al 1965 Phosphofructokinsase deficiency in skeletal muscle. A new type of glycogenosis. *Biochemical Biophysical Research Communication* **19**: 517–523

Tokya K V, Drachman D B, Pestronk K A, Kao I 1975 Myasthenia gravis: passive transfer from man to mouse. *Science* **190**: 397–399

Vincent A, Newsom-Davis H 1980 Anti-acetylcholine receptor antibodies. *Journal of Neurology, Neurosurgery and Psychiatry* **43**: 590–600

Vincent A, Newsom-Davis J, Martin V 1978 Anti-acetylcholine receptor antibodies in D-penicillamine associated myasthenia gravis. *Lancet* **i**: 1254

Walton J N, Mattrass F J 1954 On the classification, natural history and treatment of myopathies. *Brain* **77**: 169–231

Walton J N 1978 Diseases of voluntary muscle. In Bodley Scott R (ed) *Price's textbook of the practice of medicine, 12th edn*. Oxford University Press, Oxford, p 1387–1401

Walton J N, Gardner-Medwin D 1981 Progressive muscular dystrophy and the myotonic disorders. In: Walton J N (ed) *Disorders of voluntary muscle, 4th edn*. London, p 473–483

Willner J H, Wood S, Cerri C, Britt B 1980 Increased myophosphorylase in malignant hyperthermia. *New England Journal of Medicine* **303**: 138–140

Wingard D W 1974 Malignant hyperthermia: a human stress syndrome? *Lancet* **ii**: 1450–1451

Yarom R, Meyers S, More R, Liebergall M, Eldor A 1983 Platelet abnormalities in muscular dystrophy. *Thrombosis and Haemostasis* **49**: 168– 172.

Anaesthetic problems and the liver

INTRODUCTION

Soon after the introduction of chloroform into clinical practice it became apparent that anaesthetic agents could cause liver damage. Ether was always considered safer and accounted for its greater popularity in North America. Hepatitis following chloroform was first reported in Germany in 1850 and in 1894 a series was reported in Britain. However, it is only in the last 15 years that any great interest has been shown in the interaction of liver function and anaesthesia. Our understanding is far from perfect.

ANATOMY AND PHYSIOLOGY

The liver is the largest of the vital organs, approximating 1500 g, and no satisfactory replacement or support has yet been devised. It has, however, a great ability to regenerate, returning to normal size within three months of removal of 85% of functioning tissue. It is the chemical factory of the body, with important roles in the function of blood, metabolism and storage of food and biotransformation and excretion of metabolites.

The blood flow through the liver is about 1500 ml/minute, approximating 25% of cardiac output. It is from two sources: 1000 ml/minute from the low pressure portal vein draining the splanchnic vessels and 500 ml from the higher pressure hepatic artery. Over 50% of the oxygen utilised by the liver is derived from the hepatic arterial flow, which is greater than 95% saturated with oxygen. Oxygen saturation in the portal vein is 85%. The portal veins end in sinusoids, as do the capillaries of the hepatic arteries and from which the hepatic veins arise to drain into the inferior vena cava. Flow through the liver is phasic and the pressure difference between the portal veins and inferior vena cava is 5 mmHg (665 Pa).

It is difficult accurately to assess total liver blood flow and any technique is necessarily invasive. Using a modification of the Fick principle, and an agent such as bromsulphthalein, it is possible to make a relatively crude estimate of flow. More recently radioactive xenon and krypton have been used, with greater accuracy.

Changes in splanchnic and, therefore, liver blood flow, occur in response to many phsyiological variables, particularly cataecholamine release however mediated (hypercarbia, hypoxia, pain, etc.). Likewise, a reduced liver blood flow will result from a fall in the systemic blood pressure through the hepatic artery — a reason for spinal or epidural anaesthesia not being a recommended technique in liver surgery. In the normal liver, there is no real evidence to show that hypoxia or hypotension have any deleterious effect, even when the liver is stressed metabolising anaesthetic agents. This may not hold true for a liver comprised by disease. In any event, and particularly in the diseased liver, it would seem prudent to keep liver blood flow as close to normal as is physiologically possible.

The liver has two basic types of cell, the hepatocyte and the Kuppfer cell. Kuppfer cells are part of the reticuloendothelial system and are highly phagocytic cells found at intervals in the vascular sinusoids. The hepatocytes lie between the sinusoids and biliary canaliculi, neither of which have an endothelial lining. Hence the hepatocyte is in direct contact with blood and bile.

Bile is an emulsifing agent of dietary fats. It is produced in the liver and stored and con-centrated in the gall bladder. Without normal bile function, fat soluble vitamins (e.g. K) are unable to be absorbed. It is an important route of excretion of metabolites.

Carbohydrates are stored in the liver as glycogen and it is in the liver the glycogen is produced from non-carbohydrate sources. Free fatty acids produced in the liver account for 90% of the body's energy requirements.

Plasma proteins, save some of the globulins, are produced in the liver and it maintains an albumin:globulin ratio of 1·7:1.

In liver disease albumin, particularly, falls and the ratio approximates parity. Amino acids are deaminated in the liver as in other tissue, but only the liver is able to convert ammonia to urea.

PATIENT ASSESSMENT

The liver has a remarkable ability to function well in the face of severe hepatic disease. It is important to assess the degree of compensation as a patient with compensated liver disease may be regarded as no particular anaesthetic problem. Decompensation considerably increases the risks of anaesthesia or surgery. Liver function tests in isolation do not give an accurate assessment of liver damage. Serial tests will give an indication of progress in disease, but the results should always be interpreted in conjunction with clinical findings. The severity and site of surgery are important factors. Child (1966) has proposed a classification of risk, based on the patient's status, but not including the severity of surgery. This is the standard classification, Class A being a good risk, Class C poor:

	Class A	Class B	Class C
Bilirubin μmol/l	40	40–50	50
Serum albumin g/l	35	35–30	30
Ascites	None	Easy control	Poor control
Neurological disorder	None	Minimal	Advanced coma
Nutritional state	Excellent	Good	Poor—with wasting

More recently, Pugh et al (1973) have proposed a simplified, but probably more useful classification:

	1	2	3
Points per abnormality	1	2	3
Serum bilirubin μmol/l	25	25–40	40
Serum albumin g/l	35	28–35	28
Prothrombin time — prolongation sec.	4	4–6	6
Encephalopathy grade	None	1 or 2	3 or 4

Fewer than 6 points—good operative risk
    7–9 points—moderate risk
More than 10 points—poor operative risk

Routine liver function tests

Prothrombin time	12 seconds	Raised in jaundice and hepatocellular disease; 20 seconds reflects severe liver disease. Probably the most important test for the anaesthetist
Bilirubin	3–20 μmol/L	Increased in obstructive or hepato-cellular disease Clinically jaundiced 20 mol/l
Protein	total 60–80 g/L	
albumin	35–50 g/L	Reduced production in all liver disease
globulins	25–30 g/L	Raised in chronic liver disease. Includes immunoglobulins, antimitochondrial and antinuclear factors
Enzymes		
alkalinephosphatase	30–85 i.u./L	Chotestasis, but activity may be from bone, intestine or liver
aspartate transaminase	7–40 i.u./L	Non-specific. Rise seen after any tissue damage. Previously used as marker of hepatic damage caused by halothane
lactate dehydrogenase	100–300 i.u./L	Non-specific as found in many other tissues. Being replaced by H.B.D.
hydroxybutyrate dehydrogenase	100–250 i.u./L	Specific for liver disease
gamma glutamy/transpepidese	0–45 i.u./L	Pointer to effects on liver of drugs
	0–35 i.u./L	especially chronic alcohol abuse

Specific liver function tests

Alpha fetoprotein	10 ng/l	Marked rise — up to 5 000 000 with hepatoma
Ceruloplasmin	150–600 mg/l	Wilson's disease
Cholinesterase	7–20 ku/l	Low in liver disease

ANAESTHETIC CONSIDERATIONS

Most patients will have surgery for conditions unrelated to their liver disease. No ideal anaesthetic technique has evolved, though liver blood flow should be kept normal. Sears *et al* (1983) suggests that changes in liver function using four different anaesthetic techniques was very similar. Avoidance of halothane would be on emotive, rather than scientific grounds. Hepatocellular damage may lower the serum albumin with several consequences. Drugs which have an affinity to protein will have enhanced effect. Enzymes may be deficient and affect the rate of metabolism of drugs and the synthesis of clotting factors reduced. Bleeding is a common problem and perioperative use of fresh frozen plasma or specific clotting factors may be necessary.

Obstructive jaundice prevents the absorption of vitamin K, which is necessary for the production of prothrombin and factors VII, IX and X. Elevation of the prothrombin time should be treated preoperatively by using phytomenadione (K′), 10 mg parenterally until the prothrombin time approaches normal. Phytomenadione, if given intravenously, should be given slowly and not more than 40 mg in any 24-hour period.

A jaundiced patient in whom the serum bilirubin exceeds 140 μmol/litre is at risk of developing renal failure. The cause is uncertain, but renal intravascular coagulation is usually seen. The maintenance of renal function is paramount. Good perioperative hydration and the use of diuretics, e.g. mannitol or frusemide, is essential.

Anaesthesia for specific hepatic problems

Bleeding oesophageal varices

These are initially treated with vasopressin. Failing control, insertion of a Sengstaken-Blakemore tube is indicated. This occlusive oesophageal tube should be regarded only as an emergency and should not be left in place longer than 24 hours. Neither treatment requires anaesthetic involvement. Stevens and colleagues (1983) report that endoscopic sclerotherapy is back in vogue, as the long-term results of portocaval anastomosis are not as good as were expected from the short-term results. Sedation, using a benzodiazepine is the usual practice for endoscopic sclerotherapy, though general anaesthesia would be required for rigid oesophagoscopy. Doubts have been cast by Corall and Strunin (1984) on the wisdom of using strong protein binding drugs such as diazepam. It is possible to produce significant cardio-vascular depression with doses regarded as safe in most circumstances. They suggest that careful general anaesthesia may be safer as there are rarely changes in liver function associated with its administration. At some centres, transhepatic variceal sclerosis is used to occlude the oesohageal varices. The portal veins are cannulated percutaneously and trans-hepatically under X-ray control. A mixture of gel foam and thrombin is injected to occlude the portal vein. In experienced hands, sedation is feasable for this procedure, but general anaesthesia with controlled ventilation is often more comfortable for the patient and con-venient for the radiologist. General anaesthesia is always required for oesophageal tran-section, performed either with formal exposure of the oesophagus, or using a staple gun inserted through an antrostomy.

Portosystemic anastomoses are now less commonly performed than five years ago. The associated mortality is unacceptably high, particularly in an emergency situation.

It is usually possible to stop bleeding from oesophageal varices. However, the overall hospital mortality is high — about 30% — as bleeding varices are often an end stage of liver failure. Preparation for anaesthesia or sedation must include meticulous replacement of blood, fluids and electrolytes. It is advisable to avoid solutions high in sodium, as these will produce or aggravate ascites. Vitamin K should always be given, together with any clotting factors found necessary. Gastric erosions frequently complicate bleeding varices and it has become standard practice to give cimetidine. Recent experience with ranitidine, 150 mg orally, or 50 mg by slow intravenous injection, repeated at 12-hourly intervals, suggests that it is superior.

Hepatic tumours

These are usually secondary, but are occasionally primary. Treatment is feasible only if there is sufficient functioning tissue. Hepatoma is a common malignancy in black Africans in the southern part of the Continent. In whites it is rare, but when it does occur, cirrhosis or hepatitis B infection is a frequent aetiological factor. A raised serum alphafetoprotein is a diagnostic marker of hepatoma. Hepatic tumours derive the majority of their blood supply from the hepatic artery and this vessel has been the focus of attention in the therapy of these tumours. Most treatment must be regarded as palliative, rather than curative.

Hepatic resection with satisfactory liver function should pose no anaesthetic problem other than potential massive haemorrhage. At one time, laparotomy for hepatic artery ligation was popular, particularly if the tumour or tumours were confined to one lobe. However, laparotomy in patients with significant impairment of liver function is not tolerated well. It is also possible to cannulate the hepatic artery for direct infusion of cytotoxic drugs. Radiologists are now able to embolise an hepatic artery using gel foam injected through a catheter inserted into the hepatic artery via the femoral artery. A similar technique has been used by Maton *et al* (1983) to treat hepatic secondaries in carcinoid disease.

Tissue damage caused by embolisation produces toxic side effects. Patients usually develop a fever, often with rigours and vomiting is common and low sodium fluid replacement is necessary for several days.

Transplantation
Transplantation of the liver is an uncommon operation, usually performed at antisocial hours.

The one-year survival is now better than 50%. Cardiac arrest during anaesthesia is not uncommon and occurs principally when the inferior vena cava is clamped, reducing the venous return, and on revascularisation of the donor liver. Revascularisation is usually accompanied by acidosis, hyperkalcaemia, hypothermia and haemorrhage. Large quantities of blood (up to 25 litres) and clotting factors are required. Facilities must be available for frequent rapid estimation of acid base, electrolyte and serum glucose status. Recent, successful, liver transplantation has been performed in children with primary biliary atresia.

For the past decade, Kasai's procedure — a loop of intestine anastomosed to the porta hepatis – has been performed in children with this condition. These children present no anaesthetic problems other than those associated with their age. Frequently, the bilirubin is greater than 100 μmol/l, but, unlike adults with this degree of jaundice, they do not suffer any associated renal effects.

Postoperative hepatic dysfunction
For many years it has been popular to blame any postoperative hepatic dysfunction on the volatile anaesthetic agent used. Chloroform is truly hepatotoxic but problems with this agent were usually associated with hypoxia, hypotension, a concentration higher than $2 \cdot 25\%$ and in a liver low in glycogen and methionine. It was no surprise that reports of hepatic dysfunction after halothane anaesthesia in the late 1950s were recorded. 'Halothane hepatitis' has become a much abused term, an easy diagnosis for the physician, as until recently, it was impossible on clinical, biochemical and histological grounds to distinguish it from hepatic damage from other causes. Metabolites of halothane can be directly hepatotoxic, especially in a liver stressed by some other cause. Liver function changes produced by halothane have had conflicting interpretations, and recent work suggests that in most people, agents other than halothane produce similar changes. Even when definite changes in function have been seen following halothane, subsequent halothane challenge in the same patient has not repeated the liver function change or caused cell damage. The incidence of jaundice following halothane exposure is variously quoted as between 1 in 10 000 and 1 in 45 000, which makes it a very safe agent.

Recently, Neuberger *et al* (1983) has described a specific halothane related antibody. It was found in 50% of patients in fulminant hepatic failure, following halothane anaesthesia. All patients exhibiting the antibody had previous, recent, exposure to halothane. This would appear an immunologically mediated hypersensitivity reaction. The antibody is able to induce normal lymphocytes to become hepatotoxic to hepatocytes coated in antibody.

Other patients in fulminate hepatic failure, but not exhibiting the antibody, had all received halothane while their liver had been stressed by hepatitis, hepatotoxic medication or massive blood transfusion. In addition to prior exposure to halothane, hepatitis following this drug is more likely to occur in the fat and elderly, with enzyme induction in a liver stressed by other reactive metabolites and undergoing an operation or technique which will materially affect the liver blood flow.

Enflurane too is hepatotoxic, but jaundice following its use has been estimated by Lewis *et al* (1983) at about 1 in 1 000 000. This is probably a conservative estimate. The picture is identical to that seen with hepatitis following halothane: anorexia, nausea, malaise, fever, jaundice eosinophilia and occasionally a rash.

The histological and biochemical findings are identical. Of those patients developing enflurane hepatitis, almost 70% had previous exposure to enflurane or halothane. There is conflicting evidence concerning the biochemical changes produced in the liver by enflurane. Halothane and methoxyflurane have definitely been shown to enduce enzymes. This has not been demonstrated with enflurane.

Isoflorane is not hepatotoxic and does not produce hepatotoxic metabolites. It appears to have no effect on the liver of rats which have been experimentally stressed.

Viral hepatitis
This can be caused by several viruses, but is normally caused by virus A or virus B (Table 4.1). Herpes simplex, Epstein-Barr and cytomegalovirus are other viruses which are readily identifiable by laboratory testing and known to cause hepatitis. Virus non-A non-B (NA NB) has yet to be identified by simple laboratory test. Since testing for other viruses has become routine, NA NB is now the commonest cause of post-transfusion hepatitis. Hepatitis caused by A, herpes simplex, Epstein-Barr and cytomegalovirus usually runs a mild clinical course and does not lead to chronic liver disease. Hepatitis caused by virus B and NA NB is a recognised aetiological factor in cirrhosis and hepatoma.

Table 4.1 Causes and transmission of viral hepatitis

Virus	Transmission
Hb A	Faeco-oral. Poor hygiene. Associated with traveller's diarrhoea
Hb B	Close personal contact. Semen, saliva and blood products
CMV	Close personal contact. One percent neonates are seropositive
Herpes simplex	Personal contact
Epstein-Barr	Infectious mononucleosis. ? kissing, but not necessarily close contact
NA NB	Blood products

Anaesthesia in patients with viral hepatitis should be avoided at almost all cost, as fulminant hepatic failure may follow.

The risk to medical attendants is not high with hepatitis other than B and NA NB. Hepatitis surface antigen (HB$_s$Ag), previously known as Australia antigen, is a useful laboratory marker in hepatitis B. If the serum shows a core antibody (Hb$_c$Ab) an active or recent infection is indicated. The e antigen (Hb$_e$Ag) is of great importance, as it indicates that the patient is highly infectious, though may only be a carrier himself.

Protection for attendants from HB$_s$Ag should include gloves, gowns and goggles. Apparatus should be disposable, but, where necessary, sterilisation with ethylene oxide, glutaraldehyde and heat are effective.

At King's College Hospital, instruments are soaked in glutaraldehyde for 30 minutes and then autoclaved. Alternatively, 4 hours in glutaraldehyde is effective sterilisation. Where personal contamination occurs, passive immunisation should be given promptly.

Immunisation. Active immunisation is performed using inactivated HB$_s$Ag, commercially available as 'HB Vax', 20 μg of Hb$_s$Ag being absorbed on to alum. An intramuscular injection, repeated at 1 month, gives 87% protection, and a third booster injection at 6 months gives protection in 96% of individuals. Immunity lasts at least 2 years and probably 5. Mild side effects occur in 25% of people given the vaccine, but the speculation that Acquired Immune Deficiency Syndrome (AIDS) is transmitted by the vaccine, has yet to be substantiated.

Passive immunity. As fewer than 3% of the population (UK) have immunity, normal immune globulin is of little use. A specific immunoglobulin with a high titre of anti HB (HBIG) must be used. After accidental exposure to Hb$_s$Ag, HBIG should be given within 48 hours of exposure and ideally repeated at 1 month.

REFERENCES

Child C G 1966 The liver and portal hypertension. In: *Major problems in clinical surgery*, vol 1. W B Saunders Co, Philadelphia

Corall I M, Strunin L 1984 Oesophageal varices: Evaluation of sclerotherapy without general anaesthesia, using the fibreoptic gastroscope. *Annals of the Royal College of Surgeons of England* 66: 71

Lewis H, Zimmerman H J, Ishak K G, Mullick P G 1983 Enflurane hepatotoxicity. *Annals of Internal Medicine* 98: 984–992

Matron P N, Camilleri M, Griffin G, Hodgson H F, Chadwick V S 1983 The role of hepatic arterial embolisation in the carcinoid syndrome. *British Medical Journal* 287: 932–934

Neuberger J, Gimson A E S, Davis M, Williams R 1983 Specific serological markers associated with halothane anaesthesia and fulminant hepatic failure. *British Journal of Anaesthesia* 55: 15–20

Pugh R N H, Murray-Lyon I M, Dawson J L, Pietroui M C, Williams R 1973 Transection of the oesophagus for bleeding varices. *British Journal of Surgery* 60: 646–649

Sears J W, Prys Roberts C, Dye A 1983 Hepatic function after anaesthesia for major vascular reconstructive surgery — a comparison of four anaesthetic techniques. *British Journal of Anaesthesia* 55: 603–610

Steven J, Goff S C, Warren G H 1983 Endoscopic sclerotherapy for bleeding varices. Effects and complications. *Annals of Internal Medicine* 98: 900–903

Further reading

Strunin L 1977. *The liver and anaesthesia.* W B Saunders Co, London

Sherlock S 1981 *Disease of the liver and biliary systems*, 6th edn. Blackwell's Scientific Publications, London

Davis N, Tedgar J M, Williams R 1981 *Drug reactions and the liver.* Pitman Medical, London

Opioid receptors

INTRODUCTION

Studies of a variety of neurotransmitter and hormone systems have shown that, in many cases, the receptors with which the hormone interacts may be divided into sub-groups on the basis of structure–activity relationships for natural and/or synthetic ligands. Such sub-populations of receptors may reflect locational or functional differences but, in addition, they may be complementary to the various members of a whole family of chemical mediators. For example, the catecholamines (adrenaline, noradrenaline and dopamine), have subtle differences in their selectivities for particular sub-sets of receptors.

The characterisation of receptors is of fundamental importance, not only to our understanding of the physiological mechanisms underlying a particular hormone system, but also to the design of selective agonists or antagonists as potential therapeutic agents. In comparison to the long history of opioid drugs in medicine, the concept of a specific 'opioid receptor'* is a relatively recent development. During the last decade, it has become clear that there is a large number of endogenous opioid peptides. Whilst the physiological role of many of these remains largely unknown, analogy with other hormone systems in itself lends tacit support to the idea that there may be more than one sub-type of opioid receptors. This chapter is a brief overview of the progress that has been made towards confirming that proposition.

PHARMACOLOGICAL APPROACHES TO THE CLASSIFICATION OF RECEPTORS

The main approaches to the classification of receptors may be summarised as follows:

1. Relative activities of agonists in different tissues.
2. Relative activities of antagonists in different tissues.
3. Stereoselectivity of agonists and/or antagonists.
4. Selective cross-desensitisation between agonists.
5. Post-receptor mechanisms.
6. Ligand binding studies.

Each of these techniques has been used in attempts to characterise opoiod receptors although,

---

* The term *opiate* refers to compounds specifically derived from the poppy and has been used to include morphine derivatives. The term *opioid* refers to compounds that are antagonised by naloxone. (See Hughes J, Kosterlitz H W 1983 Introduction to opioid peptides. *British Medical Bulletin* **39:** 1–3.)

in common with many other systems, it was the comparison of relative activities of agonists that provided the initial leads.

Since many studies have used more than one approach, no attempt will be made to discuss them under methodological headings. A wide range of endogenous opioid peptides and their analogues, together with naturally occurring and synthetic alkaloids have been used in the work to be discussed and some key examples of these are referred to in the text.

Opioid receptor sub-types

The synthesis of nalorphine (Fig. 5.1) and the characterisation of its biological activity (Martin 1967) together represented a major turning point in opioid research. One reason for this was that, whilst it has analgesic activity in its own right, it acts as an antagonist towards morphine and so was of potential use clinically for the reversal of undesirable effects (notably respiratory depression) of morphine. Subsequently, its close analogue, naloxone, was shown to be a pure antagonist and so was adopted in preference to nalorphine.

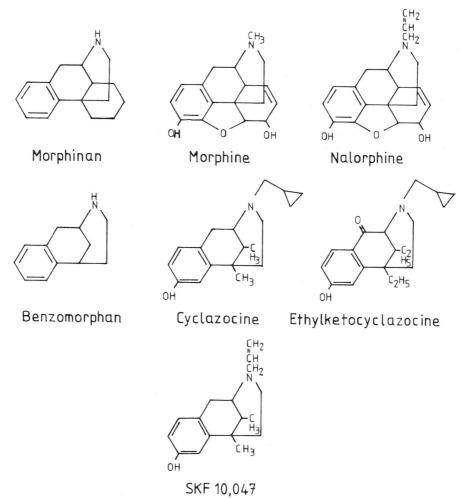

Fig. 5.1 Structures of some morphinan and benzomorphan derivatives with opioid activity.

The second important influence of nalorphine arose from recognition of the fact that its spectrum of pharmacological activity had important differences when compared to morphine (Martin 1967). This suggested that not all opioids acted through the same mechanism and one interpretation of this was that there were sub-populations of opioid receptors. In 1976, Martin laid the foundations of a classification for opioid receptors. He identified three different opioid-induced syndromes in the non-dependent spinal dog and he attributed these to three distinguishable receptor sub-types denoted μ, $\varkappa$ and σ. The prototype agonists for these sites and their respective syndromes are given in Table 5.1.

Table 5.1 Opioid receptor classification as proposed by Martin et al (1976)

Receptor type	Prototype agonist	Syndrome
μ	Morphine	Miosis, bradycardia, hypothermia, general depression of nociceptive responses, indifference to environmental stimuli
$\varkappa$	Ketocyclazocine	Pupil constriction, depression of flexor reflex to noxious stimulus (toe-pinch), sedation — but no marked change in heart rate or skin twitch reflex to heat stimulus
σ	SKF 10,047 (N-allyl normetazocine)	Mydriasis, tachypnea, tachycardia, mania (in marked contrast to μ and $\varkappa$ effects)

Each of these syndromes was considered to be an opioid receptor-mediated effect in that it could be antagonised by the opioid antagonist, naltrexone. Furthermore, chronic administration of each agonist generated tolerance to its own effects, but whilst morphine would suppress the abstinence syndrome in morphine-dependent dogs, ketocyclazocine would not. The apparent clear distinction is demonstrated in Table 5.2 (modified from Martin et al 1976).

Table 5.2

| | Receptor sub-type | | |
	μ	$\varkappa$	σ
Pulse rate	↓	0	↑
Pupil diameter	↓	↓	↑
Respiratory rate	↓	0	↑
Body temperature	↓	0	↑
Flexor reflex response to toe-pinch	↓↓	↓↓	↓
Skin twitch response to thermal stimulus	↓↓	↓	0
Suppression of morphine abstinence syndrome	+	0	0
Suppression of cyclazocine abstinence syndrome	+	+	
Behavioural effect in dog	Indifference	Sedation	Delirium

Modified from Martin et al (1976).

Some authors have questioned whether the σ site should be considered a true opioid receptor (see below), although it may mediate the psychotomimetic effects of some opioids. Nevertheless, the classification of Martin et al (1976) continues to form the basis of most current thinking on opioid receptors. That it should have been deduced from studies of complex behavioural measurements, such as antinociception, is an impressive achievement.

The discovery of the endogenous opioid peptides, [Leu^5]- and [Met^5]-enkephalin, and the subsequent reports of no less than three separate families of opioid peptides, has added a further dimension to the classification of opioid receptors since, at least some of them, are undoubtedly the endogenous ligands for those receptors (Hughes et al 1975, Hughes 1983, Akil et al 1984). Confirmation of this came from Lord et al (1977), who noted important discrepancies between two bioassays and the receptor binding of agonists as defined by their ability to displace $[^3H]$-naloxone or $[^3H]$-[Leu^5]-enkephalin from binding sites in membrane preparations from guinea-pig brain. A number of important points arose from this and a previous study (Hutchinson *et al* 1975):

1. There was good agreement between the relative potencies of many opioid agonists in depressing the electrically-evoked twitch of the mouse vas deferens or guinea-pig ileum in vitro and their analgesic potencies in man. However, certain benzomorphans (Fig 5.1), which are effective antinociceptive agents but do not substitute for morphine in dependent animals, exhibited somewhat lower potency in the vas deferens compared to the guinea-pig ileum. These are compounds which would fall into the $\varkappa$ sub-class of Martin *et al* (1976).

2. Certain benzomorphan derivatives required a higher concentration of the antagonists, naloxone or naltrexone, to reverse their actions.

3. The endogenous opioid peptides showed marked differences in the bioassays and binding studies. Thus, whereas β-endorphin was approximately equipotent in the mouse vas deferens and guinea-pig ileum, Met-enkephalin and Leu-enkephalin were relatively more potent in the mouse vas deferens than the guinea-pig ileum. Further discrepancies were found when naloxone was tested as an antagonist in the guinea-pig ileum and mouse vas deferens (Table 5.3).

Table 5.3 Dose-dependent inhibition of the twitch response to field-stimulation caused by agonists, in the guinea-pig ileum and mouse vas deferens − comparison of the effects of naloxone*

Agonist	Equilibrium dissociation constants (K_e−nM) for naloxone	
	Guinea-pig ileum	Mouse vas deferens
Normorphine	2·64	1·84
[Met^5]-enkephalin	2·45	22·6
[Leu^5]-enkephalin	2·43	21·4

* Note that there is a ten-fold discrepancy between the K_e values for the enkephalins in the mouse vas deferens compared to the values for normorphine in the same tissue or all three agonists in the guinea-pig ileum. (Data from Lord *et al* 1977.)

The conclusion from this work was that a fourth receptor should be added to the opioid receptor classification. This was considered to be the predominant sub-type in the mouse vas deferens and was designated the δ receptor.

Whilst the mouse vas deferens (at least, in some strains) appears to have predominantly δ receptors, with some μ and $\varkappa$ receptors, the rabbit vas deferens appears to have almost exclusively $\varkappa$ receptors (Oka *et al* 1980). This species variation extends to the rat vas deferens, since some compounds (e.g. ethylketocyclazocine, Mr 2034 and bremazocine), which are μ or $\varkappa$ agonists in other tissues, act as antagonists against normorphine [D-Ala^2,MePhe^4,Gly-ol^5]-enkephalin (DAGO), β-endorphin and [D-Ala^2,D-Leu^5]-enkephalin (DADLE) in this preparation (Gillan *et al* 1981). β-Endorphin is, as indicated, an agonist, and it has been suggested that the receptors in the rat vas deferens constitute a distinct population and should be designated ε (Wüster *et al* 1978,1980). However, before accepting the existence of yet another receptor sub-type, it should be noted that the apparent conversion of an agonist to an antagonist does not necessarily imply fundamental differences in receptors. Consider a low efficacy agonist (i.e. one which binds to a given receptor but is of low efficiency in effecting the conformational change which is believed to initiate the response-coupling mechanism). Such a compound may appear to be an effective agonist in a tissue which has a large pool of receptors. However, when applied to a tissue with a small pool, the compound is unable to produce a measurable response even at concentrations where it occupies a large proportion of the available receptors. Nevertheless, its ability to bind to the receptor means that it may act as a competitive antagonist towards a high-efficacy agonist. Thus, it may be that the ε receptor in the rat vas deferens is in fact a restricted population of μ receptors (Smith & Rance 1983).

The receptor sub-types discussed so far are summarised in Table 5.4. The ε receptor is included, but with the reservations referred to above.

Table 5.4 Summary of opioid receptor sub-types*

Opioid receptor sub-type	Bioassay system
μ	Field-stimulated guinea-pig ileum in vitro
κ	Field-stimulated rabbit vas deferens in vitro
δ	Field-stimulated mouse vas deferens in vitro
ε	Field-stimulated rat vas deferens in vitro
σ	Psychotomimetic effects

* The validity of the ε and σ types as genuine sub-classes of opiate receptor has been challenged. Thus, ε-receptors may be indistinguishable from μ-receptors whereas the σ-receptor may be similar to, or identical with, the 'phencyclidine receptor' (see text).

Classification of receptors is greatly assisted if selective antagonists are available. Whilst there have been considerable advances in the development of opioid antagonists, it is still not possible to define each receptor sub-type in terms of selective antagonists. Naloxone, itself, shows some selectivity for μ sites, compared to δ and κ sites, but the selectivity ratio is, at best, about 10:1 (Lord et al 1977). Naloxone is reported to inhibit the behavioural effects of the proposed σ agonist, SKF 10,047, but its binding in brain membrane preparations is not readily displaced by this antagonist. This observation has added support to the suggestion that 'σ-agonists' act through phencyclidine- rather than opioid-receptors (see Gillan et al 1981).

Naloxone also reverses the actions of opioids at the proposed ε receptor (Schulz et al 1979) but, as explained above, this may be a μ site. There is no highly selective κ antagonist, although Mr2266 shows a marginal selectivity over μ sites and a greater selectivity over δ sites (Paterson et al 1983). The most selective competitive opioid antagonists are those acting at δ receptors. A series of analogues of Leu-enkephalin is reported to have δ-antagonist activity and, the most recent of these, ICI 174,864, (N,N-diallyl-Tyr-Aib-Phe-Leu-OH) has a selectivity ratio δ:K and δ:μ of about 200 (Cotton et al 1984).

Portoghese and colleagues (see Sayre et al 1983 for references) have prepared a series of naltrexone-derived irreversible antagonists for opioid receptors and these are of potential value as affinity labels. Many of these compounds have initial agonist activity, which is reversible on washing in the guinea-pig ileum, but they tend to be partial agonists in the mouse vas deferens. The most widely reported of these compounds, β-funaltrexamine (β-FNA), and β-chlornaltrexamine (β-CNA), have proved useful in defining receptor populations involved in a particular opioid mechanism (e.g. Ward & Takemori 1983), in estimating dissociation constants for agonists and for removing a particular population of receptors (in functional terms) from a tissue having a mixture of sub-types. β-FNA has reversible κ agonist activity but irreversible μ- and δ-antagonist activity (Hayes et al 1985). β-CNA is non-selective and blocks μ, κ and δ sites.

An additional level of complexity has been added to the classification system for opioid receptors through the suggestion by some authors that further sub-divisions of the main classes may be distinguished. This has been most vigorously pursued for the μ site. In binding studies on homogenates of rat brain, Pasternak and colleagues have identified 'high' and 'low' affinity components with [³H]-normorphine and [³H]-naloxone as ligands (see

Pasternak 1982). The high affinity component appeared to be common to morphine and the enkephalins and it was suggested as being a μ-like receptor responsible for mediating the analgesic effects of the opioids. This high affinity site could be distinguished in terms of its ontogeny and phylogeny and, furthermore, naloxazone was said to be a selective, reversible antagonist. Thus, on the basis of binding studies and pharmacological experiments, a tentative classification was proposed — μl receptors mediate analgesia and catalepsy whilst other receptors ($\mu 2$?) mediate sedation and respiratory depression.

Pasternak (1982) points out that, whereas there is little evidence of cross-tolerance between μ- and δ-selective agonists in the guinea-pig ileum and mouse vas deferens preparations, it does occur when antinociception is the test under consideration. He thus argues in favour of a common mechanism for analgesia, which is sensitive to naloxazone, and that the property of an agonist which he describes as 'lethality' (i.e. respiratory depression), is mediated through a different site. However, the absence of interactions between μ- and δ-sites, in terms of analgesia or in isolated tissues in vitro, may not be as clear-cut as is envisaged here (see Vaught & Takemori 1979a b, Schulz et al 1981, Lee et al 1982). The existence of a $\mu 2$ sub-site is based largely on indirect arguments and, in many cases, cannot be clearly distinguished from the δ-site (Wood & Pasternak 1983).

The κ receptor has been a target for further sub-division also. Audigier et al (1982) have suggested that binding studies with [^{3}H]-etorphine in the guinea-pig spinal cord, under conditions whereby the μ and δ sites have been obliterated with high concentrations of DADLE, could be interpreted in terms of two κ binding sites. The authenticity of such a sub-division remains to be confirmed.

Whilst most groups have adopted the classification of Martin et al (1976), as extended by Lord et al (1977), at least as a working hypothesis, other suggestions have been made for novel classifications. Pert et al (1980) reported that opioid receptors may be sub-divided according to their sensitivity to guanosine triphosphate (GTP). Interaction of ligands with 'Type 1' binding sites was inhibited by GTP, whereas 'Type 2' sites were unaffected by this treatment. Other authors have questioned whether it is necessary to postulate a large number of receptor sub-types and have asked whether the evidence could be equated with a single receptor. For example, Smith et al (1983) have pointed out that β-endorphin is a universal ligand in biological tests and binding studies with opioids. These authors propose a model in which there is a single basic β-endorphin receptor and that different spectra of activities of selective agonists and antagonists reflect variations in receptor–response coupling at different sites. They suggest that a number of features, such as synergistic interactions between agonists, overlap of agonist effects, and mutual displacement of selective agonists from binding sites by compounds having a different selectivity, all argue in favour of their proposal. Protagonists of multiple sites would counter this by saying that many of these points are accounted for by the poor receptor selectivity ratios of most of the agonists that are used as 'selective' tools. A crucial test is the selectivity (or otherwise) of antagonists. If they can be shown to inhibit the actions of the more selective agonists in pharmacological tests and compete for specific sites in binding experiments, then a scheme of selectivities based on receptor-response coupling is severely challenged. Thus, the recent development of relatively δ-selective reversible antagonists and μ-selective irreversible antagonists argues in favour of operationally distinguishable receptor sub-types.

A further possibility has been proposed by Barnard and colleagues (see Barnard 1983). It is suggested that, whilst there are distinguishable sub-types of opioid receptor which can exist independently of one another, they may be linked together to form a receptor complex. This would take the form of two dimers*, each of which consists of two sub-units: the enkephalin dimer δ1, δ2, and the morphine dimer μ,κ. These, it is argued, are connected by disulphide bridges whose integrity is regulated by cations and by GTP. Both dimers may coexist or they may be differentially distributed. This is an inhibitory suggestion, but it poses some practical difficulties. For example, it would be necessary to invoke some form of suppressor mechanism in order to explain the predominance of one receptor sub-type in a given tissue (e.g. κ sites in rabbit vas deferens).

As a method of classifying receptors, the post-receptor mechanism (biochemical change, alteration in membrane conductance, etc.), is unlikely to be sufficiently discriminating to be considered an adequate description of receptor sub-types. However, such mechanisms may provide useful correlations to support a classification based on other factors and, in any event, the information is fundamental to an understanding of the actions of a particular compound.

A well-established action of morphine is its inhibitory effect on release of neurotransmitters in the central and peripheral nervous systems (for references, see Jordan 1983, West & Miller 1983). This forms the basis of the bioassay preparations (field-stimulated guinea-pig ileum and mouse vas deferens in vitro) which were used in the isolation and characterisation of the enkephalins (Hughes et al 1975). What is the mechanism of this effect on neurotransmitter release and is it associated with a particular receptor sub-type? Recent electrophysiological experiments suggest that there may be at least two distinguishable mechanisms:

1. *Hyperpolarisation of the neuronal cell membrane can impair the generation of action potentials, thereby altering the firing rate of the neurone.* In addition, hyperpolarisation may prevent the invasion of nerve terminals by action potentials and so prevent the release of neurotransmitter (Morita & North 1983). The release of noradrenaline from neurones having their cell bodies in the locus coeruleus is known to be inhibited by opioids. Intracellular recordings made from locus coeruleus neurones in vitro have demonstrated that normorphine and DADLE inhibit spontaneous firing and hyperpolarise the cell membrane and this is the result of an increase in potassium conductance (North & Williams 1983). These authors also found that opioids inhibit the calcium component of the action potential, but this was almost certainly a consequence of the effects on potassium conductance rather than a direct effect on calcium channels. Similar hyperpolarising responses have been observed in neurones of the myenteric plexus and in the spinal cord (Morita & North 1981, North 1982, North et al 1982).

In terms of receptor involvement in the hyperpolarising action of opiates, μ-sites are those which appear to predominate in the tissues studied so far.

2. *An inhibitory effect of opioids on calcium currents in nerve terminals is an attractive hypothesis to explain the observed reduction in release of neurotransmitters.* Inhibition of the calcium component of the action potential by opioids has been observed in a number of systems, notably in dorsal root ganglion cells (Mudge et al 1979, Werz & MacDonald 1983), and this effect appeared to be involve both μ and δ receptors. However, as indicated already, it is not always possible to distinguish this effect from one on potassium conductance — a point also noted by Werz & MacDonald (1983). Nevertheless, there is a considerable amount of electrophysiological evidence linking the action of opioids and a direct effect on calcium channels and Kamikuba et al (1983) have shown that opioids inhibit depolarisation-induced uptake of ^{45}Ca into rat brain synaptosomes. In areas where κ receptors may be important in the pharmacological actions of opioids (e.g. myenteric plexus and dorsal horn of the spinal cord), an effect on calcium channels may well be the most important mechanism.

---

* Aggregate of two large molecules.

In addition to effects on ion movements, there is evidence to suggest that biochemical changes are induced by some opioids. In the brain, adenylate cyclase activity is reduced, although it is not clear whether this is functionally linked with any particular opioid action. However, there are several cell lines in culture which have a predominance of δ receptors and in which opioids reduce CAMP activity. It is possible, therefore, that this represents an important receptor-response coupling arrangement for δ receptors.

OPIOID RECEPTORS AND THEIR INVOLVEMENT IN PARTICULAR PHARMACOLOGICAL ACTIONS OF OPIOIDS

The primary therapeutic application of opioid drugs is analgesia, although other properties such as inhibition of propulsive activity of the gut and suppression of the cough reflex are of considerable importance. A key question is whether the various desirable and undesirable effects of the opioids are separable in terms of the receptor sub-types which mediate them, since such a separation would offer the possibility of designing more selective therapeutic agents.

Receptors involved in antinociception

Whilst opioid-induced antinociception is a complex behavioural effect which results from pharmacological actions at several independent sites, it is often viewed as a unified phenomenon. However, different opioid analgesics may be distinguishable in terms of their qualitative effects and so it is important to consider the possible significance of this with respect to receptor classification. Tyers (1980) has demonstrated that, in tests involving a heat stimulus (tail-flick, hot-plate etc.), μ agonists such as morphine, pethidine and dextropropoxyphene, produce steep dose-response relationships and exhibit relative potencies similar to those observed for analgesia and bioassays in guinea-pig ileum and mouse vas deferens *in vitro*. In contrast, κ agonists such as ethylketazocine, nalorphine, Mr2034 and pentazocine, are of low activity in these tests, except in doses which produce sedation. In the writhing test (which employs a chemical stimulus), the paw pressure tests and the dog tooth-pulp test, both μ and κ agonists produce steep dose-response curves. Thus, μ agonists show little selectivity for any particular form of noxious stimulus whereas κ agonists are poorly effective in heat-based tests.

Further evidence for differences in the sites of action of opioid analgesics comes from studies in which drugs are administered directly into the csf of the ventricular system or the spinal subarachnoid space, thereby achieving a degree of localisation of their distribution. Results of experiments such as these imply that the spinal cord is an important site of action for κ agonist-induced antinociception (Wood *et al* 1981, Piercey *et al* 1982a b). However, κ receptors at other locations may be involved in antinociception also. Goodman & Snyder (1982) have suggested that cells in layer VI of the cerebral cortex (on which κ receptors are known to be located), may have a controlling influence on sensory inputs from the thalamus and so are well-placed to exert control over sensory pathways including those in arousal and, possibly, pain perception.

There is little evidence to suggest that σ receptors are involved in antinociception. SKF 10,047 is very weakly active in the phenylquinone writhing test in the mouse (Pearl & Harris 1966).

There is some uncertainty as to the degree of involvement of δ receptors in analgesic mechanisms, largely because of the relatively poor selectivity of the available agonists. There are several reports which conclude that there are genuine δ-mediated antinociceptive effects.

For example, Hynes & Frederickson (1982) concluded that there was a δ component in the effects of metkephamid in the mouse hot-plate test. Satoh *et al* (1983) have suggested that there are certain sites in the rat brain (e.g. nucleus raphe magnus and periaqueductal grey area) where δ receptors may make a major contribution to the action of opioid analgesics. Delta sites appear to be present in the spinal cord also (Goodman *et al* 1980) and may be associated with primary afferent fibres (Fields *et al* 1980). Thus, the spinal cord is a potential site for δ-mediated antinociception. The recently developed δ-selective antagonists should help to define the relative contribution of δ receptors to antinociception.

It is important to note that there are marked species differences in the relative numbers of opioid receptor sub-types (Table 5.5) and this will almost certainly determine their respective contributions to antinociception and, indeed, other actions of opioids. Thus, in the rat, the μ site appears to predominate with the κ site being a minor component. In man, as in guinea-pig, there is a marked shift towards a predominance of κ sites with a corresponding reduction in μ sites. The greater proportion of κ sites in man may have important consequences for the development of novel analgesic agents.

Table 5.5 Comparison of proportions of μ, δ and κ binding sites in the brains of different species*

Species	% binding sites as sub-type		
	μ	δ	κ
Rat	62	25	13
Pig	40	23	37
Guinea-pig	34	30	26
Human (cerebral cortex)	29	21	50

* Data from Maurer (1982). Other studies have shown similar distribution between receptor sub-types.

Receptors involved in respiratory depression

Ling *et al* (1983) have argued that respiratory depression and analgesia are mediated through different receptor populations since pre-treatment with the unsurmountable antagonist, naloxonazone, inhibited the former but not the latter effect. Ward & Holaday (1982) have found that both μ and δ antagonists inhibit the respiratory depressant effects of morphine and so, in view of this, Ling *et al* (1983) concluded that respiratory depression may be mediated through '$\mu2$' and/or δ sites. Pazos & Flórez (1984) have also found evidence for an involvement of δ receptors in respiratory depression. However, interpretation of these experiments is complicated by the relatively poor selectivity of some of the compounds used.

Ward & Takemori (1983) noted that tolerance to the respiratory depressant and anti-nociceptive effects of morphine developed at different rates. However, this does not necessarily imply a difference in receptor sub-types. In a study (in mice) of compounds with varying degrees of selectivity for μ and κ receptors, Hayes & Tyers (1983) found that undesirable effects, including respiratory depression, were most apparent in compounds acting at μ sites and least apparent in those selective for κ sites. Thus, the antinociceptive effects of μ agonists appeared to be inseparable from their undesirable effects. In contrast, κ agonists produced minimal side-effects, including respiratory depression. This latter observation concurs with the very low levels of κ receptors which appear to be present in the brainstem — the presumed site of opioid effects on respiration (Goodman & Snyder 1982).

Thus, respiratory depression appears most likely to be mediated through μ and δ receptors. The possibility that the μ sites responsible for this important action of opioids represent a sub-population distinct from those involved in antinociception remains to be confirmed.

Receptors involved in effects on the gastrointestinal tract

Inhibition of propulsive movements of the gut represents an undesirable effect of opioids when used as analgesics although it does constitute a therapeutic action in its own right. Both μ and $\varkappa$ agonists impair propulsive activity (Martin et al 1976, Porreca et al 1981, Hayes & Tyers 1983), but their sites of action may well be different. A comparison of the effects of intracerebroventricular and subcutaneous administration of μ- and $\varkappa$-selective agonists on the movement of a charcoal meal along the gastrointestinal tract in mice, suggested that μ-agonists act predominantly through sites in the c.n.s. whilst $\varkappa$ agonists act peripherally. Intrathecal administration of morphine or of δ-agonists produces inhibition of propulsive activity of the gut (Porreca et al 1983), whereas $\varkappa$ agonists, administered intrathecally or intracerebroventricularly, had no effect. This suggests that the receptors involved predominantly in the centrally mediated effects of opioids on the gut are of the μ and δ sub-types. On the basis of these experiments, the effects of $\varkappa$ agonists on the gut appear to be confined to a local action only.

Receptors involved in the sedative effects of opioids

Martin et al (1976) suggested that sedation was a $\varkappa$-mediated effect of opioids in the chronic spinal dog and, indeed, some of the recently developed $\varkappa$-selective agonists have marked sedative actions which severely limit their potential as therapeutic agents. However, others have argued that, in the conscious dog and in the mouse, there is no clear correlation between antinociceptive activity and sedation produced by $\varkappa$ agonists. Thus, if it is assumed that the antinociceptive action of these compounds is largely $\varkappa$-mediated, it may be argued that sedation is unlikely to be wholly dependent on a similar receptor population (Hayes & Tyers 1983, see also Pickworth & Sharpe 1979). However, it remains to be seen whether it will be possible to produce selective $\varkappa$ agonists which are devoid of sedative effects and hence of potential value as analgesic agents in man.

Receptors involved in the diuretic and antidiuretic effects of opioids

Morphine and other μ agonists tend to produce an antidiuretic effect which is assumed to result from an increased release of vasopressin. In complete contrast to this, selective $\varkappa$ agonists produce varying levels of diuresis (Leander 1983a b). Thus, effects on urine flow appear to be a highly discriminating measure of μ and $\varkappa$ activity. Leander (1983a) has pointed out that dynorphin appears to be co-stored with vasopressin in hypothalamic neurosecretory magnocellular neurones (see Watson et al 1982), and so it is possible that dynorphin has some autoregulatory function with respect to vasopressin-secreting cells.

Receptors involved in psychotomimetic effects of opioids

The psychotomimetic effects precipitated in man by some opioid drugs, such as nalorphine and pentazocine, represent a serious drawback to their use as therapeutic agents. This effect has been reported for a number of relatively selective $\varkappa$ agonists, but it is not clear whether it is inextricably linked to interaction with another receptor, be it designated the phencyclidine- or σ-receptor (Zukin 1982).

Prospects for the development of novel opioid analgesic agents

The aim of medicinal chemists over many years has been to produce opioid drugs with powerful analgesic effects but minimal side-effects. Whilst some major advances have been made, that aim has yet to be fully realised. The finding that there are operationally distinguishable opioid receptors offers the prospect of more selective drugs and, indeed, there is considerable interest in the potential of selective $\varkappa$ agonists as analgesics. The key question is whether the known potential side-effects of such drugs, notably diuresis, sedation and psychotomimetic manifestations are, at least quantitatively, separable from their analgesic properties.

An alternative route is that suggested by the work of Pasternak and co-workers (1982), namely, the development of a selective agonist for the '$\mu 1$' receptor sub-type (assuming this to be a discrete entity). Meptazinol has been advanced as being such a compound and is reported to be of moderate potency with marginal effects on respiration and the gut. It does not substitute for morphine in dependent animals but it acts as an antagonist towards morphine (Stephens *et al* 1978). However, this profile suggests that it may be a μ partial agonist and, in view of its known cholinomimetic properties, it has yet to be proven that this compound represents a significant advance in the development of selective opioid analgesics.

Acknowledgements

I am grateful to Dr A. G. Hayes and Dr M. B. Tyers for their helpful comments on the manuscript.

REFERENCES

Akil H, Watson S J, Young E *et al* 1984 Endogenous opioids: Biology and function. *Annual Review of Neuroscience* 7: 223–255

Audigier Y, Attali B, Mazarguil H *et al* 1982 Characterisation of ^{3}H-etorphine binding in guinea-pig striatum after blockade of μ and δ sites. *Life Sciences* 31: 1287–1290

Barnard E A, Demoliou-Mason C 1983 Molecular properties of opioid receptors. *British Medical Bulletin* 39: 37–45

Cotton R, Giles M G, Miller L *et al* 1984 ICI 174864: A highly selective antagonist for the opioid δ-receptor. *European Journal of Pharmacology* 97: 331–332

Fields H L, Emson P C, Leigh B K *et al* 1980 Multiple opiate receptor sites on primary afferent fibres. *Nature* 284: 351-353

Gillan M G C, Kosterlitz H W, Magnan J 1981 Unexpected antagonism in the rat vas deferens by benzomorphans which are agonists in other pharmacological tests. *British Journal of Pharmacology* 72: 13–15

Goodman R R, Snyder S H 1982 Autoradiographic localisation of $\varkappa$ opiate receptors to deep layers of the cerebral cortex may explain unique sedative and analgesic effects. *Life Sciences* 31: 1291–1294

Goodman R R, Snyder S H, Kuhar M J, Young S W 1980 Differentiation of δ and μ opiate receptor localisations by light microscopic autoradiography. *Proceedings of the National Academy of Science USA* 77: 6239–6243

Hayes A G, Tyers M B 1983 Determination of receptors that mediate opiate side effects in the mouse. *British Journal of Pharmacology* 79: 731–736

Hayes A G, Sheehan M J, Tyers M B 1985 Determination of the receptor selectivity of opioid agonists in the guinea-pig ileum and mouse vas deferens using β-FNA (*Submitted for publication*)

Hughes J 1983 Biogenesis, release and inactivation of enkephalins and dynorphins. *British Medical Bulletin* 39: 17–24

Hughes J, Smith T W, Kosterlitz H W *et al* 1975 Identification of two related pentapeptides from the brain with potent opiate agonist activity. *Nature* 258: 577–579

Hynes M D, Frederickson R C A 1982 Cross-tolerance studies distinguish morphine- and metkephamid-induced analgesia. *Life Sciences* 31: 1201–1204

Jordan C C 1983 Current views on the mechanism of opiate analgesia. In: Kaufman L (ed) *Anaethesia: Review 2*, Churchill Livingstone, Edinburgh, p 108–136

Kamikubo K, Niwa M, Fujimura H *et al* 1983 Morphine inhibits depolarisation-dependent calcium uptake by synaptosomes. *European Journal of Pharmacology* 95: 149–150

Leander J D 1983a A $\varkappa$ opioid effect: increased urination in the rat. *Journal of Pharmacology and Experimental Therapeutics* 224: 89–94

Leander J D 1983b Further study of $\varkappa$ opioids on increased urination. *Journal of Pharmacology and Experimental Therapeutics* 227: 35–41

Lee N M, Huidobro-Toro J-P, Smith A P, Loh H H 1982 β-Endorphin receptor and its possible relationship to other opioid receptors. *Advances in Biochemical Psychopharmacology* **33**: 75–89

Ling G S F, Spiegel K, Nishimura S L, Pasternak G W 1983 Dissociation of morphine's analgesic and respiratory depressant actions. *European Journal of Pharmacology* **86**: 487–488

Lord J A H, Waterfield A A, Hughes J, Kosterlitz H W 1977 Endogenous opioid peptides: multiple agonists and receptors. *Nature* **267**: 495–499

Martin W R 1967 Opioid antagonists. *Pharmacological Reviews* **19**: 463–521

Martin W R, Eades C G, Thompson J A, Huppler R E, Gilbert P E 1976 The effects of morphine- and nalorphine-like drugs in the non-dependent and morphine-dependent chronic spinal dog. *Journal of Pharmacology and Experimental Therapeutics* **197**: 517–532

Maurer R 1982 Multiplicity of opiate receptors in different species. *Neuroscience Letters* **30**: 303–307

Morita K, North R A 1981 Opiates and enkephalin reduce the excitability of neuronal processes. *Neuroscience* **6**: 1943–1951

Mudge A W, Leeman S E, Fischbach G D 1979 Enkephalin inhibits release of substance P from sensory neurones in culture and decreases action potential duration. *Proceedings of the National Academy of Science, USA* **76**: 526–530

North R A, Williams J T 1983 Opiate activation of potassium conductance inhibits calcium action potentials in rat locus coeruleus neurones. *British Journal of Pharmacology* **80**: 225–228

North A R, Morita K, Tokimasa T 1982 Calcium ions reduce enkephalin hyperpolarisation of myenteric neurones. *Advances in Biochemical Psychopharmacology* **33**: 333–336

Oka T, Neigishi K, Suda M *et al* 1980 Rabbit vas deferens: a specific bioassay for opioid κ-receptor agonists. *European Journal of Pharmacology* **73**: 235–236

Pasternak G W 1982 High and low affinity opioid binding sites: relationship to μ and δ sites. *Life Sciences* **31**: 1303–1306

Paterson S J, Robson L E, Kosterlitz H W 1983 Classification of opioid receptors. *British Medical Bulletin* **39**: 31–36

Pazos A, Flórez J 1984 A comparative study in rats of the respiratory depression and analgesia induced by μ- and δ-opioid agonists. *European Journal of Pharmacology* **99**: 15–21

Pearl J, Harris L S 1966 Inhibition of writhing by narcotic antagonists. *Journal of Pharmacology and Experimental Therapeutics* **154**: 319–323

Pert C B, Taylor D P, Pert A, Herkenham M A, Kent J L 1980 Biochemical and autoradiographical evidence for Type 1 and Type 2 opiate receptors. *Advances in Biochemical Psychopharmacology* **22**: 581–589

Pickworth W B, Sharpe L G 1979 EEG-behavioural dissociation after morphine- and cyclazocine-like drugs in the dog: further evidence for two opiate receptors. *Neuropharmacology* **18**: 617–622

Piercey M F, Varner K, Schroeder LA 1982 Analgesic activity of intraspinally administered dynorphin and ethylketocyclazocine. *European Journal of Pharmacology* **80**: 283–284

Piercey M F, Lahti R A, Schroeder L A *et al* 1982 U-50488H, a pure κ receptor agonist with spinal analgesic loci in the mouse. *Life Sciences* **31**: 1197–1200

Porreca F, Burks T F 1983 The spinal cord as a site of opioid effects on gastrointestinal transit in the mouse. *Journal of Pharmacology and Experimental Therapeutics* **227**: 22–27

Porreca F, Raffa R, Cowan A, Tallarida R J 1981 Ethylketocyclazocine and morphine: a comparison of their efficacies on gastrointestinal transit (GIT) after central and peripheral administration to rats. *Federation Proceedings* **40**: 288

Satoh M, Kubota A, Iwama T *et al* 1983 Comparison of analgesic potencies of μ, δ and κ agonists locally applied to various CNS regions relevant to analgesia in rats. *Life Sciences* **33 (Suppl. 1)**: 689–692

Sayre L M, Larson D L, Friers D S, Takemori A E, Portoghese P S 1983 Importance of C-6 chiralty in conferring irreversible opioid antagonism to naltrexone-derived affinity labels. *Journal of Medicinal Chemistry* **26**: 1229–1235

Schulz R, Wüster M, Herz A 1981 Differentiation of opiate receptors in the brain by the selective development of tolerance. *Pharmacology, Biochemistry and Behaviour* **14**: 75–79

Schulz R, Faase E, Wüster M *et al* 1979 Selective receptors for β-endorphin on the rat vas deferens. *Life Sciences* **24**: 843–850

Smith A P, Lee N M, Loh H H 1983 The multiple site β-endorphin receptor. *Trends in Pharmacological Sciences* **4**: 163–164

Smith F C, Rance M J 1983 Opiate receptors in the rat vas deferens. *Life Sciences* **33 (Suppl. 1)**: 327–330

Stephens R J, Waterfall J F, Franklin R A 1978 A review of the biological properties and metabolic disposition of the new analgesic agent, meptazinol. *General Pharmacology* **9**: 73–78

Tyers M B 1980 A classification of opiate receptors that mediate antinociception in animals. *British Journal of Pharmacology* **69**: 503–512

Vaught J L, Takemori A E 1979a Differential effects of leucine and methionine enkephalin on morphine-induced analgesia, acute tolerance and dependence. *Journal of Pharmacology and Experimental Therapeutics* **208**: 86–90

Vaught J L, Takemori A E 1979b A further characterisation of the differential effects of leucine enkephalin, methionine enkephalin and their analogues on morphine-induced analgesia. *Journal of Pharmacology and Experimental Therapeutics* **211**: 280–283

Ward S J, Holaday J W 1982 Relative involvement of μ- and δ-opioid mechanisms in morphine-induced depression of respiration in rats. *Neuroscience Abstracts* **8**: 389

Ward S J, Takemori A E 1983 Determination of the relative involvement of μ-opioid receptors in opioid-induced depression of respiratory rate by use of β-funaltrexamine. *European Journal of Pharmacology* **87**: 1–6

Watson S J, Akil H, Fischli W *et al* 1982 Dynorphin and vasopressin: common localisation in magnocellular neurones. *Science* **216**: 85–87

Werz M A, MacDonald R L 1983 Opioid peptides with differential affinity for μ and δ receptors decrease sensory neuron calcium-dependent action potentials. *Journal of Pharmacology and Experimental Therapeutics* **227**: 394–402

West R E, Miller R J 1983 Opiates, second messengers and cell response. *British Medical Bulletin* **39**: 53–58

Wood P L, Pasternak G W 1983 Specific μ_2 opioid isoreceptor regulation of nigrostriatal neurons: in vivo evidence with naloxonazine. *Neuroscience Letters* **37**: 291–293

Wood P L, Rackham A, Richards J 1981 Spinal analgesia: comparison of the μ agonist morphine and the κ agonist ethylketazocine. *Life Sciences* **28**: 2129–2125

Wüster M, Schulz R, Herz A 1978 Specificity of opioids towards the μ-, δ- and ε-opiate receptors. *Neuroscience Letters* **15**: 193–198

Wüster M, Schulz R, Herz A 1980 The direction of opioid agonists towards μ-, δ- and ε-receptors in the vas deferens of the mouse and rat. *Life Sciences* **27**: 163–170

Zukin S R 1982 Differing stereospecificities distinguish opiate receptor sub-types. *Life Sciences* **31**: 1307–1310

Endorphins

INTRODUCTION

The discovery by Hughes (1975) of two pentapeptides from the brain with 'opiate' like activity, has increased interest in opioid* peptides. Although the term 'endorphins' was used previously to describe those naturally occurring peptides with 'opiate' like biological activity this usage may give rise to confusion. Morley (1981) has recommended therefore that its use be confined to those opioid peptides which arise from the precursor β-lipotropin. New discoveries of various peptides have stimulated localisation studies designed to shed light on the function of neurotransmitters within the c.n.s. The accumulation of large amounts of data, the majority of which is descriptive, has led to confusion in those unfamiliar with the subject.

While there is an enormous bank of data on the localisation of various opioids, there is in contrast little information on their precise physiological roles. Thus, of necessity, this chapter must appear more 'anatomical' than 'physiological' in its orientation,

The whole range of endogenous opioids are considered briefly, and these are classified into three separate families (summarised in Table 6.1) arising from genetically determined precursors as shown in Figure 6.1. Each of the three families are reviewed separately and, in addition, the features of opioid receptors are described with a description of their clinical importance, which at present must remain largely speculative.

Table 6.1 Distribution of opioid peptides

	Major areas	Other sites
Endorphins	Pituitary Hypothalamus and its radiations	Olfactory cortex Hippocampus (GI tract & placenta)
Enkephalins	Wide c.n.s. distribution — Globus pallidus Limbic system Pre-optic nuclei Posterior pituitary GI tract Spinal cord Sympathetic ganglia Adrenal medulla	Carotid body Kidney Eye Skin Liver
Dynorphin	Pituitary Hypothalamus GI tract Spinal cord	

---

* The term *opiate* refers to compounds specifically derived from the poppy and has been used to include morphine derivatives. The term *opioid* refers to compounds that are antagonised by naloxone. (See Hughes J, Kosterlitz H W 1983 Introduction to opioid peptides. *British Medical Bulletin* **39**: 1 – 3.)

Fig. 6.1 The three opioid peptide precursors and their derived peptides.

PRECURSORS	PEPTIDES	STRUCTURES
Proopiomelanocortin	α Endorphin	Tyr-Gly-Gly-Phe-Met-Thr-Ser-Glu-Lys-Ser-Gln-Thr-Pro-Leu-Val-Thr
	γ Endorphin	Tyr-Gly-Gly-Phe-Met-Thr-Ser-Glu-Lys-Ser-Gln-Thr-Pro-Leu-Val-Thr-Leu
	β Endorphin	Tyr-Gly-Gly-Phe-Met-Thr-Ser-Glu-Lys-Ser-Gln-Thr-Pro-Leu-Val-Thr-Leu-Phe-Lys-Asn-Ala-Ile-Ile-Lys-Asn-Ala-His-Lys-Lys-Gly-Gln
Proenkephalin	Met-enkephalin	Tyr-Gly-Gly-Phe-Met
	Leu-enkephalin	Tyr-Gly-Gly-Phe-Leu
	Octapeptide	Tyr-Gly-Gly-Phe-Met-Arg-Gly-Leu
	Heptapeptide	Tyr-Gly-Gly-Phe-Met-Arg-Phe
Prodynorphin	Dynorphin A (1-17)	Tyr-Gly-Gly-Phe-Leu-Arg-Arg-Ile-Arg-Pro-Lys-Leu-Lys-Trp-Asp-Asn-Gln
	Dynorphin A (1-8)	Tyr-Gly-Gly-Phe-Leu-Arg-Arg-Ile
	α Neoendorphin	Tyr-Gly-Gly-Phe-Leu-Arg-Lys-Tyr-Pro-Lys
	β Neoendorphin	Tyr-Gly-Gly-Phe-Leu-Arg-Lys-Tyr-Pro
	Dynorphin B or Rimorphin	Tyr-Gly-Gly-Phe-Leu-Arg-Arg-Gln-Phe-Lys-Val-Val-Thr
	Prodynorphin C-terminal	Tyr-Gly-Gly-Phe-Leu-Arg-Arg-Gln-Phe-Lys-Val-Val-Thr-Arg-Ser-Gln-Glu-Asp-Pro-Ans-Ala-Tyr-Tyr-Glu-Glu-Leu-Phe-Asp-Val

Pro-opiocortin-derived peptides

Using immunoreactive staining techniques, Bloom *et al* (1978) have demonstrated that β endorphin and β lipotropin are present together with ACTH in the pituitary cells of rats, mice, pigs and frogs and Guillemin *et al* (1977) found in the rat that β endorphin and adreno-corticotrophin (ACTH) are secreted concomitantly in increased amounts by the adenohypo-physis in response to stress or adrenalectomy. Conversely, the secretion of both substances was reduced by administration of dexamethasone, suggesting the existence of a common control mechanism.

The postulated precursor molecule, pro-opiocortin was first described by Nakanishi and colleagues (1979). Its peptides are shown in Figure 6.2. The amino acid sequences of melano-cyte stimulating hormone (MSH), ACTH and β lipotropin have been elucidated using

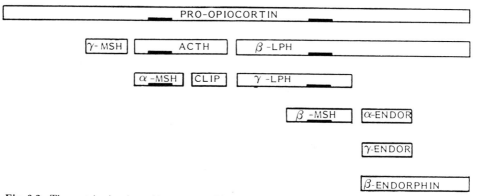

Fig. 6.2 The contained amino acid sequences within propiocortin showing: α, β, γ melanocyte stimulating hormone (MSH); adrenocorticotrophic hormone (ACTH); β/γ lipotrophic hormone (LPH); Corticotrophin-like intermediate peptide (CLIP); α/β/γ endorphin (Endor).

immunoreactive techniques in vivo and in vitro (Bertagna 1978, 1980, Nakao 1980, Hope 1981, Oki 1981, Orth 1978). β endorphin is formed from pro-opiocortin (itself derived from prepro-opiocortin).

In contrast with the wide peripheral distribution of the enkephalins, the majority of localisation studies suggest that the endorphins have a predominantly central distribution (Cuello 1983). The hypothalamus and its associated projecting radiations have been shown to be particularly rich in β endorphin containing neurones. Bloom *et al* (1978) described clusters of these cell bodies in the basal hypothalamus and arcuate nucleus, radiating to the midline structures of thalamic and pontine periaqueductal grey matter. Caudal to the Locus Coeruleus, however, β endorphin is very scarce. Other areas with significant amounts of β endorphin include the olfactory cortex and hippocampus (Bloom 1983). Generally, the respective differences in distribution between endorphins and enkephalins provide support for separate neuronal nets involving the respective families.

β endorphin immunoreactivity has been reported also in the gastrointestinal tract, viz: small intestine, pylorus, colon and pancreas (Bruni 1979, Smyth 1983, Feurle 1980, Orwoll & Kendall 1980, Vuolteenaho 1980). In addition, β endorphin, together with β lipotropin and precursors, have been described in the placenta (Nakai 1978, Odagiri 1979).

Pro-enkephalin derived peptides

Numerous enkephalin containing compounds have been isolated from adrenal chromaffin cells and the complete nucleotide sequence of bovine adrenal pro-enkephalin has been described by Gubler *et al* (1982). Pro-enkephalin contains six copies of the methionine enkephalin sequence and one copy of the leucine enkephalin sequence within its structure (Hughes 1983); various cleavages may occur, giving rise to assorted shorter chain peptides of differing biological activity.

The enkephalins are distributed both within the c.n.s. and peripherally in man. In the brain, particular areas of high concentration occur in the globus pallidus, limbic system and hypothalamic preoptic areas and lower concentrations occur in medulla and pons (Giraud 1983). It is thought that the high levels of leucine enkephalin found in the posterior pituitary correspond to fine neurone nets extending from the pars nervosa back to the supraoptic and para ventricular nuclei, which are associated with control of posterior pituitary hormone release (Rossier *et al* 1979).

Enkephalin immunoreactive neurones have cells with short fine axons and are widespread throughout the c.n.s. In contrast, endorphin-immunoreactive neurones are a relatively homogeneous cell type with larger fusiform cells and are centred on periventricular targets. Thus, there is a morphological difference between neurone types (Bloom 1983).

Peripherally the enkephalins are distributed widely in gut and nervous tissue. In the human gastrointestinal tract, immunoreactive methionine enkephalin is localised predominantly in pylorus and duedenum although it is present in smaller amounts in oesophagus, small intestine, colon, gall bladder and pancreas (Polak 1977, Uddman 1980). The enkephalins are found within the nerve fibres in gut wall nerve systems, and in the endocrine cells of antrum, duodenum and pancreas (Clement-Jones & Rees 1982).

Within the peripheral nervous system leucine enkephalin is found in the grey matter of the spinal cord (especially laminae I, II, V and VII), and sympathetic ganglia (in addition to adrenal medullae) are rich in the enkephalins and their related peptides. Lundberg (1979) reported the presence of enkephalins in the chromaffin cells of the carotid body in the cat. Many other sites including kidney, skin, liver and eye, have been reported.

Prodynorphin-derived peptides

Kakidani (1982) elucidated the sequence of a precursor protein containing β neo-endorphin, dynorphin and leucine enkephalin. Originally referred to as pro-enkephalin B, this peptide is now termed prodynorphin and is a precursor of the dynorphin-related peptides, which include rimorphin, a leucine enkephalin containing compound observed initially in the bovine pituitary by Kilpatrick (1982).

As most immunoreactive techniques for isolation of dynorphin show cross reactivity with enkephalins, reports of the localisation of this substance have been subject to some controversy. Dynorphin is highly concentrated within the neurohypophysis and hypothalamus and is present with its related peptides, rimorphin and peptide E, within the gastrointestinal system. Details of the functional role of dynorphin are still emerging. However, it has been suggested that dynorphin may be a spinal cord neurotransmitter and it is an agonist at $\varkappa$ receptors.

OPIOID RECEPTORS

The observation that nalorphine had a dual action, both antagonising the analgesic action of morphine, and also possessing its own intrinsic analgesic effect, led to the concept of multiple opioid receptors (Martin *et al* 1976). Following canine experiments using various opioid drugs, it was suggested that there were three different receptors, μ, $\varkappa$ and σ, the agonists of which were morphine, ketazocine and N-allyl normetazocine respectively (Gilbert & Martin 1976, Martin 1976).

The discovery of methionine and leucine enkephalin, and later β endorphin, made possible receptor identification using biological preparations of guinea pig ileum and mouse vas deferens. The testing of various agonists for their ability to inhibit electrically induced contractions revealed a fourth receptor δ, having a high enkephalin affinity and present in large amounts in the mouse vas deferens. In contrast, guinea pig ileum responds maximally to μ agonists and thus possesses predominantly μ receptors.

The vas deferens of the rat, however, showed a different picture of response to opioid peptides than did the mouse vas deferens (Wüster *et al* 1979, Gillan 1981) with β endorphin being more potent than the enkephalins. This prompted Wüster (1979) to postulate the existence of an epsilon (ε) receptor, which was specific for β endorphin. In contrast, work on the rabbit vas deferens has shown it to contain $\varkappa$ type receptors alone (Oka *et al* 1981), thus demonstrating a significant species difference.

Following various animal model studies which indicated that both μ and δ agonists produce analgesia, Pasternak (1982) examined the possibility of a shared receptor site mediating this response. Both high and low affinity types of binding between ligand and receptor were found and thus μ receptors were classified into high affinity μ_1 and low affinity $\mu_2 \cdot \mu_2$ and δ sites share common characteristics; the observation of Bowen *et al* (1981) that μ and δ sites could interconvert may suggest a dynamic model of a receptor existing in different binding states (vide infra). It now seems clear that analgesia as a 'desirable' effect is μ_1 or $\varkappa$ mediated (Pleuvry 1983).

The concept of receptor dualism was devised originally to explain the agonist/antagonist actions of a drug within the opioid system. It is now understood that even the endogenous ligands show a relative receptor specificity thus demonstrating dualism (i.e. able to have different actions at different receptor types). Consequently, if they are present in adequate concentrations, they may occupy non-preferred receptor sites (see Table 6.2).

Table 6.2 Relative binding affinities of common drugs at receptor subtypes

	μ	$\varkappa$	δ	
Morphine	+ + + +	+	(+)	— very low
Fentanyl	+ + + +	+	+	
Pethidine	+ + +	+	+	
Nalorphine	+ + +	+ +	+ +	
Naloxone	+ + + +	+	+	

Agonists

Agonists are drugs which bind (with varying degrees of affinity) to receptors and produce a biological response. Specific agonists at receptor subtypes are shown in Table 6.3.

However, despite these relative specificities some cross reaction may occur at other sites.

Table 6.3 Agonists at specific receptor subtypes

μ — Morphine
$\varkappa$ — Ketocyclazocine/Dynorphin
δ — D Ala, D Leu-enkephalin
σ — N-Allylnormetazocine
ε — β endorphin

Agonist-antagonists

These compounds tend to have high μ and $\varkappa$ affinities and low δ affinities (Paterson 1983). Their different efficacy at receptor types produces characteristic pharmacological effects. The new opioid nalbuphine, for example, is known to be a $\varkappa$ agonist but is a μ antagonist — to such an extent that a withdrawal response may be precipitated in morphine dependent subjects. Some agonist-antagonists, e.g. cyclazocine, share effects with powerful non-opioid analgesics such as ketamine and from this observation it has been postulated that the psychotomimetic actions may result from stimulation of a different receptor — termed the θ receptor (Adler 1981, Cowen 1981, Herling & Woods 1981).

In general, the pharmacological actions of this class of compound are complex and result from the net effect of their physiological actions at different receptors.

The finding that buprenorphine has a high affinity for μ receptors with a lower efficacy than fentanyl, has resulted in a reawakening of interest in 'sequential analgesia'. A small dose of buprenorphine, when administered after large doses of fentanyl, displaces the latter from μ receptors, and to some extent reduces unwanted effects such as profound respiratory depression. At present, this technique has little clinical support.

Antagonists

Antagonists bind to receptors and prevent occupation by an agonist drug to a degree dependent on their affinity for that particular receptor type. By definition, antagonist occupation of a receptor results in very little, or no biological response. Within the opioid system, antagonists show a preference between receptor type, for example, naloxone is relatively specific for μ but in high enough concentration occupies $\varkappa$ and δ. To date, no completely selective antagonist has been discovered, but specific antagonists for each receptor subtype would greatly aid pharmacological investigations and are being actively sought.

Receptor-ligand interaction

The 'receptor' consists of a specific site to which an appropriate ligand binds. This binding results in a biochemical event which in turn leads to a biological response (Robson et al 1983). The concentration of Na^+ and Mg^{2+} and the local concentration of guanosine triphosphate profoundly affect the specific binding characteristics of receptor subtypes. Barnard and Demoliou-Mason (1983) suggested a receptor complex of $\mu/\varkappa/\delta$ subunits connected by disulphide bridges which may be strengthened or weakened by alterations in concentration of local ions, leading to changes in behaviour of the complex.

The observations of Bowen et al (1981) using rat nervous tissue that μ and δ sites can interconvert supports this theory, and these authors suggest a dynamic model of the receptor existing within the lipid membrane of cells.

CLINICAL RELEVANCE

Cardiovascular system

There have been many reports implicating pituitary β endorphin in the pathophysiology of shock states. Using a rat model, Lemaire (1978) showed that i.v. β endorphin produced hypotension which was blocked by prior administration of naloxone. In addition, the hypotensive effect of β endorphin was greatly reduced by a serotonin depletor, and pretreatment of animals with a serotonin antagonist (mianserin) blocked the hypotensive response. However, in the presence of fluoxetine, a specific serotonin uptake inhibitor, the hypotension was more severe following β endorphin administration. These results led to the postulate of a central serotenergic mechanism for the hypotensive effect. Weissglas (1983) provided more evidence for a central mechanism by showing in isolated guinea pig papillary muscle that β endorphin has only negatively inotropic actions in extremely high (unphysiological) concentrations. In the same study, naloxone and methyl prednisolone were given (singly and combined) in a porcine septic shock model, and it was shown that the combination was superior to each drug alone as noted by increased survival and reduced hypotension. It is suggested that while naloxone blocks the peripheral effects of β endorphin methyl prednisolone suppresses the central release. Weissglas showed also that β endorphin levels in 18 patients with established hypotension (hypovolaemic, cardiogenic and septic) were greatly elevated in comparison with human volunteers.

In a rat model of hypovolaemic shock, Holaday et al (1981) demonstrated that naloxone administered i.v. elevated arterial pressure. This effect was not seen in hypophysectomised animals, indicating pituitary involvement. Using a porcine model of septic shock Gahos (1982) demonstrated that naloxone given i.v. increased cardiac output and arterial pressure, although the effect was transient.

In a canine model of endotoxic shock, Faden & Holaday (1980) investigated the effect of naloxone given either intravenously or intraventricularly, and demonstrated that the former route was associated with significantly improved haemodynamic state and survival.

In rat models, naloxone given intraventricularly has been shown to reverse the hypotension resulting from hypovolaemic or spinal shock. The effects of naloxone were shown to be specific to the levorotatory isomer. Since a parasympathetic blockade either by methyl atropine or bilateral cervical vagotomy inhibited the response to intraventricular naloxone, it was suggested that parasympathetic pathways are implicated. However, their exact role remains obscure, and other systems, such as the serotonergic, are thought to contribute.

From all this animal data, it is clear that the opioid peptides released endogenously produce hypotension and it is also known that ACTH and β endorphin are released in stress and shock states. It seems logical, therefore, to assess the effect of naloxone in the clinical treatment of patients in conditions of shock and stress. In some preliminary studies, Peters et al (1981) gave intravenous naloxone in increments of 0·4 mg (up to a maximum dose of 8 mg) to patients with prolonged hypotension and an elevation of arterial pressure was seen in those patients not receiving corticosteroids. However, three patients receiving high dose steroids and one who was hyperadrenocorticotrophic exhibited no response to naloxone. This supports the view that corticosteroids exhibit negative feedback onto the pituitary and prevent excessive release of β endorphin. The relatively low doses of naloxone used in this study have been criticised by Faden (1983) who advocates a dose of 1 mg/kg naloxone in shock states. He has suggested that δ or $\varkappa$ sites may be involved since δ and $\varkappa$ antagonists may also be effective in increasing arterial pressure in hypotensive shock.

Endogenous opioids may also be involved in normal physiological variations in arterial pressure. The normal nocturnal decrease in arterial pressure may be abolished by naloxone, and this has led to the suggestion that endogenous opioids may affect baroreceptor responsiveness either at a peripheral site or in the nucleus solitarius (Rubin 1981).

It has also been suggested that opioid peptides may regulate secretion of catecholamines at a central site of action. Van Loon (1981) observed that β endorphin administered into the cerebral ventricles of rats increased circulating catecholamine concentrations, and that this response was blocked by the prior administration of parenteral naloxone. In the adrenal gland, high concentrations of enkephalins are found in terminals of the splanchnic nerve and adrenal nerve stimulation causes release of catecholamines and enkephalins into the circulation. However, it is not certain if enkephalins are released solely from adrenal medullary chromaffin cells or also the splanchnic nerve terminals (Livett 1981).

Respiratory system

Interest has been focused particularly on the participation of opioid peptides in states of disordered respiratory function, e.g. sleep apnoea and sudden infant death syndrome (SIDS).

Kuich & Zimmerman (1981) postulated that the opioid peptides may be involved in SIDS and 'near miss' SIDS (NMSIDS). They compared features found retrospectively in patients after SIDS or NMSIDS with features expected in overactivity of the opioid system, notably hypoventilation and periodic breathing, behavioural indifference, thermal instability and decreased responsiveness to pin-prick. The presence of similar symptoms and signs in SIDS and NMSIDS suggests that over activity of central endogenous activity may be partly responsible.

At least one synthetic peptide has been shown to induce bronchoconstriction, and investigation is proceeding into the role of the opioids in nocturnal variations in airways resistance (Editorial 1982).

Yanagida & Corssen (1981) observed increased β endorphin like immunoreactivity in the plasma of patients with respiratory distress but as these patients were hypoxic and acidotic it is likely that this change resulted from a non-specific pituitary release.

The presence of opioid receptors within the respiratory centres of the brain stem suggests that endogenous opioids may be involved in respiratory control but this speculation has not yet been supported by experimental verification.

Pain modulation

Since their original discovery, the endogenous opioid peptides have been implicated in the modulation of pain. Opioid receptors are concentrated in the periaqueductal grey matter, and it is known that electrical stimulation in this area produces profound analgesia and increased c.s.f. concentrations of β endorphin (Hosobuchi et al 1979). Enkephalins and dynorphins are thought to be involved at spinal cord level in the dorsal horn where they may modulate the release of substance P from small diameter primary pain afferents, and so may alter transmission of centrally directed pain stimuli (Jessell & Iversen 1977). This could provide the basis for the classical 'pain gate' of Melzack & Wall (1965).

The modulation of pain is known to occur both neurally and hormonally via both opioid and non-opioid mechanisms. Watkins & Mayer (1982) classified multiple pain inhibiting systems into four:

1. neural opiate
2. hormonal opiate
3. neural non-opiate
4. hormonal non-opiate.

Each level of ascending pain transmission is regulated by feedback loops originating in opioid neurones in the midbrain and medulla and these modulate afferent neuronal traffic. These pathways are thought to be activated by stress and electrical stimulation in addition to analgesic drugs administered (Carr 1983).

In man, parenteral administration of β endorphin and enkephalin analogues produces only slight analgesia. However, animal studies have demonstrated that administration into the c.s.f. results in profound analgesia (Loh et al 1976). Degradation of opioid peptides occurs rapidly in blood. In addition, most of the opioid peptides are poorly lipophilic, and cross the blood brain barrier with difficulty; this may explain the relative lack of analgesic effects after parental administration.

Höllt et al (1982) found a substantial degree of analgesia from intracerebral pro-enkephalin fragments administered to mice. Further, the enkephalinase inhibiting drug thiorphan has been shown in animals to potentiate the effects of administered opioids and also to produce naloxone reversible analgesia in mice (Roques et al 1980).

With respect to analgesia resulting from electrical stimulation, it would appear that low frequency techniques are opioid mediated (Clement-Jones & Rees 1982) whereas high frequency methods may be serotonin mediated. This view is supported by the observation that only the high frequency analgesia is inhibited by a serotonin synthesis inhibitor such as parachlorophenylalanine (Cheng & Pomeranz 1979).

Neuroendocrine system

The endogenous opioids have important interactions with the hypothalamo-pituitary axis. In man, the circadian rhythm of circulatory β endorphin is identical to that of ACTH (Clement Jones & Besser 1983) but plasma methionine enkephalin concentrations do not follow the same pattern. In addition, it is well known that the opioid peptides modulate the secretion of pituitary hormones in man. Control of anterior pituitary hormone secretion occurs by modification of the release of hypothalamic regulating factors from the median eminence of the pituitary. Opioid receptor stimulation in this region leads to increases in prolactin, growth hormone and thyrotrophin secretion but reduced secretion of luteinising hormone, follicle stimulating hormone, ACTH, β lipotropin and β endorphin (Grossman & Rees 1983).

Adrenaline is known to stimulate release of pituitary β endorphin. Corroboration of this observation was provided by Berkenbosch (1983) who noted that in the rat β endorphin was released into the circulation in stress conditions, an effect which was greatly reduced by prior administration of propranolol. This propranolol-sensitive response was prevented by removal of the neuro-intermediate lobe of the pituitary but was unaffected by treatment with dexamethasone which is known to inhibit secretion of peptides by the anterior lobe. Thus release of β endorphin by stress may be mediated by β adrenoceptors located in the intermediate lobe of the pituitary.

Control of the posterior pituitary is more controversial. In summary, it would seem that opioids inhibit the osmotically stimulated release of antidiuretic hormone (ADH) by both pre- and postsynaptic effects, but they may also stimulate ADH release in response to volume mediated stimuli. There are marked species differences, but it appears most likely that each pituitary hormone has a relatively specific regulating mechanism involving a uniform receptor population. Methyl enkephalin is stored within the neurones with oxytocin, and dynorphin with vasopressin. Thus co-release after stimulation may give rise both pre- and postsynaptic effects (Martin & Voight 1981). Lightman et al (1983) have suggested that opioid receptors are present on the pituicytes themselves rather than on the neurosecretory fibres.

Behaviour

The limbic system is known to be involved in behaviour and the distribution of high concentration of opioids within this region suggests that they may be involved in mood and behaviour. In addition, the opioid system interacts with other neurotransmitter systems, and in particular with the dopaminergic which is known to be implicated in the pathology of psychiatric states (Loh 1976).

When administered to rats, β endorphin may result in 'catatonia' (Bloom 1976) and 'waxy inflexibility' (Jacquet & Marks 1976). Terenius (1976) observed increased opioid binding activity within the CSF of patients with chronic psychoses, and this finding led to trials of naloxone as treatment for schizophrenia (Watson 1978) which were inconclusive. In a double-blind study of male schizophrenics given 20 mg of β endorphin i.v. Berger et al (1980) found improvement of symptoms in eight of nine patients. Measurement of c.s.f. and blood levels of various opioids in psychiatric patients is continuing but as yet no consistent findings have been obtained. It has been suggested that des-tyr γ endorphin is an endogenous antipsychotic (De Weid et al 1980) but Emrich et al (1980) in a double-blind placebo comparison failed to find specific antipsychotic effects. The difficulties inherent in assessing psychoses are obvious.

Miscellaneous functions

Other physiological areas in which opioid function has been implicated include regulation of body temperature (Clark 1981) and regulation of appetite and satiety, particularly with respect to anorexia nervosa (Morley & Levine 1980). Decreased methyl enkephalin concentrations have been found in the globus pallidus of patients with Huntington's chorea (Emson et al 1980). Opioid peptides may be involved in the chlorpropamide-alcohol flushing syndrome. This flushing may be abolished by administration of naloxone and an early study of postmenopausal flushing showed improvement after naloxone (Lightman & Jacobs 1978). Several tumours, both endocrine and non-endocrine have been found to secrete opioid peptides, e.g. the pituitary tumours of Nelson's syndrome and Cushing's disease (Suda 1979). Elevated levels of methyl enkephalin and its precursors have been found in the plasma of patients with chronic renal failure, but the significance of this is not known.

Increased quantities of endogenous opioids have been described in a variety of other tumours. Pullan et al (1980) observed varied peptide contents including β endorphin and methyl enkephalin, associated with thymic, lung, pancreatic and gall-bladder tumours and Bertagna (1982) has described pro-opiocortin fragments in secretions from a small cell lung carcinoma. Active opioid secretion has been reported from carcinoid tumours (Bertagna 1978, Orth 1978). Enkephalins have also been observed in phaeochromocytomas in humans (Clement Jones 1980b). Thus, it has been postulated that the behaviour changes in some patients with a non-endocrine tumour may have an organic basis if sufficient endogenous opioid is liberated to affect c.n.s. mechanisms involved in mood and behaviour.

Specific binding sites for human β endorphin have been found on human complement. However, this binding is not reversed by naloxone. ACTH/β endorphin-like substances are produced by lymphocytes peripherally together with the generation of interferon in human leucocytes. Receptors for β endorphin have been also found on lymphocytes themselves but the significance of the opioid system in immunological process awaits evaluation (Carr 1983).

Panerai et al (1982) found decreased β endorphin and elevated methionine enkephalin concentrations in the plasma of patients with severe liver failure, a fact which may be of relevance in hepatic coma.

Finally, the massive release of endorphins at the approach of death has been suggested to account for vivid 'near death' experiences (Carr 1982).

THE FUTURE

Active research for specific receptor antagonists should lead to further elucidation of receptor systems and it is likely that the goal of analgesia without respiratory depression will therefore be realised. The expansion in our understanding of the physiology of pain may lead to new approaches in treatment, particularly with respect to more appropriate use of non-pharmacological methods such as acupuncture and electrical techniques,

The relevance of the opioid peptides to anaesthesia, however, must remain speculative until our knowledge of these ubiquitous compounds is more extensive.

REFERENCES

Adler M 1981 The in vivo differentiation of opiate receptors. *Life Sciences* **28**: 1543–1545

Berger P *et al* 1980 β Endorphin and schizophrenia. *Archives of General Psychiatry* **37**: 635–639

Berkenbosch F, Tilders F, Vermes I 1983 β Adrenoceptor activation mediates stress induced secretion of β endorphin related peptides from intermediate but not anterior pituitary. *Nature* **305**: 237–239

Barnard E, Demoliou-Mason C 1983 Molecular properties of opioid receptors. *British Medical Bulletin* **39**: 37–40

Bertagna X, Nicholson W, Sorenson G, Pettengill O, Mount C, Orth D 1978 Corticotropin, lipotropin and β endorphin production by a human, non-pituitary tumour in culture: evidence for a common precursor. *Proceedings of National Academy of Science USA* **75**: 5160–5164

Bertagna X, Giraud F, Seurin D, Luton J, Bricaire H, Mains R, Eipper B 1980 Evidence for a peptide similar to 16K fragment in man. *Journal of Clinical Endocrinology* **51**: 182–184

Bertagna X, Luton J, Bricaire H 1982 A new family of hormones. *Annual Medical Interne (Paris)* **133**: 145–147

Bloom F 1983 The endorphins. *Annual Review of Pharmacology and Toxicology* **23**: 151–170

Bloom F, Segal D, Ling N, Guillemin R 1976 Endorphins: profound behavioural effects in rats suggest new etiological factors in mental illness. *Science* **194**: 630–632

Bloom F *et al* 1977 Endorphins are located in the intermediate and anterior lobes of the pituitary gland, not in the neurophypophysis. *Life Sciences* **20**: 43–48

Bloom F *et al* 1978 Endorphins: cellular localisation, electrophysiological and behavioural effects. In: Costa E (ed) *Advances in biochemical psychopharmacology* **18**. Raven Press, New York, p 89–107

Bowen W, Gentleman S, Herkenham M, Pert C 1981 Interconverting μ and δ forms of the opiate receptor in rat striatal patches. *Proceedings of National Academy of Science USA* **78**: 4818–4820

Bruni F, Watkins W, Yen S 1979 β Endorphin in human pancreas. *Journal of Clinical Endocrinology and Metabolism* **49**: 649–651

Carr D 1982 Endorphins at the approach to death. *Lancet* **i**: 390

Carr D 1983 Endorphins in contemporary medicine. *Comprehensive Therapeutics* **9**: 40–45

Cheng R, Pomeranz B 1979 Electroacupuncture analgesia could be mediated by at least two pain relieving mechanisms; endorphin and non endorphin systems. *Life Sciences* **25**: 1957–1962

Clark W 1981 Effects of opioid peptides on thermoregulation. *Federation Proceedings* **40**: 2754–2759

Clement-Jones V, Besser G 1983 Clinical perspectives in opioid peptides. *British Medical Bulletin* **39**: 45–100

Clement-Jones V, Corder R, Lowry F 1980 Isolation of human met enkephalin and two groups of putative precursors from an adrenal medullary tumour. *Biochemistry and Biophysics Research Communications* **95**: 665–673

Clement-Jones V, Rees L 1982 Neuroendocrine correlates of the endorphins and enkephalins. *Clinical neuroendocrinology II*. Acadmic Press, New York, ch 4, p 139–191

Clement-Jones V, Rees L, Besser G M, Martini I (eds) 1982 In: *Clinical neuroendocrinology, vol II*. Academic Press, New York, p 134–203

Cowan A 1981 Simple in vivo tests that differentiate prototype agonists at opiate receptors. *Life Sciences* **28**: 1159–1570

Cuello A C 1983 Central distribution of opioid peptides. *British Medical Bulletin* **39**: 11–16

Emrich H, Zaudig M, Zerssen P, Herz A, Kissing P 1980 DES-TYR γ endorphin in schizophrenia *Lancet* **ii**: 1364–1365

Emson P, Arregui A, Clement-Jones V, Sandberg B, Rossor M 1980 Regional distribution of methionine enkephalin and substance P like immunoreactivity to normal human brain and in Huntington's disease. *Brain Research* **199**: 147–160

Faden A 1983 Neuropeptides. In: Chernow B, Lake R (eds) *The pharmacological approach to the critically ill patient*. Williams & Wilkins, Baltimore, ch 33, p 637–649

Faden A, Holaday J 1980 Experimental endotoxic shock. The pathophysiological function of endorphins and treatment with opiate atangonists. *Journal of Infectious Diseases* **142**: 229–238

Feurle G, Weber U, Helmstaedter V 1980 β Lipotropin like material in human pancreas and pyloric antrum mucosa. *Life Sciences* **27**: 467–473

Gahos F, Chiu R, Hinchey F, Richards G 1982 Endorphins in septic shock. *Archives of Surgery* **117:** 1053–1057

Gilbert P, Martin W 1976 The effects of morphine and nalorphine like drugs in the non dependent, morphine dependent and cyclazocine dependent chronic spinal dog. *Journal of Pharmacology and Experimental Therapeutics* **198:** 66–82

Gillan M, Kosterlitz H, Magnan J 1981 Unexpected antagonism in the rat vas deferens by benzomorphans which are agonist in other pharmacological tests. *British Journal of Pharmacology* **72:** 13–15

Giraud P, Castana E, Patey G, Oliver C, Rossier J 1983 Regional distribution of methionine-enkephalin-arg[6]-phe[7] in the rat brain. *Journal of Neurochemistry* **41:** 154–160

Grossman A, Rees L 1983 The neuroendocrinology of opioid peptides. *British Medical Bulletin* **39:** 83–88

Gubler U, Seeburg P, Hoffman B, Gage L, Udenfriend S 1982 Molecular cloning establishes proenkephalin as precursor of enkephalin containing peptides. *Nature* **295:** 206–208

Guillemin R *et al* 1977 β Endorphin and adrenocorticotrophin are secreted concomitantly by the pituitary gland. *Science* **197:** 1367–1368

Herling S, Woods J 1981 Discriminative stimulus effects of narcotics. Evidence for multiple receptor mediated actions. *Life Sciences* **28:** 1571–1584

Holaday J, O'Hara M, Faden A 1981 Hypophysectomy alters cardiorespiratory variables: central effects of pituitary endorphins in shock. *American Journal of Physiology* **241:** H479–485

Hollt V, Tulunay C, Woo S, Loh H, Herz A 1982 Opioid peptides derived from pro-enkephalin A but not that from pro-enkephalin B are substantial analgesics after administration into brain of mice. *European Journal of Pharmacology* **85:** 355–356

Hoshobuchi Y, Rossier J, Bloom F, Guillemin R 1979 Stimulation of human periaqueductal gray for pain relief increases immunoreactive β endorphin in ventricular fluid. *Science* **203:** 279–281

Hughes J 1983 Biogenesis, release and inactivation of enkephalins and dynorphins. *British Medical Bulletin* **39:** 17–24

Hughes J, Smith T, Kosterlitz H, Fothergill L, Morgan B, Morris H 1975 Identification of two pentapeptides from the brain with potent opiate agonist activity. *Nature* **258:** 577–580

Jacquet Y, Marks N 1976 The C fragment of β lipotropin — an endogenous neuroleptic or antipsychotogen? *Science* **194:** 632–634

Jessell T, Iversen L 1977 Opiate analgesics inhibit substance P release from rat trigeminal nucleus. *Nature* **268:** 549–551

Kakidani H *et al* 1982 Cloning and sequence analysis of CDNA for porcine β neo-endorphin/dynorphin precursor. *Nature* **298:** 245–248

Kilpatrick D, Wahlstrom A, Lahm H, Blacher R, Udenfriend S 1982 Rimorphin, a unique naturally occurring (Leu) enkephalin containing peptide found in association with dynorphin and neo-enkephalin. *Proceedings of National Academy of Science USA* **79:** 6480–6483

Kuich T, Zimmerman D 1981 Endorphins, ventilatory control and Sudden Infant Death Syndrome. *Medical Hypotheses* **7:** 1231–1240

Editorial 1982 Endogenous opiates and their actions. *Lancet* **i:** 305–307

Lemaire I, Tseng R, Lemaire S 1978 Systemic administration of β endorphin. *Proceedings of National Academy of Science* **75:** 6240–6242

Lightman S, Jacobs H 1979 Naloxone: Non-steroidal treatment for post menopausal flushing. *Lancet* **ii:** 1071

Lightman S, Ninkovic M, Hunt S, Iversen L 1983 Evidence for opiate receptors on pituicytes. *Nature* **305:** 235–237

Livett B, Dean D, Whelan L, Udenfriend S, Rossier J 1981 Co-release of enkephalin and catecholamines from cultured adrenal chromaffin cells. *Nature* **289:** 317–319

Loh H, Tseng L, Wei E, Li C 1976 β Endorphin is a potent analgesic agent. *Proceedings of National Academy of Science USA* **73:** 2895–2898

Van Loon G, Appel N, Ho D 1981 Regulation of catecholamine secretion by endogenous opioid peptides. In: *Physiopathology of endocrine disease and mechanisms of hormone action.* Alan Liss, New York, p 293–318

Lundberg J, Hokfelt T, Fahrenkrug J, Nilsson G, Terenius L 1979 Peptides in the cat carotid body VIP enkephalin and substance P like immunoreactivity. *Acta Physiologica Scandanavia* **107:** 279–281

Martin R, Voight K 1981 Enkephalins coexist with oxytocin and vasopressin in nerve-terminals of rat neurohypophysis. *Nature* **289:** 502–504

Martin W 1976 Opioid antagonists. *Pharmacology Reviews* **19:** 463–521

Martin W, Eades C, Thompson J, Huppler R, Gilbert P 1976 The effects of morphine and nalorphine like drugs in the non-dependent and morphine dependent chronic spinal dog. *Journal of Pharmacology and Experimental Therapeutics* **197:** 517–531

Melzack R, Wall P 1965 Pain mechanisms. A new approach. *Science* **150:** 971–979

Morley J S 1981 Synthetic endorphins. In: Eberle A, Greiger R, Welland T (eds) *Perspectives in peptide chemistry.* S Karger, Basel, p 329–343

Morley J S 1983 Chemistry of opioid peptides. *British Medical Bulletin* **39:** 9–10

Morley J, Levine A 1980 Stress induced eating is mediated through endogenous opiates. *Science* **209:** 1250–1260

Nakai Y, Nakao K, Oki S, Imura H 1978 Presence of immunoreactive β lipotropin and β endorphin in human placenta. *Life Sciences* **23:** 2013–2018

Nakanishi S, Inoue A, Kita T, Nakamura M, Chang A, Cohen S, Numa S 1979 Nucleotide sequence of cloned CDNA for bovine corticotrophin-β-lipotropin precursor. *Nature* **278:** 423–427

Nakao K, Oki S, Tanaka I, Nakai Y, Imura H 1980 Concomitant secretion of MSH with ACTH and β endorphin in humans. *Journal of Clinical Endocrinology and Metabolism* **51:** 1205–1207

Noda *et al* 1982 Cloning and sequence analysis for CDNA for bovine adrenal preproenkephalin. *Nature* **259:** 202–206

Odagiri E, Sherrell B, Mount C, Nicholson W, Orth D 1979 Human placental immunoreactive corticotrophin, lipotropin and β endorphin. *Proceedings of the National Academy of Science USA* **76:** 2027–2031

Oki S *et al* 1981 Concomitant secretion of adrenocorticotrophin, β endorphin and melantropin from perfused cells of Cushing's disease: effects of lysine vasopressin, rat median eminence extracts, thyrotrophin releasing hormone and luteinising hormone-releasing hormone. *Journal of Clinical Endocrinology and Metabolism* **52:** 42–49

Oka T, Nagishi K, Suda M, Sawa A, Fujino M, Wakimasu M 1981 Evidence that dynorphin 1-13 acts as an agonist on opioid x receptors. *European Journal of Pharmacology* **77:** 137–139

Orth D, Guillemin R, Ling N, Nicholson W 1978 Immunoreactive endorphins, lipotropins and corticotrophins in a human non pituitary tumor. *Journal of Clinical Endocrinology and Metabolism* **46:** 849–852

Orwoll E, Kendall J 1980 β Endorphin and adrenocorticotrophin in extrapituitary sites. *Endocrinology* **107:** 438–442

Panerai A, Martini A, De Rosa A, Salerno F, Guilio A, Mantegazza P 1982 Plasma β endorphin and met-enkephalin in physiological and pathological conditions. In: Costa E, Trabucchi M (eds) *Regulatory peptides: from molecular biology to function.* Raven Press, New York, p 139–149

Pasternak G W 1982 High and low affinity opioid binding sites: relationship to μ and δ sites. *Life Sciences* **31:** 1303–1307

Paterson S, Robson L, Kosterlitz H W 1983 Classification of opioid receptors. *British Medical Bulletin* **39:** 31–36

Peters W, Johnson M, Friedman P, Mitch W 1981 Pressor effect of naloxone in septic shock. *Lancet* **ii:** 1529–1532

Pleuvry B 1983 An update on opioid receptors. *British Journal of Anaesthesia* **55 (Suppl. 2):** 1435–1465

Polak J, Sullivan S, Bloom S, Facer P 1977 Enkephalin like immunoreactivity in the human gastrointestinal tract. *Lancet* **i:** 972–974

Pullan P, Clement-Jones V, Corder R, Lowry P, Besser G, Rees L 1980 ACTH LPH and related peptides in the ectopic ACTH syndrome. *Clinical Endocrinology* **13:** 437–445

Robson L, Paterson S, Kosterlitz H 1983 Opiate receptors. In: Iversen L, Iversen S, Snyder S (eds) *Handbook of psychopharmacology, vol 17.* Plenum Press, New York, ch 2

Roques B, Fourme-Zaluski M, Soroca E, Lecomte J, Malfroy B, Llorens C, Schwartz J 1980 The enkephalinase inhibitor thiorphan shows antinocioceptive activity in mice. *Nature* **288:** 286–288

Rossier J *et al* 1979 Hypothalamic enkephalin neurones may regulate the neurohypophysis. *Nature* **277:** 653–655

Rubin P, Blaschke T, Guilleminault G 1981 Effect of naloxone on blood pressure fall during sleep. *Circulation* **63:** 17–121

Smyth D 1983 β Endorphin and related peptides in pituitary, brain, pancreas and antrum. *British Medical Bulletin* **39:** 25–30

Suda T, Abe Y, Demura H, Demura R, Shizume K, Tamahashi N, Sasano N 1979 ACTH, β LPH, and β endorphin in pituitary adenomas of patients with Cushing's disease. *Journal of Clinical Endocrinology and Metabolism* **49:** 475–477

Terenius L, Wahlstrom A, Lindstrom L, Widerlov E 1976 Increased CSF levels of endorphins in chronic psychosis. *Neuroscience Letters* **3:** 157–162

Uddman R, Alumets J, Hakanson R, Sundler F, Walles B 1980 Peptidergic enkephalin innervation of the mammalian eosophagus. *Gastroenterology* **78:** 732–737

Vuolteenaho O, Vakkuri O, Leppaluoto J 1980 Wide distribution of β endorphin like immunoreactivity in extrapituitary tissues of rat. *Life Sciences* **27:** 57–65

Watkins L, Mayer D 1982 Organisation of endogenous opiate and non opiate pain control systems. *Science* **216:** 1185–1192

Watson S, Berger P, Akil H 1978 Effect of naloxone on schizophrenia. *Science* **201:** 73–75

Weissglas I 1983 The role of endogenous opiate in shock: experimental and clinical studies in vitro and in vivo. *Advances in Shock Research* **10:** 87–94

De Wied D, van Ree J, Verhoven W, van Praag H 1980 Antipsychotic effects of γ DES-TYR endorphins in schizophrenia. *Lancet* **ii:** 1363–1364

Wuster M, Schulz R, Herz A 1979 Specificity of opioids toward the μ, δ and ε opiate receptors. *Neuroscience Letters* **15:** 193–198

Wuster M, Schulz R, Herz A 1980 Opiate activity and receptor selectivity of dynorphin 1–13 and related peptides. *Neuroscience Letters* **20:** 79–83

Yanagida H, Corssen G 1981 Respiratory distress and β endorphin like immunoreactivity in humans. *Anesthesiology* **55:** 515–519

The new muscle relaxants

HISTORICAL DEVELOPMENT

Although news of the South American arrow poison reached Europe in the 16th century, it remained a scientific curiosity largely because of the impure nature of the alkaloids extracted from early specimens. The chemical structure of the potent alkaloid (+)-tubocurarine was studied by Harold King in 1935, who deduced that it was a bisquaternary ammonium compound with two tetrahydroisoquinoline bases joined together by an ether bridge. In 1938 Richard Gill (1940), who had settled on a ranch in Ecuador, obtained sufficient crude curare from the bark of *Chondrodendron tomentosum* to allow McIntyre to purify the drug. From this material Wintersteiner & Dutcher (1943), working in the Squibb Laboratories in America, were able to produce a standardised preparation. This product was used by Griffith & Johnson (1942) to produced muscle relaxation during cyclopropane anaesthesia in man. In 1942 they published their experience with the use of this drug in 25 patients and opened the door to what has probably been the most significant advance in the practice of anaesthesia in the last 50 years. In 1943, Wintersteiner & Dutcher purified (+)-tubocurarine and the pure alkaloid was marketed for clinical use.

The similarities in the chemical composition of acetylcholine (Fig. 7.1) and the subunits in

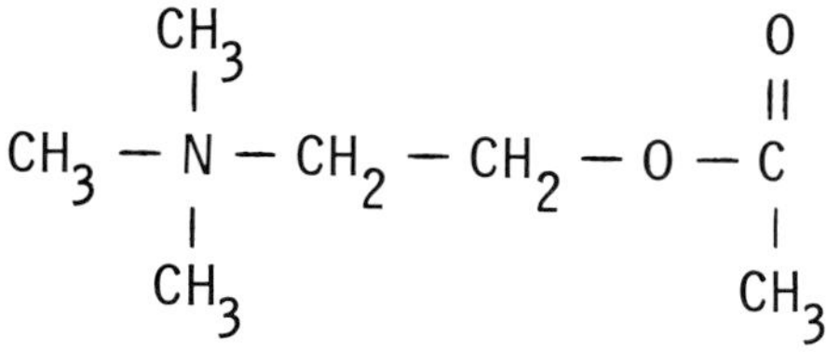

$$CH_3 - \underset{\underset{CH_3}{|}}{\overset{\overset{CH_3}{|}}{N}} - CH_2 - CH_2 - O - \underset{\underset{CH_3}{|}}{\overset{\overset{O}{||}}{C}}$$

Fig. 7.1 Structural formula of acetylcholine.

the King structure of d-tubocurarine (Fig. 7.2), where quaternary ammonium group is near to an esteric group, led to the concept that curare acted by fitting into the acetylcholine receptor. This was supported by the finding that neuromuscular blocking potency was related to charge density on the ammonium moiety (Holmes *et al* 1947). From this proposition the concept developed that a bisquaternary ammonium compound was necessary for potent neuromuscular blockade. Following the studies of Barlow & Ing (1948) on the poly-methylene bis quaternary compounds of general formula $(CH_3)_3 N^+ - (CH_2)_n - N^+(CH_3)_3$ and the finding of Paton & Zaimis (1949) that when $n=6$ (hexamethonium) nicotinic block was maximal whereas when $n=10$ (decamethonium) the compound was a potent neuro-muscular blocking agent, gave support to the concept that, for potent neuromuscular blocking activity, it was necessary to have two quaternary ammonium groups separated by an interonium distance about 1 nm.

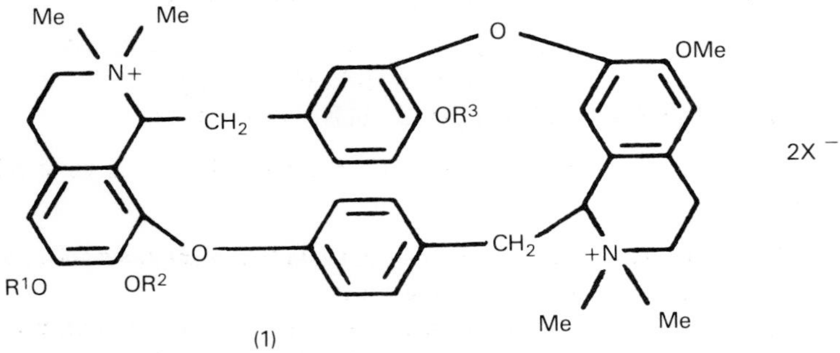

Fig. 7.2 Structural formula ascribed to d-tubocurarine by King 1935.

This concept has dominated the approach to the development of new neuromuscular blocking drugs although β erythroidine, an active neuromuscular blocking drug, is not a bis-quaternary compound. Indeed in 1970 Everett *et al*, using the then new nuclear magnetic resonance spectroscopy technique demonstrated that at physiological pH (+)-tubocurarine is a monoquaternary compound even though the second nitrogen atom is heavily protonated (Fig. 7.3). Recently the importance of the stereoisometric relationship of the various groups have been demonstrated, and the importance of visualising the topography of the chemical structures in three-dimensional terms has been emphasised by Savage (1983), as compounds that may appear similar in a two-dimensional form may have markedly different properties due to differences in the rotational angles of these groups, within the molecule.

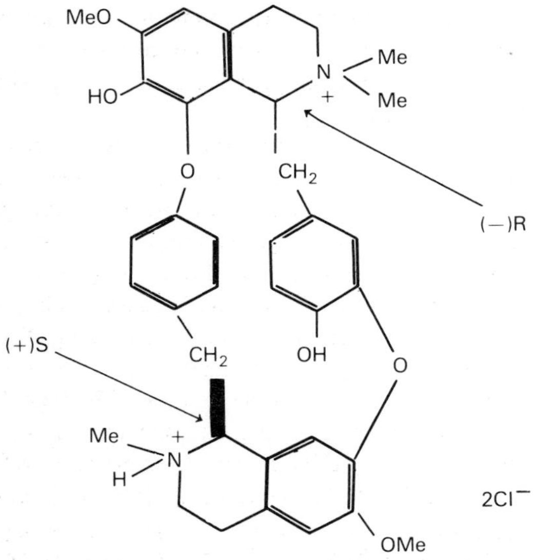

Fig. 7.3 Structural formula of d-tubocurarine elucidated by Everett *et al* 1970.

PROPERTIES OF THE IDEAL NEUROMUSCULAR BLOCKING AGENT

In an editorial reviewing the need for new muscle relaxants in 1975, Saverese and Kitz suggested that there was a need for three types of muscle relaxant:

1. Short acting non-depolarising agent.
2. Intermediate duration non-cumulative non-depolarising agent.
3. Long duration non-depolarising agent devoid of c.v.s. effects.

In 1979 Feldman proposed that the ideal neuromuscular blocking agent should have the following properties:

1. It should be non-depolarising in action — to avoid the inherent side effects and lack of pharmacological reversability of depolarising drugs.

2. It should be completely and safely reversible within 10 minutes of administration — this requires a large rapid initial distribution volume for the drug.

3. It should be non-cumulative upon successive repeated equipotent doses — this requires relatively rapid redistribution, metabolism and/or excretion of the drug.

4. It should be specific for the neuromuscular junction — this would result in a lack of cardiovascular or cerebral side effects in doses up to 20 times the ED_{90} *.

5. It should be rapid in onset — the great convenience of suxamethonium is largely due to its rapid onset.

6. It should not release histamine.

In addition, it may be added that it should not be associated with sensitivity or allergic reactions on repeated exposure and it should not be a potent anti-cholinesterase.

Various means have been attempted to achieve these ends and by reviewing them one can better understand the advantages of the new neuromuscular blocking drugs.

Non-depolarising

From past experience with structure activity relationship, it was assumed that for a potent non-depolarising agent one needed a bulky, rigid molecule with two quaternary ammonium ions placed about 1 nm apart. Indeed even with tubocurarine which is a monoquaternary monotertiary compound quaternising the second ammonium to produce the King chemical structure increases the potency markedly.

In 1960 Quévauviller and Lainé demonstrated neuromuscular blocking properties of the steroid malouetine. This led to the use of the steroidal androstane molecule as rigid skeleton on which to insert or drape quaternary ammonium and esteric groups.

Pancuronium was the result of draping two acetylcholine-like molecules on the 2–3 position and 16–17 positions (Fig. 7.4) (Buckett & Bonta 1966, Buckett et al 1973). This drug was introduced into clinical practice in 1967 by Baird and Reid. The success of this approach has led to the study of various derivatives and analogues including ORG 6368, a short-acting relatively fat-soluble relaxant which produced marked tachycardia (Surgrue et al 1975) and dacuronium, a shorter acting drug than pancuronium with about 1/10. Its potency and vagolytic properties that were more evident than pancuronium at $2 \times ED_{95}$ (Feldman & Tyrrell 1970, Norman & Katz 1971). Of all the analogues prepared by Savage at the Organon Laboratories in Scotland, ORG NC45 vecuronium (Fig. 7.5), most closely meets the

* ED_{90} and ED_{95} are doses that correspond to those that produce 90% or 95% depression of the twitch response under light general anaesthesia in man. The information is usually obtained using a 'culmulative' dose response curve and as a result the exact dose accepted varies slightly according to the detailed methodology.

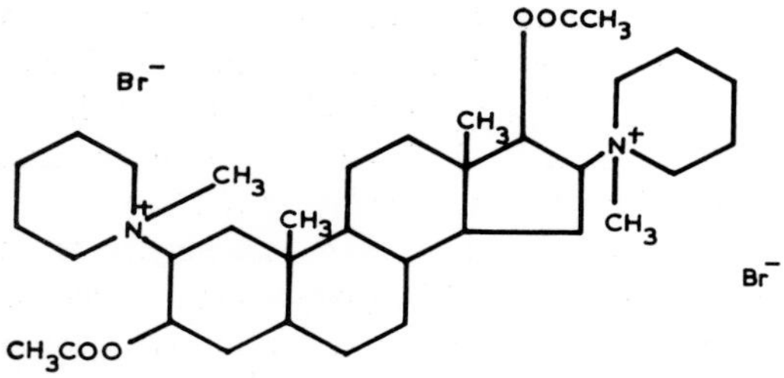

Fig. 7.4 Structural formula of pancuronium bromide.

requirements of the ideal drug. Pipecuronium, a Hungarian drug described by Boros *et al* (1980) and Newton *et al* (1982) also uses the steriod nucleus as a rigid skeleton on which acetyl and quaternary ammonium groups are based at a longer interonium distance than in pancuronium.

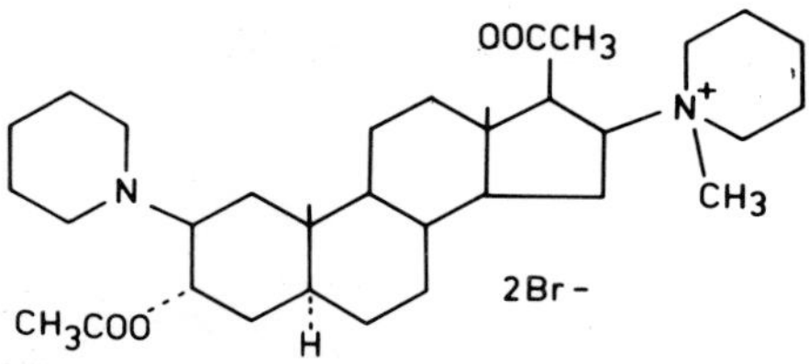

NC 45

Fig. 7.5 Structural formula of vecuronium bromide (ORG NC45).

Singh and his co-workers (1972) used the alternative technique of inserting one or two quaternary ammonium groups into the steroidal ring. Of the series of drugs produced, Chandonium (Fig. 7.6) received clinical trials as a potent short-acting neuromuscular blocking agent; unfortunately it produced tachycardia at a dose of about $2 \times ED_{95}$ (Gandiha *et al* 1975, Feldman 1980). Recently Biro & Karpati (1981) have produced a new drug Duador (Fig. 7.7a), this drug is said to have less vagolytic effect and is undergoing clinical trials in Hungary.

An alternative approach has been to use the bulky bisquaternary benzoisoquinoline structure to produce drugs without the side effects of tubocurarine and with a shorter duration of action (Fig. 7.8).

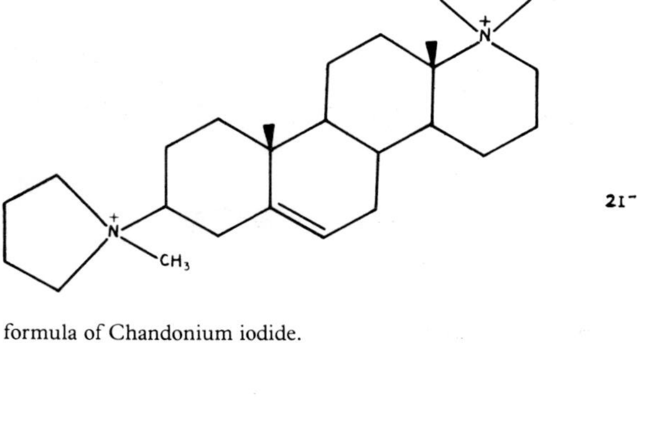

Fig. 7.6 Structural formula of Chandonium iodide.

Savarese & Wastella (1979) have studied a series of esters which are susceptable to hydrolysis by plasma cholinesterase, whilst Stenlake *et al* (1978) developed similar compounds which undergo Hofmann degeneration, a process which involves electron transfer at alkaline pH of blood to break the N–H bond producing an inactive tertiary metabolite. Atracurium (Fig. 7.9) uses this method of metabolism (Stenlake *et al* 1981).

Other drugs using a similar basic structure have been reported in the Russian literature but clinical data is limited. Danilov *et al* (1978) reported that tercuronium, which has a rigid structure and was synthesised in Russia, has been used without apparent side effects in man.

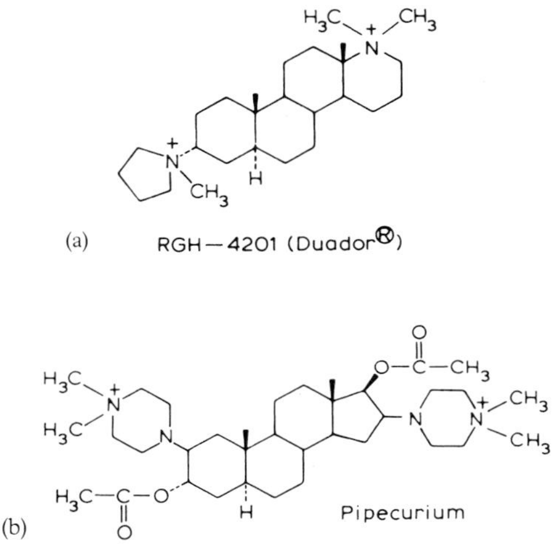

(a)   RGH—4201 (Duador®)

(b)   Pipecurium

Fig. 7.7   Structural formulae of Duador (a) and pipecurium (b).

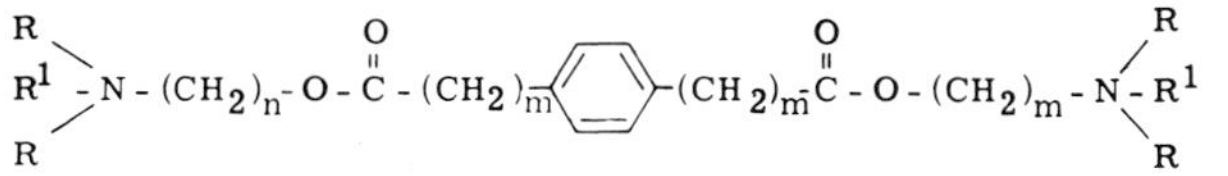

Fig. 7.8   Genetic formula of the bulky esters.

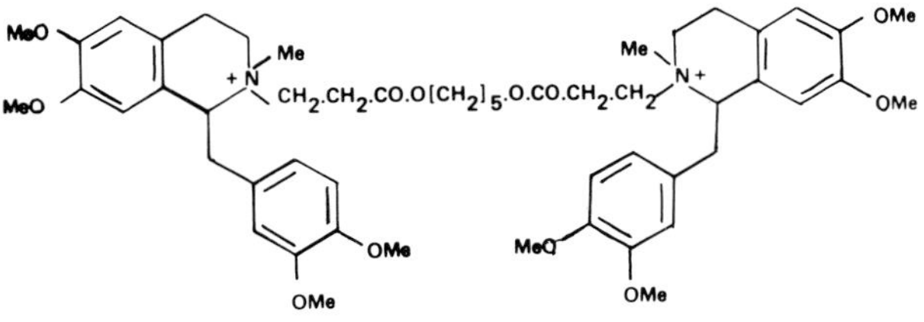

Fig. 7.9   Structural formula of atracurium.

Short duration of activity and lack of cumulative effect

For a neuromuscular drug to be reversible, either as a result of spontaneous recovery of neuromuscular function or following the administration of neostigmine, the plasma level must fall below that required to produce 70% receptor occupancy or 90% depression of twitch height (Katz & Katz 1967). It follows that for short duration of action a drug must have a short half-life and a large rapid distribution volume. Various approaches have been made to achieve this:

1. *Metabolism of the drug* by one of the following methods:

   a. splitting the bisquaternary compound into monoquaternary metabolites by plasma cholinesterase as with suxamethonium and the bulky esters described by Savarese and Ginsberg

   b. splitting an azo linkage as in Fazadinium by means of azo reductase — NADPH (Fig. 7.10). Unfortunately this process does not occur to any significant extent in humans

   c. Hofmann alkali degradation and ester hydrolysis, as with atracurium

   d. deacetylation of the ester groups in pancuronium and probably vecuronium — the extent of this varies according to conditions of study but is unlikely to account for more than 30% of the drug.

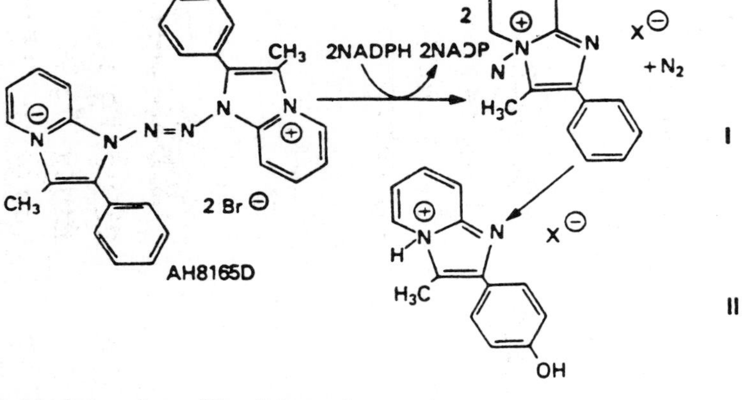

Fig. 7.10 Metabolic pathway of Fazadinium under azo-reductase.

2. *Rapid uptake by liver and other acceptor sites.* The ability of the liver to sequestrate large quantities of quaternary ammonium salt was demonstrated by the radiostope auto-radiographs of Cohen *et al* (1968). Generally, plasma clearance by the liver increases with increasing fat solubility (although none of the bisquaternary compounds is truly fat soluble). ORG 6368 showed a remarkable hepatic clearance (Fig. 7.11) and there is evidence from animal studies that vecuronium also demonstrates an important rapid hepatic clearance.

Rapid onset

All attempts to achieve a suxamethonium-like onset time with a non-depolarising drug have failed. It may well be that this is the result of an inherent difference in the nature of the binding of the drug to the receptor that is necessary to produce a non-depolarising effect. The greater the dose of drug and the higher the plasma-receptor concentration gradient, generally

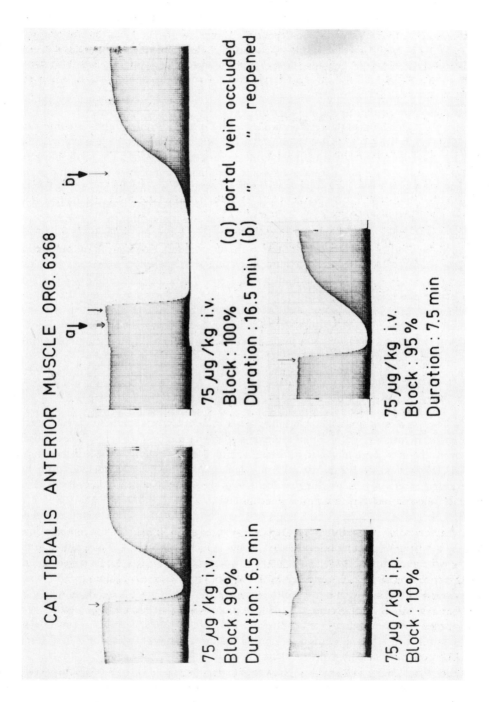

Fig. 7.11 Demonstrating the importance of hepatic elimination of ORG 6368. i.p. = intrapartal injection. Note drug inactive when administered by this route. (By permission of S Agoston.)

the more rapid the onset, but even this effect is limited and with $3-4 \times ED_{90}$ dose, maximum onset time has usually been achieved. Foldes (1983) suggested an ingenious way of overcoming the slow onset of the non-depolarising drugs. By giving 10% of the dose of drug 5 minutes before induction of anaesthesia, a subclinical degree of receptor occupancy can be established and when the remaining 90% of the drug is given some minutes later the onset of relaxation is rapid.

Specificity for neuromuscular junction

Savage (1983) has studied the relationship between the esteric groups in pancuronium and vagolytic effect. He has proposed that the 17-ester group is associated with neuromuscular blocking potency whilst the 3-ester group is the cause of the vagolytic action and the blocking of nor-adrenaline receptor[2] reuptake. In vecuronium the stereoisometric relationship of the acetyl group to the tertiary onium group at the 2 position is radically altered, causing a destabilising effect that results in spontaneous ester hydrolysis, which is especially rapid if it is in high concentrations in solution (hence the preparation is presented in freeze-dried form to achieve stability). The alteration in the position of 3 acetyl group results in an absence of vagolytic and other cardiovascular effects with vecuronium. However, if the side chain length is increased, i.e. to a butyl derivative, then this favourable effect is lost (Savage 1982).

No histamine release

Although absence of histamine release is ideal, histamine release at low levels is of minor clinical significance except in atopic individuals, and is better avoided. Histamine release appears to be associated with the benzylisoquinoline structure found in tubocurarine, atracurium and the bulky esters of Savarese and co-worker.

THE NEW RELAXANTS

Of all the new neuromuscular blocking agents that have been synthesised, two are of particular importance. Vecuronium bromide and atracurium besylate are both new muscle relaxants that have been marketed in Western Europe and are shortly to be launched in the USA. In spite of their attractive pharmacological profiles, however, neither drug has succeeded in seriously encroaching on the sales of the established neuromuscular blocking agents tubocurarine, pancuronium and alcuronium.*

Both drugs are short acting, both drugs are free of cardiovascular effects in clinical dosage, and neither drug is markedly cumulative upon repeated doses. It is difficult to compare doses of the new drugs with that of established agents in a clinical context. Thus, although the ED_{90} of vecuronium is between 30 and 40 µg/kg compared with 50 µg/kg for pancuronium, at this dose level the recovery of neuro-muscular block following vecuronium to 50% twitch depression is less than 10 minutes and the relaxation produced inadequate for most surgical procedures, whereas that produced by pancuronium is adequate for operations lasting 30 to 40 minutes. The same is true of atracurium: the ED_{90} of 150–200 µg/kg produces insufficient relaxation which is too short-lived for clinical usefulness unless the patient is first deeply anaesthetised with halothane or enflurane.

As a result, it is necessary to use a bolus dose of the new agents to produce a rather greater initial block than with tubocurarine or pancuronium if useful relaxation is to be achieved. An

---

*Recent information suggests that sales of atracurium are comparable with those of alcuronium and pancuronium.

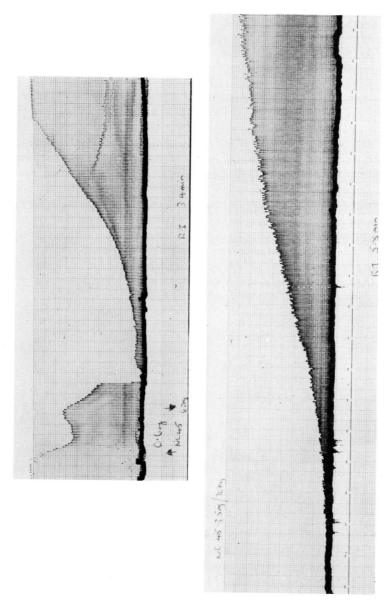

Fig. 7.12 Recovery index of vecuronium. Top trace: isolated arm — recovery index (25–75% recovery) at 3·4 min. Bottom trace: 6 injection — recovery index 5·8 min.

initial dose of 100 µg/kg of vecuronium ($3 \times ED_{90}$) or 500 µg/kg of atracurium ($2\frac{1}{2}-3 \times ED_{90}$) is usual.

Vecuronium bromide (Norcuron — Organon) ORG NC45

Due to the instability of the 3-acetyl group in high concentrations in solution the preparation is presented as freeze-dried buffered powder with water in a separate ampoule of solvent. The powder can be kept on the shelf at room temperature without deterioration.

The ED_{90} of the drug is between 40 to 50 µg/kg (Crul & Booij 1980, Crul 1983, Agoston *et al* 1980, Agoston & Richardson 1983), being lower if given after suxamethonium, halothane or enflurane anaesthesia. At this dose the duration to complete recovery is about 20 minutes with a recovery index (from 25% to 75% recovery of twitch response) of 7–8 minutes (Fig. 7.12). If given in a clinically effective dose at 100 µg/kg, it produces about 10–15 minutes of complete twitch suppression followed by recovery in 25 minutes with a recovery index of 9–10 minutes; with this dose complete reversal of the neuromuscular block by edrophonium 30 mg or neostigmine 2·5 mg is possible after about 15 minutes (Baird *et al* 1982, Foldes *et al* 1981). For a prolongation of action, supplementary doses of 20 µg/kg are adequate every 12–15 minutes. However, once neuromuscular recovery starts the time to inadequate surgical relaxation can be so brief that it is necessary to give the 'top up dose', when post-tetanic potentiation can be clearly demonstrated. For this reason it is necessary to monitor neuromuscular condition if this technique is to be used without inconvenience to the surgeon (Feldman 1983, Baird 1983). The cumulative effect of repeated doses is minimal if this regime is followed (Buzello/Fahey *et al* 1981, Nolge 1982). However, although cumulation is minimal, it is present once the 3rd or 4th supplementary dose is given if one does not allow twitch recovery greater than 5% of control to occur (Fig. 7.13).

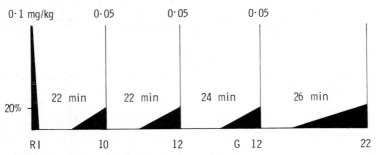

Fig. 7.13 Repeated doses of vecuronium show very modest cumulative effect. Note: G = gentamicin 40 mg i.v. caused prolonged recovery time.

Because of the absence of any cardiovascular or cerebral side effects from this drug (Barnes & Brindle-Smith 1982, Morris *et al* 1981), until about $60 \times ED_{90}$ dose it is possible to extend the duration of action by increasing the size of the bolus dose. Doses up to 150–200 µg/kg ($4–5 \times ED_{95}$) produce good relaxation for 60–90 min (Hollway & Feldman 1982, Agoston & Richardson 1983). The recovery index is slightly prolonged at these high dose levels, but is still shorter than an equivalent dose of tubocurarine or pancuronium (Fig. 7.14).

d'Hollander *et al* (1982, 1983) have advocated a bolus dose followed by a continuous infusion to obtain a steady state with equilibrium between plasma and receptor. In our hands

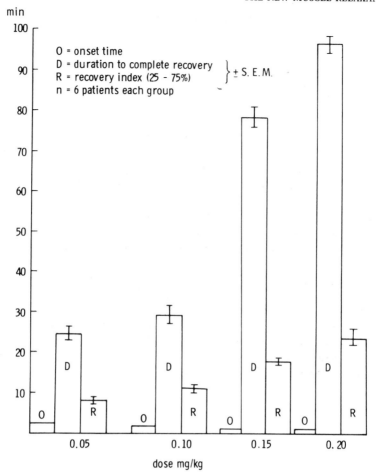

min

O = onset time
D = duration to complete recovery
R = recovery index (25 - 75%) } ± S. E. M.
n = 6 patients each group

dose mg/kg

Fig. 7.14 Effect of multiples of the ED$_{90}$ dose of vecuronium upon onset, duration and recovery of twitch (from Hollway & Feldman 1982).

this technique is cumbersome and produces less good surgical conditions than bolus injection. Continuous monitoring necessitates some degree of twitch response to be present, the constant attention to the i.v. infusion is distracting and therefore dangerous and, when the infusion is stopped after operations over 90 minutes, the recovery index is prolonged compared to the large bolus technique (Fig. 7.15). Although this technique has considerable pharmacokinetic appeal, it reduces the utility of this very useful drug and ignores the great pharmacological flexibility resulting from the absence of side effects consequent upon its high specificity for the neuromuscular junction.

Onset of action
Although it was originally claimed to produce good intubating conditions rapidly (Crul & Booij, Fahey *et al* 1980), this has not proved to be the case. Harrison & Feldman (1981) found intubating conditions at 100 μg/kg to be similar to those of pancuronium 100 μg/kg and only when the dose was increased to 150 μg/kg was it possible to intubate more rapidly with

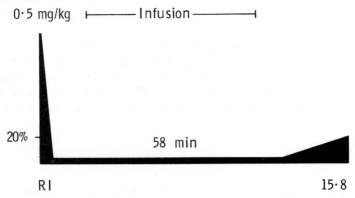

Fig. 7.15   Continuous injection of vecuronium produces a small prolongation of recovery index.

vecuronium. Clarke (1983) found that at 100 μg/kg excellent intubating conditions were present in only 50% of patients at 120 seconds, although intubation could be achieved in a further 30% with some minor difficulties. Schiller & Feldman (1984), in a double-blind study, have confirmed that there is little difference in the intubating conditions between pancuronium 100 μg/kg and vecuronium 100 μg/kg, although in terms of the ED_{95} the latter was 50% more potent.

Specificity of action
Vecuronium is the most specific neuromuscular blocking drug. Only when the dose exceeds $60 \times ED_{90}$ can any effect on cardiac vagus or autonomic ganglia be demonstrated (Savage 1983, Bowman 1983, Sutherland *et al* 1983). In doses $10 \times ED_{95}$ no effect on reuptake[1] of noradrenaline can be demonstrated.

Histamine release and anticholinesterase effect
Vecuronium does not release histamine. In equipotent doses it has less inhibition of choline-sterase than pancuronium. In large doses (200 μg/kg) the anticholinesterase effect will be greater than with a similar dose of pancuronium producing a neuro-muscular block of similar duration. However, as this effect appears to be short-lived due to rapid plasma clearance of the drug, it does not produce any difficulty at the time of reversal.

Pharmacokinetics
Vecuronium is rapidly cleared from the plasma. In three-compartment models, the second compartment, the effective rapid distribution volume, is some four times greater than with pancuronium (Bencini 1983). It is probable that rapid distribution to the liver is an important part of this distribution volume. Fahey *et al* (1981) and Upton *et al* (1982) have demonstrated rapid liver uptake in animals (up to 45% of injected dose in rats) but in man only about 10–15% of an injected dose has been recovered from the bile. However, because of the nature of the experimental design, excretion occurring in the first 15–30 minutes after injection might have been missed. Urinary excretion of vecuronium totals about 20–25% of an in-jected dose principally in the 4 hours following injection and this is about half the urinary excretion of pancuronium (Durrant *et al* 1979). For this reason vecuronium may be safely administered to patients with oliguria or anuria and only minor prolongation (up to 10%) of

the duration of action is observed (Fahey *et al* 1981, Shanks 1983, Morris *et al* 1980, Buzello 1983).

Vecuronium is metabolised principally to the 3-hydroxy derivative. Up to 10% of an injected dose may appear as this form in the urine. Small amounts of the 3-H derivative are also found together with trace amounts of 17 and 17–3 hydroxy derivatives (Bencini 1983).

Because of the rapid plasma clearance, the half-life of drug is shorter than that of pancuronium (Fig. 7.16) and cumulation is not normally a problem. It also allows early complete

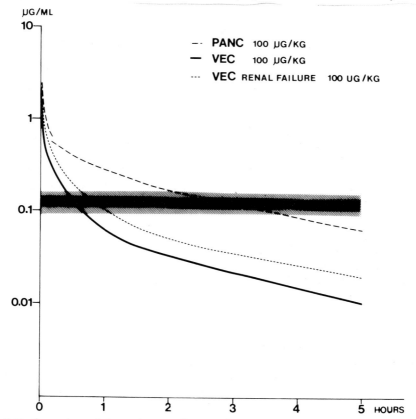

Fig. 7.16 Comparisons of plasma clearance of pancuronium, vecuronium and vecuronium in patients with renal failure. (Permission of S Agoston.)

and safe reversal to be achieved. However, as this process depends upon hepatic clearance, it is reduced in the presence of jaundice (Westra *et al* 1981).

Placental transfer

According to Duveldestin *et al* (1983), in spite of the greater lipophilicity of vecuronium the placental transfer rate was lower than with pancuronium. Using doses of 100 µg/kg or less the ratio of umbilical vein concentration to maternal plasma concentrate was about 1:10 and always well below the level to produce a clinical effect in the fetus.

Neonates and infants

The differences in the relative size of the fluid compartments in the neonate and adult (e.c.f.

44% of body weight of neonate at birth compared with 22% at 1 year) the reduced renal clearance and hepatic metabolism combine to affect the drug requirements of neonates. In children, however, dose response curves show a shift to the right indicating resistance to both vecuronium and atracurium. Nishan & Goudsozian (1983) found an ED_{95} at 60 µg/mg for vecuronium compared to 45 µg/kg in adults and young children.

Atracurium

Atracurium is presented as a solution in an acidic medium. It should be kept at 4°C as it slowly deteriorates at room temperature. Because of its acidity it is painful on i.m. injection. As it is inactivated at alkaline pH it should not be mixed with thiopentone in the same syringe and, when using sequential injections through a butterfly needle, the thiopentone should be cleared with saline before the atracurium is injected.

The ED_{90} of atracurium depends upon the background anaesthesia and whether suxamethonium has been used for intubation: it is in the range of 150 to 300 µg/mg and, like vecuronium, recovery from this bolus dose is so rapid that the duration of relaxation is too short to be clinical useful. The recovery index of atracurium in our studies was fractionally shorter than vecuronium (Fig. 7.17), being the order of $6-7 \cdot 5$ minutes. Complete reversal is possible with edrophonium or neostigmine at any time after 10 minutes. It is in the dose range of 400–500 µg/kg that atracurium is a useful neuromuscular blocking agent. Clinical reports of experience in patients using atracurium have been presented by Hughes & Payne (1983) and Payne & Hughes (1981).

Like vecuronium relaxation, atracurium neuromuscular block should be continuously monitored and supplementary doses of 100–150 µg/kg administered at the first sign of recovery. If one waits for clinical evidence of recovery then an unacceptable degree of muscle rigidity is likely to develop before the supplement takes effect. Because of the rapid metabolism of the drug there is no cumulative effect when successive 'top up' doses are administered (Hughes & Chapple 1981, Payne & Chapple 1981).

Atracurium is very suited to continuous infusion techniques and, once the administration of the drug is stopped, recovery occurs in a predictable period, whether relaxation has been obtained for 2 hours or 4 hours (Hughes et al 1983).

However, because of its propensity to release histamine, atracurium cannot be administered in multiples of its ED_{95} to give the flexibility of duration of action associated with vecuronium, resulting from the ability to use a large single bolus dose for a moderately prolonged operation. Thus, for operations of 60–90 minutes, either multiple supplements or a continuous infusion is required. With both techniques monitoring neuromuscular conduction is required and both reduce the general utility of drug for prolonged procedures. Although atracurium has been used in cardiac surgery by Flynn (1982) and associates, it is in short procedures that its relatively rapid onset, short duration of action and rapid recovery are most useful.

Onset of action

Until 10 times the ED_{95} is administered, no vagolytic action can be detected, making atracurium less pharmacologically specific for nicotinic receptors than vecuronium. In clinically recommended doses it does not affect autonomic ganglia or the cardiac vagus (Hughes & Chapple 1981). Reports of bradycardia up to 1 hour following its administration (Carter 1983, Skinner 1983) are likely to be due to the unmasking of the vagotonic properties of morphine, fentanyl or halothane when a neuromuscular drug lacking vagolytic effects is

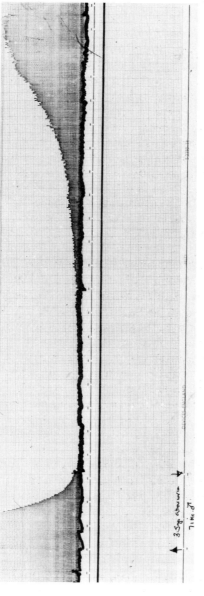

Fig. 7.17 Recovery slope following paralysis with atracurium.

used. Similar bradycardia has also been reported following the use of vecuronium. In sensitive individuals histamine release may cause a transient hypotension, but it is less dramatic and less consistent than with tubocurarine unless doses in excess of 600 µg/kg are used.

Histamine release
Atracurium, like virtually all the benzoyl isoquinolines, does cause histamine release (Basta 1983, Moss *et al* 1982, Basta *et al* 1982). This response is log/dose related and only becomes consistently high when 600 µg/kg are exceeded. It has about one-third the histamine releasing properties of tubocurarine. Nevertheless it would be prudent to avoid the use of this drug in atopic individuals, although the manufacturers maintain it is not contraindicated in asthmatic patients. The most common sign of histamine release is flushing of the arm or face but bronchospasm and severe hypotension have occurred when higher doses than at present recommended were used.

Pharmacokinetics
Rapid Hofmann degradation and slower spontaneous hydrolysis (Fig. 7.18) at the pH of blood produces a monotertiary and monoquaternary derivative. Both products are inactive at the neuromuscular junction and are free of cardiovascular effects.

The half-life of this process in vitro at physiological pH and temperature (Payne & Hughes 1983) is about 26 minutes in man and 19 minutes in cats. Coupled with the uptake by liver, kidney and other tissues, this produces a rapid plasma clearance and an apparent large rapid

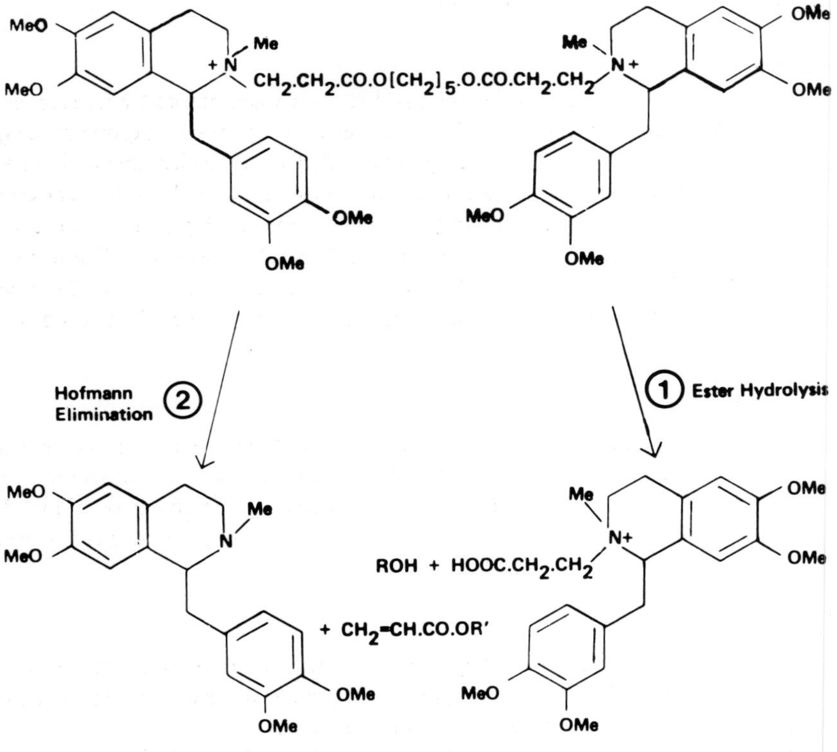

Fig. 7.18 Metabolic pathways of atracurium.

distribution volume. Because of this, the Hofman degradation process does not need an enzyme system. It retains a linear relation between dose of drug and rate of metabolism irrespective of the substrate load. As neither process involves liver metabolism or renal excretion it would be anticipated that the duration of block would be unaffected by hepatic disease or anuria. Atracurium has been used in patients with renal failure (Hunter *et al* 1982) and in patients with acute hepatic failure without any prolongation of the neuromuscular block (Ward & Neill 1983). Although anephric patients appear to have resistance to the drug, this is probably due to an increase in the rapid distribution volume.

Some concern has been expressed regarding a possible central nervous system action of the tertiary metabolite of atracurium. This drug, laudanosine, does penetrate the blood-brain barrier and, in higher concentrations than are likely to be produced with clinical doses in normal patients, it can cause analeptic and convulsant effects. However, no reports of side effects attributable to laudanosine have been described in humans.

Placental barrier
Atracurium has been passed by the Committee on Safety of Medicine (UK) as safe for use in Caesarian section.

Neonates and infants
The drug has been widely and safely used both in neonates and infants in a dose of 400 μg/mg without any reported serious side effects. Relatively higher doses on a body weight basis compared to adults were required (Brandon *et al* 1983). The flushes seen in adults are rare in neonates but not unusual in older children.

Bulky esters

Savarese *et al* (1973), working with Burroughs Wellcome Laboratories USA, have produced a series of bulky diester compounds with a two quaternary ammonium group of the general structure shown in Figure 7.8. These drugs are readily hydrolysed by plasma cholinesterase into inactive monoquaternary compounds. Although the rate of hydrolysis may exceed that of suxamethonium, the duration of neuromuscular block invariably exceeds that of suxamethonium. The neuromuscular block is reversable with anticholinesterases. Unfortunately all the drugs so far used in clinical trials release too much histamine for safe use. However, the concept of a non-depolarising drug with a plasma half-life measured in seconds is very attractive.

Pipecuronium

This steroid neuromuscular blocking agent has been investigated in Hungary by Karparti & Biro (1980) and Boros (1983). It is longer acting than atracurium and vecuronium and appears to be free of cardiovascular side effects at a clinically effective dose of 60-80 μg/kg (Newton *et al* 1982). As it is not widely available outside Eastern Europe, it is of less clinical interest than vecuronium and atracurium.

Duador

Like pipecuronium this Hungarian drug based on the steroid nucleus has undergone clinical investigation in Eastern Europe. Initial reports suggest it is shorter acting than pipecuronium but more likely to produce vagolytic effects at higher doses.

Bowman (1983) has pointed out that the very success and safety of the quaternary-based neuromuscular blocking agents has limited the search for alternative methods of producing muscle relaxation or alternative types of drugs. A polypeptide similar to the snake venoms may be an alternative to the quaternary bases as potential neuromuscular blocking drugs. Calcium channel blockers specific for the presynaptic site at the motor nerve, possibly acting in a manner similar to the aminoglycoside antibiotics, might be useful in producing neuromuscular block reversible by a drug like 4 aminopyridine.

Finally dantrolene-like drugs, acting upon the contractile process of the muscle itself, could prove a fruitful alternative to pure nicotinic blocking agents. However, for a drug to replace the present neuromuscular blocking agents in clinical use it must either offer an enormous advantage in safety or in general utility.

REFERENCES

Agoston S, Richardson F J 1983 Clinical use of vecuronium. *Report to International Symposium on Clinical Neuromuscular Pharmacology*, Boston

Agoston S, Salt P, Newton D, Bencini A, Boornsova P, Erdmann W 1980 The neuromuscular blocking action of ORG NC45, a new pancuronium derivative in anaesthetised man. *British Journal of Anaesthesia* **52:** 53S

Baird W L M 1983 Present day practice with muscle relaxants. *Geneva Symposium*, to be published by Excerpta Medica

Baird W L M, Bowman W C, Kerr W J 1982 Some actions of ORG NC45 and of endrophonium in anaesthetised cat and man. *British Journal of Anaesthesia* **54:** 375

Baird W L M, Hewett C L, Savage D S 1973 Pancuronium bromide and other steroidal neuromuscular blocking agents containing acetylcholine fragments. *British Journal of Anaesthesia* **39:** 775

Baird W L M, Reid A M 1967 The neuromuscular blocking properties of a new steroid compound, pancuronium bromide; a pilot study in man. *British Journal of Anaesthesia* **39:** 775

Barlow R B, Ing H B 1948 Curare-like action of polymethylene bisquaternary ammonium salts. *British Pharmacology and Chemotherapy* **3:** 298

Barnes P K, Brindle-Smith G 1982 Comparison of the effects upon heart rate and arterial pressure of pancuronium and ORG NC45 in anaesthetised man. *British Journal of Anaesthesia* **55:** 666

Basta S J 1983 Release of endogenous histamine by non-depolarising neuromuscular blocking agents. *Report to International Symposium on Clinical Neuromuscular Pharmacology*, Boston

Basta S J, Savarese J J, Ali H *et al* 1982 Clinical pharmacology of atracurium (BW33A). A new neuromuscular blocking agent. *Anesthesiology* **57:** A261

Bencini A 1983 Clinical pharmacokinetics of vecuronium bromide. In: Agoston S (ed) *Clinical experiences with Norcuron*. Excepta Medica, p 25

Biro K, Karpati E 1981 The pharmacology of a new short acting non-depolarising muscle relaxant steroid (RGH 4201). *Amzneimethal-Forschung Drug Research* **31:** 1918

Boros M 1983 More information about pipecuronium, a new neuromuscular blocking agent. *Anesthesiology* **58:** 108

Boros M, Szenohradsky J, Marosi G, Toth J 1980 Arzneim Forsh/Drug Research **30:** 389

Bowman W C 1983 A preclinical pharmacology of vecuronium bromide. In: Agoston S (ed) *Clinical Experience with Norcuron*. Excepta Medica, p 7

Bowman W C 1983b Peripherally acting muscle relaxants. *Psychology and Neuropharmacology* **1:** 106

Buckett W R, Hewe C L, Savage D S (1973) Pancuronium bromide and other steroidal neuromuscular blocking agents containing acetylcholine fragments. *Journal of Medical Chemistry* **6:** 116

Burke H W R, Bonta I L 1966 Pharmacological studies with NA97 (R, 16 dipiperidine 5 androstane. 3a17

Burke H W R, Hewett C L, Savage D S 1973 Pancuronium bromide and other steroidal neuromuscular blocking agents containing ace-tylocholine fragments. *Journal of Medicine and Chemistry* **6:** 1116

Buzello W 1983 The use of continuously infused vecuronium. *Report to International Symposium on Clinical Neuromuscular Pharmacology*, Boston

Buzello W, Nolge G 1982 Repetitive administration of pancuronium and vecuronium (ORG NC45 Norcuron) in patients undergoing long-lasting operation. *British Journal of Anaesthesia* **54:** 1151

Carter M L 1983 Bradycardia after the use of atracurium. *British Medical Journal* **287:** 6387

Clarke R S J 1983 Intubating conditions and neuromuscular effects following administration of vecuronium bromide. Comparison with suxamethonium and pancuronium. In: Agoston S (ed) *Clinical experiences with Norcuron*. Excepta Medica, p 60

Cohen E N, Hood N, Golling R 1968 Use of whole body autoradiography for determination of uptake and distribution of labelled muscle relaxants in the rat. *Anesthesiology* **21:** 987

Crul J F 1983 Clinical pharmacology of vecuronium. *Report to International Symposium on Clinical Neuromuscular Pharmacology*, Boston

Crul J F, Booji L M D J 1980 First clinical experiences with ORG NC45. *British Journal of Anaesthesia* **52:** 49S

Danilov A, Malygin V, Starshinova L 1978 7th International Congress of Pharmacology, Paris. Pergamon Press, Exford. *Abstract* p 153

Duvaldestin P, Agoston S, Henzel E, Kerten V N, Desmonts J H 1978 Pancuronium pharmacokinetics in patients with liver cirrhosis. *British Journal of Anaesthesia* **50:** 1131

Duvaldestin P, Demetrion M, Depoix J P 1983 Use of vecuronium bromide and ancuronium bromide drug anaesthesia for caesarian section. In: Agoston S (ed) *Clinical experiences with Norcuon*. Excepta Medica, p 92

d'Hollander A 1982 Stable muscle relaxation during abdominal surgery using combined intravenous bolus and demand infusion. *Canadian Anaesthetic Society Journal* **29:** 136

d'Hollander A, Bomblet J P, Esselen M 1983 Administration of vecuronium bromide by intravenous infusion during long lasting operations, Effect of age and interaction with suxamethonium chloride, In: Agoston S (ed) *Clinical experience with Norcuron*. Excepta Medica

Durant N N, Honwertjes M, Agoston S 1979 Hepatic elimination of ORG NC45 and pancuronium. *Anesthesiology* **51:** N3 supplement 267

Everett A J, Lowe L A, Wilkinson S 1970 Revision of structure of (+)-tubocurarine chloride and chandrocurarine. *Chemical Communications*, p 1020

Fahey M R, Morris R B, Miller R D, Nguyen T L, Upton L A 1981a Pharmacokinetics of ORG NC45 (Norcuron) in patients with and without renal failure. *British Journal of Anaesthesia* **54:** 1049

Fahey M R, Morris R B, Miller R D, Sohn Y J, Cronelly R 1980 Can Norcuron be used for intubation? *Anesthesiology* **53:** n3 273

Fahey M R, Sohn Y J, Cronelly R, Gencarelli P 1981b Clinical pharmacology of ORG NC45 (Norcuron). *Anesthesiology* **55:** 6

Feldman S A 1979 In: *Muscle relaxants*, 2nd edn. W B Saunders & Co Ltd, London

Feldman S A 1983 Forty years on. *Report to symposium on Clinical Neuromuscular Pharmacology*, Boston

Feldman S A, Tyrrel M F 1970 NB68. A new steroid muscle relaxant. *Anaesthesia* **25:** 349

Flynn P J, Hughes R, Walton B, Jothilingham S 1982 Paper 5.7 Atracurium Symposium, Royal College of Surgeons, London. Hughes R (ed)

Foldes F F 1983 Personal communication of International Symposium. *Clinical Neuromuscular Pharmacology*, Boston

Foldes F F, Yun H, Radnay P A, Bodola R P, Kaplan R, Nageshima H 1981 Antagonism of neuromuscular effect of ORG NC45 by edrophonium. *Anesthesiology* **55:** N3A, A201

Gandila A, Marshall I G, Paul D, Rodger I W, Scott W, Singh M 1975 Some actions of chandonium iodine, a new short-acting muscle relaxant in anaesthetised cats and in isolated muscle preparations. *Clinical and Experimental Pharmacology and Physiology* **2:** 159

Gill R 1940 White water and black magic. Henry Holt & Co, New York

Griffith H R, Johnson G E 1942 The use of curare in general anesthesia. *Anesthesiology* **3:** 418

Harrison P, Feldman S A 1981 Intubating conditions with ORG NC45. *Anaesthesia* **36:** 874

Hollway T, Feldman S A 1982 Use of multiple of ED $_{90}$ dose of ORG NC45 in anaesthetised man. *Report to European Congress of Anaesthesiology*, London

Holmes P E B, Jenden D J, Taylor D B 1947 *Nature* **159:** 86

Hughes R 1983 Clinical pharmacology and special uses of atracurium — report to the international symposium on Clinical Neuromuscular Pharmacology, Boston

Hughes R, Chapple D J 1981a The pharmacology of atracurium a new neuromuscular blocking agent. *British Journal of Anaesthesia* **53:** 31

Hughes R, Chapple D J 1981b The pharmacology of atracurium a new competitive neuromuscular blocking agent. *British Journal of Anaesthesia* **53:** 31

Hughes R, Payne J P 1983 Clinical assessment of atracurium using the tetanic and single twitch responses of adductor pollucis muscle. *British Journal of Anaesthesia* **55:** Supp. to be published

Hughes R, Flynn P J, Eagar B 1983 Administration of atracurium by continuous infusion for long surgical procedures. To be published

Hunter J M, Jones R S, Utting J E 1982 The use of atracurium in patients with no renal function. *British Journal of Anaesthesia* **54:** 1251

Karparti E, Biro K 1980 Pharmacological study of a new competitive neuromuscular blocking steroid; pipecuronium bromide. *Drug Research* **30(1):** 346

Katz R L, Katz G 1967 Clinical use of muscle relaxants. In: *Advances in anesthesiology — muscle relaxants*. Excepta Medica, New York

King H 1935 Curare alkaloids 1. Tubocurarine. *Journal of Chemistry Society* 1381

Kirkwood I, Duckworth R A 1983 An unusual case of sinus arrest. *British Journal of Anaesthesia* **55:** 1273

McIntyre A R 1947 Curare, its history, nature and clinical use. University of Chicago Press, Chicago III

Marrlett R A, Thompson C J, Webb F E 1983 In vitro degradation of atracurium in human patients. *British Journal of Anaesthesia* **55:** 61

Morris R, Fahey, Muller M D, Connelly R, Nguyen T L, Upton R 1980 The pharmacokinetics of Norcuron in patients with normal and impaired renal function. *Anesthesiology* **IV53:** 5267

Morris R B, Wilkinson P L, Miller R D, Caholan M, Quasha A, Robinson S 1981 Cardiovascular effects of ORG NC45 (norcuron) in patients undergoing coronary artery bypass grafting. *Anesthesiology* **55:** A205

Moss J, Philbin D M, Roscow C E 1982 Histamine release by muscle relaxants in man. *Klinische Wochenschrift* **60:** 891

Neill E A M, Chapple D J 1982 Metabolic studies in cat with atracurium; a neuromuscular blocking agent designed for non-enzymatic inactivation at physiological pH. *Xenobiotica* **12:** 203

Newton D E F, Richardson F J, Agoston S 1982 Preliminary studies in man with pipecuronium bromide (Arduan). A new steroid neuromuscular blocking agent. *British Journal of Anaesthesia* **54:** 789

Nishan G, Goudsouzian N 1983 Short-acting muscle relaxants in children. In: International Symposium on Clinical Neuromuscular Pharmacology, Boston

Norman J, Katz R L 1971 Some effects of the steroidal muscle relaxant dacuronium bromide in anaesthetised patients. *British Journal of Anaesthesia* **43:** 313

Paton W D M, Zaimis E 1949 The pharmacological actions of the polymethyline bis methylammonium salts. *British Journal of Pharmacology and Chemotherapy* **4:** 381

Payne J P, Hughes R 1981 Evaluation of atracurium in anaesthetised man. *British Journal of Anaesthesia* **53:** 45

Savage D S 1983a Development of vecuronium — lecture to International Symposium on Clinical Neuromuscular Pharmacology, Boston

Savage D S 1983b Neuromuscular blocking agents. In: Horn A S, de Ranter C J (eds) *X-ray crystallography and drug action.* Oxford University Press, Oxford

Savage D S 1983c The discovery of vecuronium bromide. In: Agoston (ed) *Clinical experiences with Norcuron.* Excepta Medica, New York, p 1

Savarese J J *et al* 1973 The pharmacology of new short-acting non-depolarising ester neuromuscular blocking agents: clinical implications. *Anesthesia and Analgesia (Cleveland)* **52:** 982

Savarese J J, Ginsberg S, Braswell L, Kitz R J 1979 Actions at neuromuscular and esteratic cholinoreceptive sites of some phenylene disacrylol bis-cholinium esters. *Journal of Pharmacology and Experimental Therapy* **208N3:** 436

Savarese J J, Kitz R J 1975 Does clinical anaesthesia need new neuromuscular blocking agents? *Anesthesiology* **42:** 236

Savarese J J, Wastilla W B 1979 BW444U. Intermediate-duration non-depolarising neuromuscular blocking agent with significant lack of cardiovascular and autonomic effect. *Anesthesiology* **51N3:** 279

Schiller D W, Feldman S A 1984 Comparison of intubating conditions with atracurium, vecuronium and pancuronium. *Anaesthesia* **39:** 1188

Shanks C A 1983 Relaxants in renal failure. Report to International Symposium on Clinical Neuromuscular Pharmacology, Boston 1983

Singh M, Paul D, Parashar V V 1972 Abstracts 10 PAC. Symposium on the chemistry of natural products, New Delhi, p 247

Skinner A C 1983 Bradycardia after the use of atracurium. *British Medical Journal* **287:** 6401

Stenlake J B 1978 Biodegradable neuromuscular blocking agents. In: Stoclet J C (ed) *Advances in pharmacology and therapeutics, vol 3.* Pergamon Press, Oxford, p 303

Stenlake J B, Waigh R D, Dewar G H, Hughes R, Chapple D J, Coker G G 1981 Biodegradable neuromuscular blocking agents. Part 4. Atracurium besylate and related polyalkaline di-esters. *European Journal of Medicine and Chemistry* **16:** 515

Sugrue M F, Duff N, McIndewar I 1975 On the pharmacology of ORG 6368 (2B, 16B dipiperidine 5α-androstane. 3 acetate demethobromide) a new steroidal neuromuscular blocking agent. *Journal of Pharmacy and Pharmacology* **27:** 721

Sutherland G H, Squire I B, Gibb A J, Marshall I G 1983 Neuromuscular blocking and autonomic effects of vecuronium and atracurium in the anaesthetised cat. *British Journal of Anaesthesia* **55:** 1119

Upton R A, Nguyen T L, Miller R D, Castagna N 1982 Renal and biliary elimination of vecuronium (ORG NC45) and pancuronium in rats. *Anesthesia and Analgesia* **61:** 313

Ward S, Neill E A M 1983 Pharmacokinetics of atracurium in acute hepatic failure with acute renal failure. *British Journal of Anaesthesia* **55:** 1169

Westra P, Houwertjes M C, Wessling H, Myer D F K 1981 Bile salt and neuromuscular blocking agents. *British Journal of Anaesthesia* **53:** 407

Wintersteiner O, Dutcher J D 1943 Curare alkaloids from chondrodendron tomentosum. *Science* **97:** 467

Functional assessment of the normal brain during general anaesthesia

INTRODUCTION

One of the skills acquired by anaesthetists early in their training is the ability to evaluate the effects on the brain of general anaesthetic agents and procedures. This is to ensure that the patient's brain is protected from the damaging effects of impaired oxygen delivery due to hypoxia, arterial hypotension or intracranial hypertension, and that the patient is sufficiently anaesthetised to be unaware of the operative procedure.

Prevention of awareness during surgery depends upon observation of certain vital signs, and in current practice the anaesthetist relies on changes in heart rate and blood pressure, pupil size, sweating, lachrymation and, where appropriate, respiratory patterns, to assess consciousness during anaesthesia. Some of these signs are directly related to depth of anaesthesia but changes in others are due to side effects of the particular anaesthetic agent. Three factors in modern anaesthetic practice make an objective measure of the depth of anaesthesia more difficult than hitherto.

These are (1) the use of neuromuscular blockade, (2) anaesthetic drugs which have few side effects and (3) the use of continuous intravenous anaesthesia.

Neuromuscular blockade is combined with drugs with few side effects in 'balanced anaesthesia', the opiate–relaxant–IPPV sequence. The lack of muscular movement, in particular the respiratory movement, and the minimal cardiovascular side effects of this technique has severely curtailed the signs available for assessing depth of anaesthesia. This has led to an increasing incidence of awareness during anaesthesia.

Total intravenous anaesthesia poses other problems. While it is relatively easy to regulate the uptake and elimination, and thus the dose, of inhalation anaesthetics sufficiently to be able to use these drugs, the use of intravenous agents is not so convenient. This is because the only factor available for manipulation is the infusion rate, and there is no control of the metabolic/excretion rate, nor any clear definition of the dilution volumes, so that standard infusion rates based on weight result in widely differing concentrations of the drug in the blood and hence the brain. This can cause delayed recovery on the one hand or an increased incidence of awareness on the other. These two factors combine to make an objective measure of the depth of anaesthesia a desirable aim.

These two topics, the *assessment of brain function during anaesthesia* and the *assessment of depth of anaesthesia*, while clearly related, can be considered separately. Firstly, consideration will be given to methods of assessing brain cell function, some of which have applications only in the laboratory, but nevertheless they provide information which can be used to develop techniques suitable for everyday use in the operating theatre.

ASSESSMENT OF BRAIN FUNCTION

Physiological considerations

In conscious man clinical examination provides a great deal of information about the function of the central nervous system (c.n.s.). During general anaesthesia, however, this is of limited value and other methods should be applied. Techniques are now being developed which permit the study of brain function, and therefore the graded effects of anaesthetics on this function, even in deeply anaesthetised subjects. These fall into three interrelated areas of study: (1) regional brain blood flow, (2) metabolic rate of brain tissue and (3) electrical activity of the brain.

It might be thought that measuring brain blood flow is an unusual way of obtaining information about brain cell function. However, in many organs of the body, and the brain is no exception, there is a very close relationship between metabolic function and blood flow. It was originally suggested almost 100 years ago by Roy & Sherrington (1890) that the brain possesses an intrinsic mechanism whereby its blood supply can be varied locally in proportion to local changes in function. A major part of this chapter will review the evidence that there is a very close linkage between cerebral *blood flow*, *metabolism* and the *electrical activity* of brain cells measured with scalp electrodes. The aim is to explore the possibility that the measurement of one or other of these variables will accurately reflect the change in activity of different functional groups of neurones during the transition from the conscious state to deep stages of anaesthesia.

Interrelationship between brain activity, metabolism and blood flow in animals

The first demonstration of close correlation between regional blood *flow* and neuronal *metabolism* in the normal brain used autoradiography of rat brain slices (Sokoloff *et al* 1977, Sakurada *et al* 1978). This technique employed ^{14}C deoxyglucose (a metabolic marker) and [^{14}C] iodo-antipyrine (a blood flow marker) to examine metabolism and blood flow in more than 25 discrete anatomical and functional regions of the brain.

In conscious rats, the regional cerebral metabolic rate for glucose (rCMRG$_L$) varies in different brain structures, the rate in grey structures being three times greater than that in white structures. The highest values are in the auditory pathways, and it is possible to alter those values by a variety of methods. For example, bilateral auditory deprivation markedly reduces metabolism only in auditory pathways, but with general anaesthesia with thiopentone there was a reduction in rCMRG$_L$ in all structures of the brain, although the greatest reduction was in the grey structures of the primary sensor pathways, particularly the auditory pathways.

Using the [^{14}C] iodo antipyrine method for measuring *blood flow* in the same regions of the brain (rCBF), Sakurada *et al* (1978) have related blood flow to metabolism. There was a highly significant correlation between rCMRG$_L$ and rCBF in different functional regions of the brain in conscious animals and this correlation continued to hold during thiopentone anaesthesia when regional function was dramatically reduced. Conversely, in the awake animal, when rCMRG$_L$ was increased by stimulating the auditory or visual pathways, rCBF increased to match the rCMRG$_L$. These observations emphatically confirm the predictions of Roy and Sherrington (Sokaloff 1981), at least in rats.

Measurement of cerebral blood flow and metabolism in man

Global flow and metabolism

Autoradiography of brain slices is not applicable to man, so other methods have had to be applied. Initially, global techniques were applied, but latterly regional information is coming to light. The Kety-Schmidt arteriovenous difference method is the original technique for measuring global CBF in man. In outline, this involves breathing 15% N_2O for 10–15 minutes and measuring the N_2O concentration in repeated blood samples from the jugular bulb and a peripheral artery. The difference in the rate of change of the two concentrations allows CBF to be calculated. This principle can be applied less invasively by substituting [133]xenon or [85]krypton for N_2O and measuring radioactivity extracranially. Methods for measuring cerebral blood flow and metabolism are well described by Todd et al (1981) and Lassen (1982).

If the cerebral arteriovenous (A-V) oxygen or glucose concentration gradients are measured simultaneously with CBF, the cerebral metabolic rate for oxygen ($CMRO_2$) or glucose ($CMRG_L$) can be calculated. This approach provides information about the blood flow and metabolism of the brain as a whole but cannot detect poorly perfused regions. Therefore this method cannot test the hypothesis that cerebral metabolism and blood flow in man are closely interrelated in a particular part of the brain because of the lack of uniformity of metabolic activity and blood flow.

Regional cerebral blood flow

The first approach to differentiating blood flow to grey and white regions of the brain was to inject a bolus of [85]krypton or [133]xenon into the carotid artery and measuring the clearance from the brain with one external scintillation detector. This allowed discrimination between slow and fast clearance regions by analysis of the shape of the clearance curve (Mallett & Veall 1965, Lassen & Christensen 1976) showing the relative proportions of grey and white matter; the former had three times greater blood flow per unit mass than the latter. A development of this method places more than 250 scinitillation detectors extracranially and gives more detailed information about regional blood flow. This technique showed that voluntary movement of the hand produced an increase in blood flow in the contralateral cortical hand motor area (Raichle et al 1976). Although of some use clinically, it provides no direct information about metabolism, and the superimposition of tissue layers limits the discrimination of the technique.

Regional cerebral blood flow and metabolism in man using computerised tomography

The problem of superimposition is solved by the use of *computerised tomography (CT)*. Besides X-ray CT there are three other tomographic techniques of interest: (1) nuclear magnetic resonance (NMR) tomography, (2) single photon γ-emission tomography and (3) positron emission tomography.

NMR is an exciting new development for looking at regional brain structure (Smith 1983) giving images with much more precise resolution even than X-ray CT. The great potential of NMR is to measure metabolic function in vivo, using small topical surface coils placed over regions of interest, but so far the technique has not been applied to anaesthetised man.

Single photon γ-emission tomography is used to study regional brain function (Coleman et al 1982) by rotating the gamma camera around the head just as the X-ray apparatus is rotated for X-ray CT scans. Using radioactive xenon it has been shown that visual perception augments regional cerebral blood flow (rCBF) in the visual cortex by about 35%, and unilateral hand movements increase rCBF by 20–50% in the contralateral primary sensory-motor areas (Henriksen et al 1981, Lauritzen et al 1981). However, the xenon tracer gives no direct information about regional brain metabolism, and application of the technique to study the linkage between rCBF and metabolism must await the development of suitable radiolabelled metabolic presursors. This is important because some general anaesthetic drugs interfere with the link between metabolism (brain cell function) and blood flow (Todd *et al* 1982).

Positron emission tomography (PET) is one of the most exciting developments in studying regional brain metabolism and blood flow in man. A comprehensive review is presented by Phelps *et al* (1982) and only a brief outline is given here. At present, this technique is only available in a few centres because of the enormous cost and because a cyclotron is required to generate the tracers.

The development of PET allows CT scanning for position (β^+) emitting tracer molecules such as 15-oxygen, 18-fluorine, 11 or 15 carbon. These are very short-lived tracers which are made on site in a cyclotron particle accelerator and can be used for metabolic as well as flow studies (Wolf & Fowler 1983). This non-invasive technique has a much higher resolution than single photon γ emission tomography, and enables measurements to be made in man in discrete regions throughout the brain of cerebral blood flow (rCBF), metabolic rate for oxygen (rCMRO$_2$) and glucose (rCMRG$_L$), oxygen extraction ratio (rOER) and cerebral blood volume (rCBV) (Wise 1983, Phelps *et al* 1982, Hawkins *et al* 1983, Crosby & Sokoloff 1983).

Interrelationship of cerebral metabolism and blood flow in man using PET

The normal brain. PET has been used to show that there is a very close interrelationship between regional brain function and blood flow in the normal human brain (Phelps *et al* 1982). Although the technique does not give information about as many regions of the brain as the autoradiographic method it certainly confirms, in a spectacular way, the close coupling between rCBF, rCMRO$_2$ and rCMRG$_L$.

The extraordinary sensitivity of the technique to the most subtle changes in brain function is illustrated by observations following visual or auditory stimulation. Increasing the complexity of the visual stimulus progressively increased the rCMRG$_L$ of the visual cortex, as follows: progressively changing patterns of rCMRG$_L$ were seen first with white light, eyes closed, then one eye open, two open, then black and white checkerboard and finally a complex outdoor scene.

Using the rCMRG$_L$ technique in normal man to examine the function of the *auditory system* Phelps *et al* (1982) showed that verbal stimuli (a Sherlock Holmes story) produced diffuse predominant left-sided activities whereas musical stimulation (a Brandenburg Concerto) gave diffuse right-sided activation in musically naive subjects but left-sided activation in the musically sophisticated!

These observations demonstrate the astonishing ability of the PET technique to measure the most subtle changes in regional function within the brain of conscious man. So far no studies using this technique have been reported in anaesthetised patients. Nevertheless its application to the anaesthetised man in the laboratory is needed to provide confirmation in man of the autoradiographic studies in animals (Sokoloff *et al* 1977).

The abnormal brain. Lassen (1966) observed that some regions of the injured brain have rCBF in excess of normal and called this phenomenon 'luxury perfusion'. The loss of the normal close coupling between cerebral metabolism (rOER, rCMRO$_2$ and rCMRG$_L$) and blood flow has been described in patients with intracranial pathology (Ackerman *et al* 1981, Baron *et al* 1981). Baron (1981) showed that two types of focal disruption of flow occurred. In 20% of patients with cerebrovascular disease rCBF was reduced below the metabolic demands (misery perfusion). In 80% of these patients rCBF was in excess of metabolic demand (luxury perfusion) despite the fact that rCBF was actually less than normal in about half of these cases.

It was concluded from these studies that measurements of *brain cell metabolism* is very highly correlated with *brain cell function* in health and disease. Although rCBF was also closely coupled to brain cell function in normal man, this coupling could break down following brain injury and measurements of rCBF in these circumstances gives quite misleading information about cerebral function. This might also be the case in anaesthesia where anaesthetics with powerful effects on vascular control, e.g. halothane, may produce dissociation between metabolism and blood flow (Todd *et al* 1982).

These techniques are useful at present mainly for laboratory studies of the basic physiology and pathophysiology of brain cell function. For monitoring brain function in the operating theatre or intensive care unit the most readily available device appears to be the electroencephalogram (e.e.g.). What is the relationship between the e.e.g. and metabolic activity of brain cells?

Correlation of electroencephalography with regional brain function

Most of our knowledge of neurophysiology has been derived from studies of the electrical activity from within discrete parts of the brain (Sokoloff 1981). This section explores the use of electroencephalography, measured from the skin surface, as an index of brain cell function.

Paulson & Sharborough (1974) have reviewed the relationship between the e.e.g. on the one hand and CBF and $CMRO_2$ on the other. The problem is divided into two components *analysing* the e.e.g. signal and measuring rCBF and $rCMRO_2$ in *discrete parts* of the brain. Ten years ago signal processing provided *quantitative* frequency analysis but the anatomical resolution of the e.e.g. was limited to superficial brain structures whereas CBF and $CMRO_2$ measurements reflected total brain blood flow and O_2 consumption. Despite these

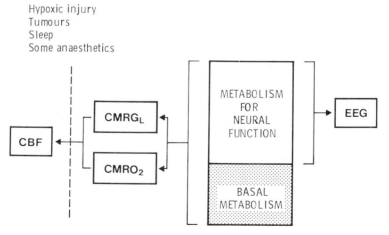

Fig. 8.1   The relationship between cerebral blood flow (CBF), cerebral metabolic rate ($CMRO_2$, $CMRG_L$) and neuronal activity (e.e.g.). Regional CBF is proportional to the total CMR whereas e.e.g. activity correlates with only a part of the CMR. There is a residual basal metabolic rate even when there is complete absence of e.e.g. activity. The normal linkage between CMR and CBF is broken in a number of circumstances indicated in the figure. Volatile anaesthetics cause a reduction in metabolism but by dilating cerebral vessels they increase CBF. Halothane in particular produces marked dissociation of metabolism and flow (Todd *et al* 1982).

limitations it could be shown that in normal awake people, regardless of age, there was close coupling of e.e.g. activity and CBF and $CMRO_2$, a decrease in activity corresponding closely to a decrease in CBF and $CMRO_2$.

These observations have been confirmed by Fitzpatrick *et al* (1976) and Ingvar *et al* (1976). Furthermore, there were an appreciable number of clinical abnormalities of cerebral function, including epilepsy and various metabolic comas, where this coupling was maintained. However, during sleep or in childhood there appeared to be some uncoupling of the link between CBF and $CMRO_2$ and uncoupling is also found in cerebral hypoxic damage and in some tumours. They also made a very important observation that it is the activity but not the number of grey cells that is the key determinant of the amount of e.e.g. activity.

This implies that in the adult it *is possible to interpret the mean frequency of a given e.e.g. in terms of $CMRO_2$* (Obrist 1963). However, a further 'translation' of the e.e.g. into CBF terms should be avoided since dissociation of $CMRO_2$ and CBF may occur following anoxia or various general anaesthetic drugs. The general relationship between CBF, $CMRO_2$, $CMRG_L$ and e.e.g. are shown in Figure 8.1. Note that the metabolic function ($CMRO_2$ or $CMRG_L$) is subdivided into basal metabolic function and specialised, neuronal, function. The latter function is measured by the e.e.g. This concept is discussed below.

Partitioning of $CMRO_2$ and e.e.g. during anaesthesia

At this point it must be emphasised that the metabolic activity ($CMRO_2$) of the brain cell may be subdivided into that required for electrical activity and that for basal cellular integrity (Michenfelder & Theye 1975, Michenfelder 1983). This is of relevance both to the interpretation of the relationship between e.e.g. and $CMRO_2$ and to an understanding of possible

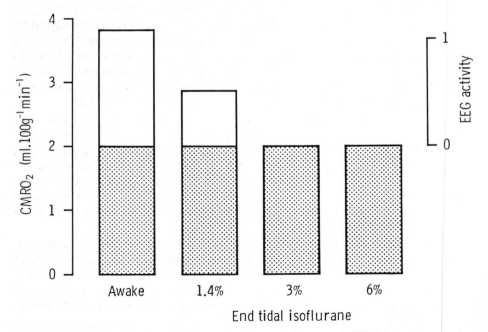

Fig. 8.2 The effect of increasing end-tidal concentrations of isoflurane on $CMRO_2$ (after Newberg *et al* 1983). The clear areas represent the part of metabolism serving the specialised, neuroelectrical, component of CMR; the dotted areas represent the unspecialised, basal, component of CMR. This component is reduced only by hypothermia.

mechanisms of brain cell protection after hypoxic injury. They suggested that general anaesthetics such as thiopentone, halothane or isoflurane depress electrical activity, and thus metabolism, until electrical activity ceases and only basal metabolism persists. It is the supra basal, or specialised neuronal, function which is demonstrable as e.e.g. activity and there is a close relationship between e.e.g., $CMRO_2$ and, for example, thiopentone-concentration up to the point where the e.e.g. is abolished. It is not surprising that further large increments of thiopentone, up to twice the concentration necessary to achieve isoelectric conditions, does not reduce $CMRO_2$ further and the cell remains at basal metabolic levels. Isoflurane (Newberg et al 1983) has a similar dose related effect on $CMRO_2$ until the e.e.g. becomes iso-electric (2·4% end-tidal isoflurane in man) and increasing the end expired isoflurane to 6% has no further effect on $CMRO_2$ (Fig. 8.2). In contrast, progressive hypothermia continues to reduce $CMRO_2$ after the e.e.g. has become isoelectric which implies that the basal meta-bolism of the cell is reduced by cooling but not by drugs such as thiopentone or isoflurane (Newberg & Michenfelder 1983).

Thus, as far as some commonly used anaesthetic drugs are concerned there is a close relationship between $CMRO_2$, e.e.g. activity and anaesthetic concentration up to the point of an isoelectric e.e.g.

Effects of other anaesthetic drugs on $CMRO_2$ and CBF

Because of the close link between the e.e.g. and $CMRO_2$ and the fact that changes in the e.e.g. with many anaesthetic drugs have not been reported in detail we infer changes in the e.e.g. from changes in $CMRO_2$. *Halothane* (3%) increased CBF by 140%, but at 1 and 3% $CMRO_2$ and $CMRG_L$ were reduced by 40 and 70% respectively (Pellegrino et al 1982). In contrast, *nitrous oxide (70%)* increased CBF (200%), $CMRO_2$ (160%) and $CMRG_L$ (120%) in one study in goats (Pellegrino et al 1982) but had little effect in other studies (Carlsson et al 1976). This increase in cerebral metabolism with nitrous oxide has also been reported by Ingvar et al (1980) and was attributed to the excitatory phase or stage II anaesthesia. *Enflurane* at 0·6 MAC in man produced no change in $CMRO_2$ or CBF compared to the awake state but at 1·2 MAC $CMRO_2$ was reduced and CBF increased (Sakabe et al 1983).

Morphine 1 mg/kg intravenously in dogs reduced $CMRO_2$, $CMRG_L$ and CBF (Matsumiya & Dohi 1983). This effect was reversed by naloxone. Similar effects on spinal cord blood flow (SCBF) were seen after i.v. but not spinal subarachnoid injection. Naloxone, by itself, had no effect on CBF, SCBF, $CMRO_2$ or $CMRG_L$. *Fentanyl* (Michenfelder & Theye 1971) and *pethidine* (Messick & Theye 1969) have similar effects to morphine. *Lorazepam* (Rockoff et al 1980) decreases CBF and $CMRO_2$ with minimal changes in blood pressure. *Midazolam* and *diazepam* (Forster et al 1982, Nugent et al 1980) both produce a decrease in CBF and $CMRO_2$.

Ketamine (Crosby et al 1982) has a fascinating effect on regional cerebral metabolism. There appears to be a system specific effect, some regions having decreased metabolism and others increased metabolism. Of particular interest was the marked metabolic *depression* in the auditory pathway (auditory cortex, medial geniculate and inferior colliculus) and sensory motor area. In contrast there was *increased* metabolism in the visual cortex, and some parts of the limbic system.

An important limitation of these metabolic studies is that they do not discriminate between direct and indirect action of anaesthetic drugs (Crosby et al 1982). An entire neuronal path-way may be affected even though the anaesthetic agent acts at only one end of the pathway.

However, reduced neuronal activity, manifest as a change in the e.e.g., is always followed by reduced energy consumption (Sokoloff 1977).

Summary

It is now known that in most circumstances there is good correlation between cerebral metabolic rate ($CMRO_2$ or $CMRG_L$) and cerebral blood flow (CBF) and, within limits, a good correlation between cerebral electrical activity and metabolic rate. A number of pathological conditions may upset the correlation of metabolism and flow, in particular cerebral ischaemia and raised intracranial pressure, and these upsets may be further disturbed by the addition of some anaesthetic drugs. There is thus some danger of ischaemia progressing during anaesthesia by increasing cerebral blood volume, increasing intracranial pressure and reducing blood flow.

The reduction of neuronal metabolic rate with anaesthetic drugs is limited to the component of metabolism concerned with electrical activity. Anaesthesia alone will not switch off cerebral metabolism completely, only reduce it by 50–70%. This has crucial implications in application to brain protection after head injury or cerebral infarction.

MEASUREMENT OF THE DEPTH OF ANAESTHESIA

So far we have reviewed the evidence that brain function is well represented by $CMRG_L$ and $CMRO_2$ and above basal levels of metabolism there is a close correlation between these variables and the e.e.g. Apart from observations of the vital signs, the electroencephalograph provides the only non-invasive method that may be applied by the anaesthetist to assess brain function directly during anaesthesia. Clark & Rosner (1973) provide an early review of the role of the e.e.g. for routine monitoring of depth of anaesthesia in man. The problem is twofold: (1) standardising the definition of depth of anaesthesia, (2) producing an e.e.g. derivative which is universally affected by anaesthetics.

Difficulties in defining depth of anaesthesia

This subject presents difficulties because of the absence, so far, of any continuous scale of depth of anaesthesia. Most anaesthetists would agree that awareness of a surgical incision, recalled post operatively, represents a lighter stage of anaesthesia than that at which movement occurs in response to incision, but there is *no* recall postoperatively. Does the response of an 'anaesthetised' patient to the spoken word, but without subsequent recall, fall mid-way between awareness and movement in response to incision? Even if there were agreement on the order of responses it could not be assumed that these responses held any fixed relationship to one another. Finally if a patient is aware, but forgets about it, has he come to any harm because of the awareness? This last problem is particularly relevant since the introduction of amnesic drugs like lorazepam. It would seem to us to be preferable that patients should be anaesthetised, without the use of amnesic drugs, to a stage where they are unaware of surgical stimuli. At present, this problem is unresolved.

Development of e.e.g. techniques suitable for clinical anaesthesia

Can the e.e.g. be used to demonstrate graded changes in brain function with increasing concentration of anaesthetic? If so can this be used to indicate the likelihood of the patient being so lightly anaesthetised that awareness, in one form or the other, becomes a probability?

The limitations of the conventional method electroencephalography has been reviewed by

Gevins (1980) and Simons & Pronk (1983). The e.e.g. activity of the brain is characterised on the conventional polygraph trace by its frequency, amplitude and wave morphology and by its spatial and temporal distribution. The standard e.e.g. analysis is a 'by-eye' report based on a visual identification of individual components in complex e.e.g. records. This, however, is often very difficult, requires considerable training and is therefore not applicable to routine use by anaesthetists. Other more structured methods have been applied, but they are all unsatisfactory as there is wide variability in e.e.g. patterns with different anaesthetic agents at comparable levels of anaesthesia. Thus, if the e.e.g. is to be useful in this role, there is a requirement (a) that the complex information contained in the e.e.g. is processed to a simple form, (b) the processed output is consistently affected by anaesthetics, (c) the output is easily understood, (d) the whole process is convenient and inexpensive.

This means some form of computer processing (Greenberg et al 1981) and so far this has been either (1) frequency domain analysis, or (2) time domain analysis.

Frequency domain analysis

In one form of frequency domain analysis the e.e.g. signal is separated into groups based on frequency by subjecting the digitised e.e.g. to fast fourier transformation. One popular presentation of the result of this analysis is the *compressed spectral array* (CSA) (Bickford 1971). This is a plot of power against frequency over a 1 to 40 Hz frequency range. This can be further divided into β (13–27 Hz), α (7·5–13 Hz), θ (3·5–7·5 Hz) and δ (1–3·5 Hz) wave bands.

Bart et al (1971) have reviewed the effects of a number of volatile anaesthetics on the CSA. He concluded that there were widely different effects of common anaesthetics which must limit its usefulness as a universal indicator of the graded effects of these anaesthetics.

An attempt to circumvent this problem has been suggested by Rampil et al (1980). This is the use of the *spectral edge frequency* (SEF) which is the highest frequency in the power spectrum at which a significant amount of energy is present in the e.e.g.: this is around 25–30 Hz in awake animals and man. Rampil et al (1980) showed that in dogs the SEF falls rapidly in response to increases in inspired concentrations of enflurane or halothane. The change in SEF frequency in response to incremental changes in halothane concentration in dogs was 8 Hz/MAC whereas with enflurane it was 20 Hz/MAC. It was found that an infusion of thiopentone in man (150 mg/min for 4 min) produced a shift in SEF from an awake value of 25 Hz down to a mean of 13 Hz during thiopentone and this returned towards control levels as the subjects woke up (Stanski et al 1982). Using a similar technique in man Hudson et al (1983) showed that there was no acute tolerance to three sequential infusions of thiopentone given 20–25 min apart.

The effects of fentanyl (150 μg/min for 5 min) compared to alfentanyl (1500 μg/min for 4 min) on SEF has been examined in man by Scott & Stanski (1984). They found that SEF fell from an awake value of about 19 Hz to 12 Hz following administration of either drug to conscious volunteers. It may be important that drugs not considered to be general anaesthetics should produce effects on the SEF similar to those seen with both intravenous and inhalation anaesthetic agents.

So far there is insufficient information available to decide whether the changes in SEF with different anaesthetic agents provides a good method of measuring depth of anaesthesia with different anaesthetic agents. However, different affects of different drugs on SEF, as with the CSA itself, suggest that it may not fit the part.

Another approach employed at the London Hospital is the *Cerebral Function Analysing*

Monitor (Maynard 1979, Sebel *et al* 1983). This provides a display of the weighted amplitude (μV) of the e.e.g. signal between 1·5–27 Hz and the amplitude of each of the above mentioned frequency bands (β, α, δ and θ). Using this technique it has been shown that N_2O at 30% and 50% produced significant *reductions* in weighted amplitude but no consistent changes in the different frequency bands (Williams *et al* 1984). Thiopentone produces an *increase* in the weighted amplitude with quite different patterns of changing amplitude in the frequency bands (Sebel *et al* 1983). This method does not, so far, avoid the problem of different patterns of e.e.g. activity with different anaesthetics.

Time domain analysis

The e.e.g. techniques described so far have evolved to the point of providing an easily recognised signal which may be proportional to the effect of a number of 'anaesthetic' drugs on the brain although the effects on the e.e.g. may be specific to a particular anaesthetic agent. Furthermore this approach does not provide localisation of action of these drugs in different parts of the brain. An example of time domain analysis is the *evoked responses in the e.e.g.* An attractive feature of the evoked potential (EP) technique is that it provides information about the function of specific anatomical structures and their interconnections within the brain (see reviews by Chiappa & Ropper 1982, Aminoff 1980 and Grundy 1983). Three clinically useful EP techniques have been developed: *visual, auditory* and *somatosensory* EPs. The anatomical pathways in each of the three techniques have been very well worked out and the tests have been used to localise tumours, the lesions of multiple sclerosis, the effects of operative procedures (Symon *et al* 1984) and as an index of brain injury in intensive care patients (Taylor *et al* 1983).

Basic principles in recording EPs

The technique differs from conventional e.e.g. recording in that repetitive stimuli are applied either to the eyes, ears or peripheral nerves. The potentials evoked in the e.e.g. by these stimuli are then extracted from background activity by electronic processing. The EPs appear at fixed time intervals following the stimulus and summing the e.e.g. following the stimulus reveals the evoked response from the jungle of random background activity.

Each of the three techniques has a characteristic wave form and there is a close relationship between the waves and the anatomy of each sensory tract from sensor to cortex. General anaesthetic drugs may diminish the amplitude of the waves or delay their appearance (increase latency).

Visual EP (VEP)

The usual stimulus used to examine the visual pathways is the reversing checkerboard pattern with constant light output (Sokol 1980). The major feature in the processed e.e.g. signal is a wave whose peak, P100 (sometimes called P1) appears 100 ms after the stimulus onset has a neural source in the visual cortex and is derived from the e.e.g. measured at occipital and parietal locations. Uhl *et al* (1980) found a close relationship between end-tidal halothane concentration and increased latency of P100 in man. Increasing concentrations of N_2O produce a reduction in amplitude and increase in latency of the VEP (Sebel *et al* 1984). Further studies are required to establish the role of this technique in measuring depth of anaesthesia.

Somatosensory EP (SEP)

These potentials are elicited by transcutaneous electrical stimulation of the median, peroneal or tibial nerves using a square wave stimulus $0 \cdot 2$–2 ms in duration at 5 impulses per second. After upper limb stimulation negative and positive potentials 11 and 13 ms later (N11 P13) are recorded over the neck (dorsal column nuclei). Subsequently wave N19 originating from the thalamus and P22 from the contralateral parietal sensory cortex, are recorded from surface electrodes 19 and 22 ms after the stimulus.

Increasing concentrations of nitrous oxide produce a progressive decrease in amplitude of the SEP in man (Jordan *et al* 1983). The effects of enflurane on SEP were reported to be quite variable by McPherson *et al* (1983). Studies of the effects of anaesthetics on SEP in man are too limited to draw conclusions about the role of this technique in measuring depth of anaesthesia.

Auditory evoked potentials (AEP)
The anatomical pathway of the auditory evoked potential has been particularly well studied. Following an acoustic stimulus there is sequential activation of the cochlear nuclei (low pons), superior olives (lower third to upper two-thirds pons), lateral lemnisci (mid- to upper pons), inferior colliculi (mid-brain), medial geniculate (thalamus) and radiation to the auditory cortex (Chiappa & Ropper 1982). We have already pointed out that there is a very high level of metabolic activity in this pathway and that anaesthetic agents such as thiopentone and ketamine cause a highly significant reduction in its metabolism. This being the case it might be expected that the AEP would be a sensitive indicator of depth of anaesthesia.

Recording the auditory evoked potential
The auditory stimulus is a series of clicks at a rate of 6 Hz presented binaurally using headphones. The e.e.g. is recorded at the mastoid, inion and vertex. The response over the 0–80 ms period following the stimulus was obtained by averaging 2048 consecutive click stimuli (Jones *et al* 1983). This produces a series of waves representing the transmission of the stimulus through the brain stem and up to the auditory cortex. Wave I (2 ms) is generated by the auditory nerve, wave II (3 ms) originates in the cochlar nuclei in man. Wave III (4 ms) originates in the superior olive. Wave IV (5 ms) is thought to originate in the lateral lemnisci and wave V (6 ms) in the inferior colliculus. Waves VI (7 ms) and VII (9 ms) are thought to arise in the medial geniculate body and auditory radiations. Waves Pa (25 ms) and Nb (40 ms) represent positive and negative waves reaching the auditory cortex.

Effects of general anaesthesia on AEP in man
Previous workers have commented on the effects of various anaesthetic drugs on the brain stem part of the AEP, i.e. only up to 10 ms after the stimulus (Stockard *et al* 1980). *Isoflurane* anaesthesia reduced the amplitude of wave V but had little effect on latency despite the absence of spontaneous e.e.g. activity. *Enflurane* produced a prolongation of interpeak latency but in contrast they found that clinically used doses of *halothane, pethidine, nitrous oxide, barbiturates* and *diazepam* did not alter latencies of brainstem EPs although the amplitude of the later peaks (up to peak V) were reduced. Despite these unpromising reports we decided to investigate the effects of a number of volatile and intravenous anaesthetics on the auditory EP in man.

This investigation was initiated for a number of reasons: (1) to measure graded effects of general anaesthetics on the c.n.s. as a guide in the administration of anaesthesia, (2) to study the effects of different general anaesthetics on particular pathways in the human brain, (3) as an index of awareness. So far we have no information on (3).

Effects of volatile anaesthetics

We studied patients before and after induction of general anaesthesia but prior to surgery. In contrast to Stockard et al (1980) we have shown that halothane, enflurane (Thornton et al 1983, 1984) and isoflurane (unpublished) in nitrous oxide all produced dose related changes both in the brainstem (up to peak V) and in the early cortical (Pa, Nb) waves in every subject studied (Fig. 8.3). Graded increases of anaesthetic concentration caused a graded slowing of transmission through the brainstem (III and V), and signals arriving at the primary auditory cortex were both delayed and reduced in amplitude. These effects could not be attributed either to changes in carbon dioxide tension or to changes in body temperature (Samra & Lilly 1983). We have previously presented arguments discounting the suggestion that nitrous oxide could affect middle ear pressure so as to produce changes in the AEP (Thornton et al 1984), and disproved the suggestion in a double-blind study (Navaratnarajah et al 1984).

The concentration ranges of volatile agents used in these studies were approximately equipotent based on their MAC values. The slopes of the lines relating anaesthetic concentration to its effect on the AEP were greater for halothane than for enflurane and isoflurane, which correlates with the greater potency of the former drug.

Effects of intravenous anaesthetics

The intravenous anaesthetic agents etomidate and althesin showed both differences and similarities in the effects on AEP compared with the effect of the volatile agents. The important difference was that these two intravenous agents had *no effect* on the brainstem AEP. In contrast the amplitude and latencies of the early cortical waves Pa and Nb were affected in just the *same way* as they were by the inhalational agents and there was a close linear relationship between graded increases in anaesthetic concentration and the change in the early cortical waves of the AEP (Navaratnarajh et al 1984, Heneghan et al 1984 (Fig. 8.3).

This finding is remarkable in that it is the first clear demonstration in man that different anaesthetics exert their effects on different parts of the central nervous system. The absence of effect on the brainstem portion of the auditory pathway suggests that other brainstem structures may be resistant to the effects of these drugs. The effect of thiopentone on the brainstem responses in man has not been well studied but it does affect the early cortical waves up to 2·5 minutes after a single induction dose (Pacelli et al 1983) whereas ketamine had a minor and much more transient effect. We have previously commented on the marked regional differences in the effects of ketamine on the brain in animals. It will be of great interest to look in man at the correlations between regional effects of anaesthetic agents using evoked potentials and PET techniques.

All the anaesthetics that we have studied so far produce a reduction in amplitude and increase in latency of waves corresponding to early cortical activation. This suggests an equivalence between loss of consciousness and these changes in the auditory evoked response. Other workers have shown that nitrous oxide in oxygen produces changes in the visual and somatasensory response but not the brainstem components of the AEP (Sebel et al 1984). Our studies of the effects of anaesthesia on the AEP have all been completed prior to surgery, so as yet we have no information regarding the influence of painful surgical procedures on the AEP in anaesthetised man. Nevertheless we have shown similar graded effects of a number of quite different general anaesthetics on the early cortical part of the AEP. It remains to be seen whether this can be used as an index of awareness.

CONCLUSIONS

Modern anaesthetic agents pose problems for the anaesthetist in regulating the depth of

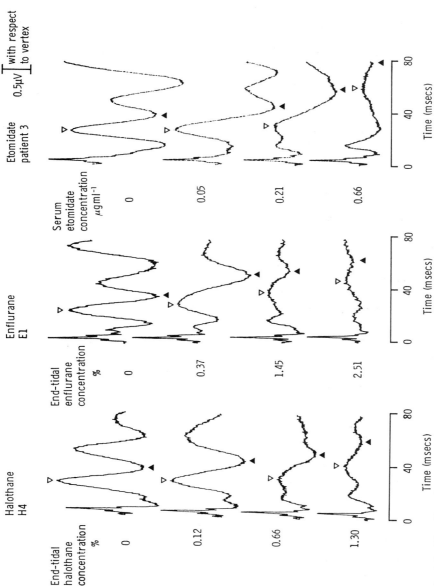

Fig. 8.3 The effect of anaesthetic agents on the auditory evoked potential (AEP) of three patients who received either halothane (*left*), enflurane (*middle*) and etomidate (*right*), with end-tidal or serum anaesthetic concentrations, as appropriate, listed to the left of each panel. △ = Pa, ▲ = Nb. In each case, there is a dose-related increase in latency and reduction in amplitude of both waves, and this occurs to a similar extent over approximately equipotent concentration ranges of anaesthetic.

anaesthesia. The state of general anaesthesia itself makes it extremely difficult to make a clinical assessment of the effect of central nervous system function. In this chapter we have reviewed the interrelationship between the metabolism, blood flow, specialised function and electrical activity of different regions of the brain. Although regional brain metabolism (CMRO$_2$ or CMRG$_L$) shows wide variation, almost certainly due to different specialised activity, there is very close coupling of all these variables in the normal brain. There may be dissociation of blood flow from metabolism in brain injury and with some anaesthetics, however, the association between function, metabolism and electrical activity maintains its close coupling. The electroencephalogram (e.e.g.) is likely to be the most useful monitoring device for measuring graded effects of general anaesthetics on the brain. The most appropriate form of e.e.g. signal processing remains to be established. Currently, the early cortical components of the auditory evoked potential seems to provide one of the most reliable techniques for demonstrating graded effects on brain function of a variety of inhalational or intravenous general anaesthetic drugs.

REFERENCES

Ackerman R H, Correia J A, Alpert N M et al 1981 Positron imaging in ischaemic stroke disease using compounds labelled with oxygen 15. Archives of Neurology 38: 537–543

Aminoff M J 1980 Electrodiagnosis in clinical neurology. Churchill Livingstone, New York, Edinburgh & London

Baron J C, Bousser M G, Comar D, Soussaline F, Castaigne P 1981 Noninvasive tomographic study of cerebral blood flow and oxygen metabolism in vivo. European Neurology 20: 273–284

Bart A J, Homi J, Linde H W 1971 Changes in power spectra of electroencephalograms during anesthesia with fluoroxene, methoxyflurane and ethrane. Anesthesia and Analgesia 50: 53–63

Bickford R G, Billinger T W, Flemming N I, Stewart L 1972 The compressed spectral array CSA — a pictorial e.e.g. Proceedings of the San Diego Biomedical Symposium 11: 365

Carlsson C, Hägerdal M, Siesjö 1976 The effect of nitrous oxide on oxygen consumption and blood flow in the cerebral cortex of the rat. Acta Anaesthesiologica Scandinavica 57: 7–17, 1

Chiappa K H, Ropper A H 1982 Evoked potentials in clinical medicine. New England Journal of Medicine 306: 1140–1150, 1205–1211

Clark D L, Rosner B S 1973 Neurophysiologic effects of general anesthetics. Anesthesiology 38: 564–582

Coleman R E, Drayer B P, Jaszczak R J 1982 Studying regional brain function: A challenge for SPECT. Journal of Nuclear Medicine 23: 266–270

Crosby G, Crane A M, Sokoloff L 1982 Local changes in cerebral glucose utilisation during ketamine anesthesia. Anesthesiology 56: 437–443

Crosby G, Sokoloff L 1983 Potential pitfalls in measuring regional cerebral glucose utilisation. Anesthesiology 58: 292–292

Fitzpatrick J H, Gilboe D D, Drewes L R, Betz A L 1976 Relationship of cerebral oxygen uptake to e.e.g. frequency in isolated canine brain. American Journal of Physiology 231: 1840–1846

Forster A, Juge O, Morel D 1982 Effects of midazolam on cerebral blood flow in human volunteers. Anesthesiology 56: 453–455

Gevins A S, Schaffer R E 1980 A critical review of electroencephalographic (e.e.g.) correlates of higher cortical functions. CRC Critical Reviews in Bioengineering 4: 113–164

Greenberg R P, Ward J D, Lutz H, Miller J D, Becker D P 1981 In: Grenvick A & Safar P (eds) Advanced monitoring of the brain in brain failure and resuscitation. Churchill Livingstone, Edinburgh, p 67–90

Grundy B L 1983 Intraoperative monitoring of sensory-evoked potentials. Anesthesiology 58: 72–87

Hawkins R, Hass W, Ransohoff J 1983 Potential pitfalls in measuring regional cerebral glucose utilisation. Anesthesiology 58: 290–291

Heneghan C P H, Thornton C, Navaranarajah M, Jones J G 1984 The effect of althesin on the auditory evoked response in man. British Journal of Anaesthesia 56: 792 P

Henriksen L, Paulson O B, Lassen N A 1981 Visual cortex activation recorded by dynamic emission computed tomography of inhaled xenon 133. European Journal of Nuclear Medicine 6: 487–489

Hudson R J, Stanski D R, Saidman L J, Meath E 1983 A model for studying depth of anesthesia and acute tolerance to thiopental. Anesthesiology 59: 301–308

Ingvar D H, Sjölund B, Ardo A 1976 Correlation between dominant e.e.g. frequency, cerebral oxygen uptake and blood flow. Electroencephalography and Clinical Neurophysiology 41: 268–276

Ingvar M, Abdul-Rahman A, Siesjö B K 1980 Local cerebral glucose consumption in the artificially ventilated rat: influence of nitrous oxide analgesia and of phenobarbital anesthesia. *Acta Physiologica Scandinavica* **109:** 177–185

Jones J G, Thornton C, Heneghan C P H, James M F K, Navaratnarajah M 1983 The use of the auditory evoked response to measure graded effects of general anaesthetics. In: Beneken J E W, Lavelle S M (eds) *Objective medical decision-making; systems approach in acute disease.* Springer-Verlag, Berlin, Heidelberg, p 57–64

Jordan W S, Grahn A R, Roberts L S, Wong K C, Dunn H 1983 Nitrous oxide suppression of spinal evoked e.e.g. potentials in surgical patients. *Anesthesia and Analgesia* **62:** 267

Lassen N A 1966 The luxury perfusion syndrome and its possible relation to acute metabolic acidosis localised within the brain. *Lancet* **ii:** 1113–1115

Lassen N A 1982 Measurement of cerebral blood flow and metabolism in man. *Clinical Science* **62:** 567–572

Lassen N A, Christensen M S 1976 Physiology of cerebral blood flow. *British Journal of Anaesthesia* **48:** 719–734

Lauritzen M, Henriksen L, Lassen N A 1981 Regional cerebral blood flow during rest and skilled hand movements by xenon-133 inhalation and emission computerised tomography. *Journal of Cerebral Blood Flow and Metabolism* **1:** 385–387

Mallett B L, Veal N 1965 Measurement of regional cerebral clearance rates in man using Xe-133 inhalation and extracranial recording. *Clinical Science* **29:** 179–191

Matsumiya N, Dohi S 1983 Effects of intravenous or subarachnoid morphine or cerebral and spinal cord hemodynamics and antagonism with naloxone in dogs. *Anesthesiology* **59:** 175–181

Maynard D E 1979 Development of the CFM: the cerebral function analysing monitor (CFAM). *Annales de l'Anesthesiologie Francaise* **20:** 253–255

McPherson R W, Mahla M, Traystman 1983 Effects of anaesthetic gases on somatosensory evoked potentials during narcotic anesthesia. *Anesthesiology* **59:** A319

Messick J M, Theye R A 1969 Effects of pentobarbital and meperidine on canine cerebral and total oxygen consumption in rats. *Canadian Anesthetists' Society Journal* **16:** 321–330

Michenfelder J D 1983 Brain hypoxia: current status of experimental and clinical therapy. *Seminars in Anaesthesia* **2:** 81–90

Michenfelder J D, Theye R A 1971 Effects of fentanyl, droperidol and innovar on canine cerebral metabolism and blood flow. *British Journal of Anaesthesia* **43:** 630–636

Michenfelder J D, Theye R A 1975 The influence of anaesthesia and ischaemia on the cerebral energy state. In: Whisnat J P, Sandok B A (eds) *Cerebral vascular diseases.* Grune & Stratton, New York, p 243–250

Navaratnarajah M, Thornton C, Heneghan C P H, Bateman P E, Jones J G 1983 The effect of etomidate on the auditory evoked response in man. *British Journal of Anaesthesia* **55:** 1157–1158A

Newberg L A, Michenfelder J D 1983 Cerebral protection by isoflurane during hypoxemia or ischaemia. *Anesthesiology* **59:** 29–35

Newberg L A, Milde J H, Michenfelder J D 1983 The cerebral metabolic effects of isoflurane at and above concentrations that suppress cortical electrical activity. *Anesthesiology* **59:** 23–28

Nugent M, Artru A A, Michenfelder J D 1980 Cerebral effects of midazolam and diazepam. *Anesthesiology* **53:** 5–8

Obrist W D 1963 The e.e.g. of healthy males. In: Birren J E, Butler R N, Greenhouse S W, Sokoloff L, Yarrow M R (eds) *Human aging: A biological and behavioural study (Public Health Service Publications 986).* Government Printing Office, Washington DC, p 77–93

Pacelli G D, Cullen B F, Starr A 1983 Effects of thiopental and ketamine on middle latency auditory evoked responses. *Anesthesiology* **59:** A366

Paulson O B, Sharborough F W 1974 Physiologic and pathophysiologic relationship between the e.e.g. and the regional cerebral blood flow. *Acta Neurologica Scandinavica* **50:** 194–229

Pellegrino D A, Miletch D J, Hoffman R F 1982 Regional CBF and $CMRO_2$, CMRgl and brain metabolite levels during N_2O or halothane: Comparison to the awake state. *Anesthesiology* **57:** A249

Phelps M E, Mazziotta J C, Huang S-C 1982 Study of cerebral function with positron computed tomography. *Journal of Cerebral Blood Flow and Metabolism* **2:** 113–162

Raichle M E, Grubb R L, Gado M H, Eichling J O, Ter-Pogossian M M 1976 Correlation between regional cerebral blood flow and oxidative metabolism. *Archives of Neurology* **33:** 523–526

Rampil I J, Sasse F J, Smith N T, Hoff B H, Flemming D C 1980 Spectral edge frequency — A new correlate of anesthetic depth. *Anesthesiology* **53:** 512

Rockoff M A, Naughton K U H, Shapiro H M et al 1980 Cerebral circulatory and metabolic responses to intravenously administered Lorazepam. *Anesthesiology* **53:** 215–218

Roy C S, Sherrington C S 1890 On the regulation of the blood supply of the brain. *Journal of Physiology (London)* **11:** 85–108

Sakabe T, Maekawa T, Fuji S, Ishikawa T, Tateishi A, Takeshita H 1983 Cerebral circulation and metabolism during enflurance anaesthesia in humans. *Anesthesiology* **59:** 532–536

Sakurado O, Kennedy C, Jehle J, Brown J D, Carbin G L, Sokoloff L 1978 Measurement of local cerebral blood flow with [¹⁴C] iodoantipyrine. *American Journal of Physiology* **234**: H59-H66

Samra S K, Lilly D J 1983 Effect of hypothermia on human brain-stem auditory evoked potentials. *Anesthesiology* **59**: A170

Scott J C, Stanski D R 1984 Comparative pharmacodynamics of fentanyl and alfentanil using the e.e.g. *Anesthesiology* **61**: A376

Sebel P S, Maynard D E, Major E, Frank M 1983 The cerebral function analysing monitor (cFAM) — A new microprocessor based devise for on-line e.e.g. and evoked potential analysis. *British Journal of Anaesthesia* **55**: 1265–1270

Sebel P S, Flynn P J, Ingram D, 1984 The effect of nitrous oxide (N₂O) on visual auditory and somatosensory evoked potentials. *British Journal of Anaesthesia* **56**: 1403–1407

Simons A J R, Pronk R A F 1983 E.e.g. analysis in monitoring anaesthesia. In: Beneken J E W, Lavelle S M (eds) *Objective medical decision-making: systems approach in acute disease.* Springer-Verlag, Berlin **22**: 65–67

Smith F W 1983 Nuclear magnetic resonance in the investigation of cerebral disorder. *Journal of Cerebral Blood Flow and Metabolism* **3**: 263–269

Sokol S 1980 Visual evoked responses. In: Aminoff M J (ed) *Electrodiagnosis in clinical neurology.* Churchill Livingstone, Edinburgh, p 348–369

Sokoloff L 1977 Relation between physiological function and energy metabolism in the central nervous system. *Journal of Neurochemistry* **29**: 13–26

Sokoloff L 1981 Localisation of functional activity in the central nervous system by measurement of glucose utilisation with radioactive deoxyglucose. *Journal of Cerebral Blood Flow and Metabolism* **1**: 7–36

Sokoloff L, Reivich M, Kennedy C et al 1977 The [¹⁴C] deoxyglucose method for the measurement of local cerebral glucose utilisation: theory, procedure and normal values in the conscious and anesthetised albino rat. *Journal of Neurochemistry* **28**: 897–916

Stanski D R, Hudson R J, Meathe E, Saidman L J 1982 Estimation of brain sensitivity to thiopental with the e.e.g. *Anesthesiology* **57**: A502

Stockard J J, Stockard J E, Sharbrough F W 1980 Brainstem auditory evoked potentials in neurology: methodology, interpretation, clinical application. In: Aminoff M J (ed) *Electrodiagnosis in clinical neurology.* Churchill Livingstone, Edinburgh, p 370–413

Symon L, Wang A D, Silva I E C-E, Gentili F 1984 Perioperative use of somatosensory evoked responses in aneurysm surgery. *Journal of Neurosurgery* **60**: 269–275

Taylor M J, Houston B D, Lowry N J 1983 Recovery of auditory brainstem responses after a severe hypoxic ischaemic insult. *New England Journal of Medicine* **309**: 1169–1170

Thornton C, Heneghan C P H, James M F M, Jones J G 1984 Effects of halothane or enflurane with controlled ventilation on auditory evoked potentials. *British Journal of Anaesthesia* **56**: 315–323

Thornton C, Catley D M, Jordan C, Lehane J R, Royston D, Jones J G 1983 Enflurane anaesthesia causes graded changes in the brainstem and early cortical auditory-evoked response in man. *British Journal of Anaesthesia* **56**: 479–486

Todd M M, Shapiro H M, Obrist W D 1981 Cerebral blood flow measurements in the critically ill patient. In: Grenvick A, Safar P (eds) *Brain failure and resuscitation.* Churchill Livingstone, Edinburgh, p 125–154

Todd M M, Drummond J C, Shapiro H M 1982 Comparative cerebrovascular and metabolic effects of halothane, enflurane and isoflurane. *Anesthesiology* **57**: A332

Uhl R R, Squires K C, Bruce D L, Staer A 1980 Effect of halothane anaesthesia on the human cortical visual evoked response. *Anesthesiology* **53**: 273–276

Wise R S J 1983 Regional cerebral blood flow and oxygen metabolism in acute stroke. In: Sarner M (ed) *Advanced medicine 18.* Pitman Medical, London, p 302–311

Williams D J M, Morgan R J M, Sebel P S, Maynard D E 1984 The effect of nitrous oxide on cerebral electrical activity. *Anaesthesia* **39**: 422–425

Wolff A P, Fowler J S 1983 Labelled compounds for positron emission tomography. In: Heiss W-D, Phelps M E (eds) *Positron emission tomography of the brain.* Springer-Verlag, Berlin, New York, p 52–64

Neurosurgical anaesthesia

In reviewing recent developments in neurosurgical anaesthesia attention will be directed to two areas in which the introduction of new drugs and recent research may make the anaesthetist reflect on current practice. The introduction of new inhalational anaesthetic drugs, particularly isoflurane, suggests that the place of volatile agents in intracranial surgery has to be reappraised. Secondly the continued use of the sitting position for posterior fossa surgery generates controversy as to how the risks of this position and the possibility of air embolism should be managed or indeed if they are so great that this position should not be used at all. The background and current research in relation to these two subjects will be assessed.

VOLATILE ANAESTHETIC AGENTS IN NEUROSURGICAL ANAESTHESIA

The brain is enclosed within a box, the skull, and an increase in the volume of the contents of the box will produce a rise in pressure inside it. In this simple concept is contained the essence of the problem that confronts the anaesthetist when he induces anaesthesia in a patient with raised intracranial pressure (ICP). In the normal patient dilation of the cerebral circulation produced by inhalational anaesthetic agents can be compensated for by the movement of c.s.f. through the foramen magnum into the spinal subarachnoid space and, over a longer period, by a decrease in c.s.f. production leading to a fall in volume. In the patient with a space-occupying lesion such compensatory mechanisms will already be in operation. This relationship between pressure and volume is usually represented graphically as in Fig. 9.1.

If an inhalational anaesthetic agent produces dilatation of the cerebral arterioles and increases cerebral blood flow (CBF) then in the normal patient this should do no harm, and might even be considered beneficial, but if the patient has a raised ICP and is on the steeper slope of the pressure-volume curve an increase in CBF will lead to an increase in ICP. The significance of such a rise in ICP will depend on both the magnitude and also on the level of the mean arterial pressure (MAP). The pressure driving blood through the cerebral circulation is the cerebral perfusion pressure (CPP). This will be the MAP less the pressures acting against it within the skull and these include the ICP and the venous pressure at the outlet of the skull. The latter will normally be approximately zero and may be ignored but the level of the ICP is vitally important. The balance of the pressures may be represented as follows:

$$CPP = MAP - ICP$$

The effect of volatile anaesthetic agents on this relationship should be kept in mind at all times during neurosurgical procedures.

When metabolism is increased in an area of the brain the cerebral metabolic requirement

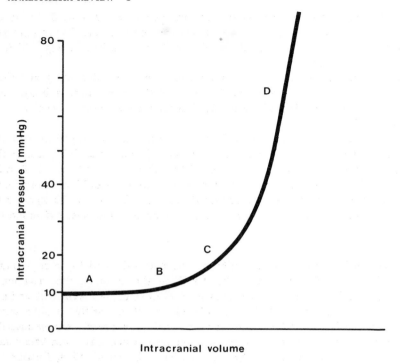

Fig. 9.1. The effect of increasing intracranial volume on intracranial pressure. In the initial part of the curve between A and B, compensation is taking place. In the steep part of the curve from C to D, compensatory mechanisms have ceased and small changes in volume lead to large changes in pressure.

for oxygen (CMR_{O_2}) will rise in that area. The cerebral arterioles will dilate, presumably due to the fall in pH of the extracellular fluid caused by the products of metabolism and this will lead to dilatation which will increase CBF. The increased CBF will lead to more oxygen and glucose being delivered to the active area and thus aerobic metabolism can continue. When metabolism is reduced the reverse process occurs and local CBF falls.

Halothane
Inhalational anaesthetic agents reduce cerebral metabolism and hence CMR_{O_2}. With halothane the normal relationship between CMR_{O_2} and CBF becomes uncoupled and instead of falling the CBF rises (Smith & Woollman 1972) because halothane dilates the cerebral arterioles. This is believed to be a direct action of the drug on the cerebral vessels and results in a dose-dependent decrease in cerebrovascular resistance as the concentration of halothane is increased from $0 \cdot 5\%$ to $4 \cdot 0\%$ (McDowall 1967). At concentrations of 1% and with normocapnia maintained throughout the study (Christensen *et el* 1967) halothane increased CBF by 27% and decreased CMR_{O_2} by 26% compared with awake values.

Concentrations of halothane up to $0 \cdot 5\%$ have been studied in monkeys (Morita *et al* 1977) and a fall in CMR_{O_2} was demonstrated with $0 \cdot 5\%$ halothane, but at this concentration the CBF also decreased by 17%. To explain this difference in the response of CBF to halothane administration the authors postulated that initially with low concentrations of halothane the normal physiological mechanisms continued to apply, and that as CMR_{O_2} decreased CBF also fell. However once the concentration of halothane increased above 0·5% the direct vasodilatation it produced on the cerebral arterioles predominated, leading to a progressive increase in CBF despite the continued reduction of $CMRo_2$, the latter falling to 50% at 2% halothane concentrations.

Autoregulation has also been shown to be impaired by halothane depending on the level of the administered concentration. It is still present at 0·5% halothane although slightly impaired but at concentrations of 1% and 2% it is completely absent (Miletich *et al* 1976, Morita *et al* 1977).

Halothane leads to an increase in CBF leading to a rise in ICP. In patients with space-occupying lesions this increase may be accentuated (Jennett *et al* 1972) and could be extremely hazardous for as well as increasing ICP halothane will also lower MAP and may also compromise CPP. It has been suggested that hyperventilation for 10 minutes prior to the administration of halothane can prevent such rises in ICP (Adams *et al* 1972) but it is not certain that this effect occurs when a space-occupying lesion is also present (Gordon 1970).

Enflurane

Cerebral metabolism decreases with enflurane anaesthesia the $CMRo_2$ in dogs falling by 35% at 1MAC (1·7% enflurane). This has been shown to be the maximum fall (Michenfelder & Cuccharia 1974). In man falls in $CMRo_2$ of 50% occur with an inspired concentration of 3% enflurane (Wollman *et al* 1969). The fall in CBF that would be expected to accompany this fall in metabolism does not occur in the presence of enflurane anaesthesia. In dogs the CBF has been shown to rise but to a lesser extent than with halothane, the maximum being between 12% and 20% (Michenfelder & Cucchiaria 1974, Takasaki 1974). In man measurements of CBF in normal subjects have shown that 2% enflurane has no effect (Rolly & Van Aken 1979) and although enflurane may cause a small degree of cerebral vasodilatation (McKay *et al* 1976) the decrease in MAP it also produces may help to prevent the consequent increase in CBF.

These results with CBF would suggest that enflurane should have little effect on ICP. In a recent investigation in 10 patients with cerebral tumours anaesthetised with a standard technique and controlled arterial Pco_2, no significant changes in ICP were demonstrated with the administration of 2% enflurane (Moss *et al* 1983). Previously rises in ICP of 9–15 mmHg had been demonstrated in patients presenting with a high ICP but not in those with a near normal ICP, given 1–2% enflurane (Zattoni *et al* 1974).

Two other factors are important in considering the use of enflurane in neurosurgical anaesthesia and these include its action on MAP and hence CPP and also its recognised ability to produce epileptiform activity on the e.e.g. In Moss's study previously referred to, the CPP fell to low levels in four of the ten subjects and the administration of 2% enflurane had to be discontinued before the specified 15 minute period of the investigation had been reached. In two other patients it was below 40 mmHg at the end of this period.

With higher concentrations of enflurane high amplitude spikes or spike and wave complexes, or both, may appear on the e.e.g.; these are indicative of epileptic activity and when they are present CBF and ICP will be greatly increased as will $CMRo_2$. Although hypocarbia has been shown to lower the threshold for this activity, it is unlikely to occur if the concentrations of enflurane is less than 2·5% (Neigh *et al* 1971).

Isoflurane

Isoflurane also reduced cerebral metabolism and it has been shown in the dog that $CMRo_2$

fell by 23% at 1 MAC (1·3%) and by 30% at 2 MAC (Cucchiara *et al* 1974). Thus the reduction in metabolism is non-linear being greater initially.

Changes in CBF with isoflurane have been assessed in man using volunteers who were paralysed with d-tubocurarine and had their MAP maintained at normal levels by infusion of phenylephrine. No signifcant change in CBF from awake values was demonstrated at isoflurane concentrations of 0·6% or 1·1%, while a further increase to 1·6% led to a doubling of CBF. These changes were considerably less than those seen with halothane whereas enflurane produced intermediate results (Murphy *et al* 1974). In dogs Cucchiara *et al* (1974) obtained similar results there being no significant change in CBF at 1 MAC but a 60% increase at 1·7 MAC. In addition these investigators found evidence of continuing autoregulation at 1 MAC isoflurane anaesthesia and the cerebral circulation remained responsive to the effects of changes in arterial $P\text{CO}_2$.

As CBF rises with higher concentrations of isoflurane it is to be expected that ICP will also rise, particularly in patients with a space-occupying lesion. Adams *et al* (1981) have demonstrated increases in ICP in 5 normocapnic patients but this can be abolished by decreasing the Pa_{CO_2}. When a further series of 15 patients with raised ICP were ventilated and the Pa_{CO_2} lowered before isoflurane was administered a fall in ICP occurred. In dogs anaesthetised with isoflurane this ability of hypocapnia to prevent increases in ICP has been confirmed (Schettini & Mahig 1973) and even at normocarbia the same authors have shown a rise of only 25% in the ICP with isoflurane as compared with 100% at similar levels of enflurane and halothane anaesthesia.

Although isoflurane, in common with halothane and enflurane produces a dose related fall in MAP when concentrations up to 2 MAC are administered to normocapnic volunteers, the mechanism by which this occurs with isoflurane differs from that with the other two drugs. With isoflurane cardiac output is maintained and peripheral resistance falls. The stimulation provided by surgery tends to reduce this fall in MAP at lighter levels of isoflurane anaesthesia in the operating theatre (Eger 1981). These changes in MAP will effect CPP, but because the ICP is more stable with isoflurane they should be easier to assess with this agent than with halothane or enflurane, provided MAP is carefully monitored. Advantage has been taken of this fall in blood pressure in cerebral aneurysm surgery where isoflurane has been used successfully as the hypotensive agent (Lam & Gelb 1982).

Adrenaline containing solutions are often used for infiltration in neurosurgical operations to reduce bleeding, for example when scalp flaps are raised or in the trans-sphenoidal approach to the pituitary. Isoflurane has been shown to have a greater margin of safety than halothane in relation to the incidence of cardiac dysrhythmias (Johnson *et al* 1976). Isoflurane is an isomer of enflurane but appears to show no evidence of convulsive activity even with hypocapnia or deep levels of anaesthesia (Stockard & Bickford 1975).

Summary

Although general anaesthesia can be administered to neurosurgical patients using a total intravenous technique, many anaesthetists find that inhalational agents are still preferable for smooth anaesthesia. Amongst the volatile anaesthetics halothane concentrations above 0·5% appear to have clear disadvantages in patients with raised ICP while enflurane concentrations below 2% seem to be acceptable provided that care is taken to avoid excessive falls in MAP that may compromise CPP. Isoflurane at the moment appears to be potentially the most suitable volatile agent for neurosurgical anaesthesia, but the high commercial price may limit its use unless more economical methods of administration are employed.

PROBLEMS WITH THE SITTING POSITION FOR POSTERIOR FOSSA SURGERY

Correct positioning of patients on the operating table is particularly important in neuro-surgical procedures. Obstruction of the venous outflow from the skull will cause a high venous pressure and increased intraoperative haemorrhage. Elevating the head will reduce the ICP by decreasing the hydrostatic pressure. The logical extension of this principle is to have the patient in the sitting position: this posture is frequently used for posterior fossa exploration (it may also be used for cervical laminectomies). Additional advantages are the good access and view afforded to the surgeon particularly when operating on midline or cerebello-pontine angle lesions and when visualisation of the fourth ventricle is necessary. The fall in arterial pressure that occurs can also be beneficial in reducing haemorrhage. These advantages must be set against the additional risks of excessive arterial hypotension and air embolism that can occur with the patient in the sitting position.

Opinion is sharply divided as to whether the advantages outweigh the disadvantages (Walters & Torrens 1982, Campkin 1982) but in a survey of neurosurgical centres in the United Kingdom published in 1978 it was shown that the sitting position was used routinely for infratentorial surgery in just over half the units (Campkin 1978). The decision must rest on the choice of the surgeon, the experience of the anaesthetist and the suitability of the patient but if the sitting position is chosen the anaesthetist carries a heavy responsibility in preventing an increase in morbidity or mortality.

Arterial hypotension

Moving an anaesthetised patient into the sitting position leads to pooling of blood in the dependant parts of the body which in turn reduces venous return, cardiac output and hence arterial pressure: these effects are further accentuated by positive pressure ventilation. A fall of 20–30 mmHg in MAP may be expected but any decrease more than this must be avoided as the resultant fall in CPP may be detrimental. In this respect it must be borne in mind that when the patient is sitting the MAP at the level of the head will be approximately 10–15 mmHg lower than that measured at the arm.

Patients with poor cardiac reserve should be anaesthetised in the horizontal position. Patients may be hypovolaemic due to inadequate fluid intake because of their poor physical state or due to restriction of intravenous fluid replacement in order to reduce ICP. It may be necessary to correct possible hypovolaemia prior to inducing anaesthesia. Arterial pressure must be carefully monitored during elevation of the patient to the sitting position and direct intra-arterial monitoring of blood pressure is mandatory. Placing the transducer at head level to obtain a zero base line removes the influence of hydrostatic pressure and allows a more realistic estimate of CPP.

Patients should be slowly positioned in the sitting posture with the arterial pressure monitored continuously. It is preferable to keep the legs in the near horizontal position rather than to employ the full chair position. Atropine is best avoided for although it may help to maintain the blood pressure by blocking vagal activity it may mask the effects of surgical stimulation of vital brain stem functions. Compressive bandages applied from the ankle to the groin can also be used to reduce venous pooling.

Air embolism

Pathophysiology

When posterior fossa surgery is performed in the sitting position air embolism is likely to occur as there is a large hydrostatic pressure gradient between the occiput and the heart and because veins within the skull and in the dura and the venous sinuses tend to remain open if they are incised. The result is that air is intrained into the circulation and passes through the heart to the pulmonary circulation, lodging in the arterioles. Intense pulmonary vasoconstriction results leading to ventilation-perfusion mismatch, a fall in CO_2 excretion and a decrease in oxygen uptake. Intestitial pulmonary oedema developes while cardiac output is reduced following the increase in pulmonary vascular resistance (Adornato et al 1978).

Incidence

The incidence of this complication during posterior fossa surgery varies and is influenced by the skill of the surgeon and precautions taken to prevent air entry by increasing the venous pressure. Michenfelder et al (1972) suggested that the incidence may be as high as 93%. Early detection is essential as a small amount of air may cause no harm but larger amounts can lead to a fatal outcome.

Monitoring methods

The entry of air into the circulation may be detected either by monitoring for the physical presence of air in the blood or by noting the onset of the pathological changes it produces. The methods available and their relative advantages will be discussed in detail.

Doppler ultrasonic monitor. The Doppler ultrasonic probe is the most sensitive monitor currently available for the detection of air embolism (Michenfelder et al 1972). It relies on the reflection of an ultrasonic beam from the interface between blood and air. Correct positioning of a probe is important and it should be placed over the right atrium close to the tricuspid valve, that is to the right of the sternum in the third to the sixth intercostal space. The correct position can be can be confirmed, for if a right atrial line is in situ an injection of 5 ml of saline will result in a change in the Doppler signal (Tinker et al 1975). In animal studies it has been shown that less than 1 ml of air can be detected by a correctly positioned probe.

The Doppler probe should be part of the standard monitoring especially where there is any likelihood of air embolism. It is non-invasive, relatively inexpensive but is not a quantitative indicator of air entry. However, it is not infallible and there have been instances where there were no changes in the Doppler signal when air was shown to be in the circulation. On the other hand the technique may be too sensitive and there may be frequent interruptions of the operation when only small amounts of air have entered the circulation. Problems can occur if the probe is not secured, in fat patients or instances when there is mediastinal shift due to lung pathology. A directional Doppler probe which can be inserted into the oesophagus has recently been described and would overcome these problems (Martin & Colley 1983). The diathermy causes severe interference and some form of suppression is necessary but this means that air entry may be missed when the diathermy is being used.

Capnograph. With air embolism, air trapping occurs in the pulmonary circulation and there is a fall in the CO_2 reaching the pulmonary capillaries with a corresponding drop in the alveolar and end tidal CO_2 ($ETCO_2\%$). The fall in $ETCO_2\%$ is related to the degree of air embolism and therefore the use of a capnograph is an additional non-invasive method of monitoring (Bethune & Bechner 1968). The capnograph is not as sensitive as the Doppler probe. Calibration is not essential as only qualitative changes in $ETCO_2\%$ are required.

Circulatory collapse due to manipulations in the posterior fossa involving the medulla may also cause a sudden fall in $ETco_2\%$. $ETco_2\%$ and arterial blood pressure fall simultaneously during manipulation in the medulla whereas with air embolism the $ETco_2\%$ usually falls first. Continuous recording of arterial pressure and $ETco_2\%$ is advantageous.

Central venous catheterisation. The routine use of a central venous catheter for patients in the sitting position has achieved wide acceptance following the report of its value in aspirating air from the right side of the heart when air embolism had occurred (Michenfelder et al 1969) but an increase in right atrial pressure is of limited diagnostic value as it is a late sign of the complication. Jackson (1978) has recently questioned the need for central venous catheterisation in view of the possible hazards. Mogos et al (1982) reviewed 200 cases and could find no advantage in right atrial catheterisation and reported 3 instances of pneumothorax. Munson (1979) and Albin et al (1979) do not endorse this view and recently Merrill et al (1982) reported the case where air was clearly seen entering the circulation and although the surgeon was unable to find the offending open vein, over 300 ml of air was aspirated through the central line.

The correct positioning of the catheter tip is essential if air is to be successfully aspirated. Bunegin et al (1981) have shown that the maximum recovery of air is achieved when the catheter tip is placed approximately 3 cm above the junction of the superior vena cava and the right atrium and that the catheter should preferably be multiorificed. Campkin (1982) recommended routine chest X-ray but Michenfelder (1981) felt that this was too imprecise and recommended more elegant methods of placement. (See also Martin 1970.)

The use of the central line may be used in the control of preoperative fluid management as well as during operation. The measurement of central venous pressure helps to assess blood loss and the success of measures taken to raise the venous pressure.

Pulmonary artery pressure (PAP). The use of a Swan-Ganz catheter to measure the PAP and diagnose air embolism was first described by Munson et al (1975). When air enters the pulmonary circulation the PAP increases proportionally to the amount of air entering, thus quantifying the severity of the embolism. Good correlation has been demonstrated between changes in the $ETco_2\%$ and PAP with the latter being perhaps slightly more sensitive but the Swan-Ganz catheter was not very successful for the recovery of air from the circulation (Bedford et al 1981).

Two advantages exist for PAP monitoring as compared with other methods of air embolism detection. Firstly as described in relation to the capnograph, PAP measurement will enable circulatory collapse to be differentiated from air embolism and secondly patients at risk from paradoxical (systemic) embolism can be identified. In 20–30% of the general population the foramen ovale will allow the passage of a probe; thus the potential exists for air to pass from the right to the left artrium if the right atrial pressure is higher than the left and for dangerous systemic air embolism to occur. If this happens the outcome is likely to be fatal as cases reported in the literature testify (Buckland & Manners 1976, Gronert et al 1979). With a Swan-Ganz catheter right atrial pressure and left atrial pressure (as pulmonary capillary wedge pressure) can be measured with the patient in the sitting position and the risk of this complication anticipated. In their prospective investigation of 100 patients Bedford and his colleagues found 29 in whom the right atrial pressure exceeded pulmonary artery wedge pressure (Bedford et al 1981).

Heart sounds. When air enters the heart, the heart sounds change becoming metallic, resonant and then drum like in character. There may be the sudden onset of a systolic murmur before progressing to the characteristic grinding mill-wheel murmur. These changes can be monitored precordially or more conveniently with an intraoesophageal stethoscope. Although the method is simple and cheap it does not detect changes produced by small amounts of air. Buckland & Manners (1976) in a comparative study were only able to detect air embolism in 1 patient using the stethoscope whereas the Doppler probe detected this in 10 patients.

Blood pressure and e.c.g. Monitoring of both intra-arterial pressure and e.c.g. are standard practice in posterior fossa surgery. Arterial hypotension occurs when the cardiac output falls following the reduction in the output of the right ventricle due to rising pulmonary vascular resistance. In late stages air embolism causes mechanical embarrassment to ventricular function. The arrhythmias and right ventricular strain may confirm the presence of air embolism but these changes are invariably late.

Prevention

With the patient in the sitting position and where there is an open vein at the site of operation in the posterior fossa there will be considerable negative pressure tending to draw air into the circulation, especially if the pressure in the right atrium is zero. If steps are taken to raise the venous pressure it is possible to reduce the rate of inflow of air and if the venous pressure were raised to the pressure of the incision the open vein would bleed and the risk of air embolism would be eliminated. Attention should be paid to rehydrating patients prior to anaesthesia using colloid as well as crystalloid solutions to ensure that venous pressure is maintained.

Positive end expiratory pressure (PEEP) is frequently advocated for these patients. Levels of up to 10 cmH$_2$O are used leading to a rise in the venous pressure. Unfortunately PEEP may lead to a fall in cardiac output.

The antigravity g-suit as used by fighter pilots can be fitted to the lower half of the anaesthetised patient to apply pressure to the veins and thus raise venous pressure. The g-suit can be rapidly inflated to a pressure of 40–60 mmHg and if applied firmly to the abdomen venous pressure will immediately rise (Logue & Hewer 1962).

By the careful use of all three methods together marked rises in venous pressure can be achieved to limit the risks of air embolism.

Treatment

As soon as air embolism is detected the surgeon must be alerted to pack the wound with wet swabs, thus preventing further air entering the circulation. The anaesthetist should manually compress both internal jugular veins in the neck to raise the venous pressure in the skull. This will stop air entering the circulation and should produce venous bleeding which will help the surgeon to identify the open vein. Nitrous oxide must be discontinued for this gas diffuses into the air. Attempts to recover air through a central venous catheter should be instituted. By these measures the further entry of air should be prevented, and the situation stabilised. If deterioration continues and, in particular, if the arterial blood pressure falls or arrhythmias develop, the patient must be lowered to a horizontal position.

Once the acute episode has been controlled the monitoring equipment should be carefully watched to ensure that the open vein or veins have in fact been closed. If all appears stable it is useful to obtain some indication as to whether air remains in the circulation or if it has been absorbed. If the ET co$_2$% again falls when nitrous oxide is reintroduced, it can be assumed that significant amounts of air remain in the pulmonary circulation (Shapiro *et al* 1982).

In considering the use of nitrous oxide for posterior fossa surgery another complication of its use has been pointed out in the recent literature. During surgery in the seated position c.s.f. leaks out of the subarachnoid space and the cerebral hemispheres tend to collapse. Air enters through the craniotomy and passes up to accumulate over the cortex. Once the skull is closed, c.s.f. accumulates more rapidly than air is absorbed, and if nitrous oxide is still being administered, this will diffuse into the air and a tension pneumocephalus develops (Artru 1982, MacGillivray 1982). If the development of this situation is not recognised cardiac arrest can ensue (Thiagarajah *et al* 1982). Diagnosis can be rapidly made with a plain skull X-ray and the air can be released through a simple twist drill burr hole.

Summary

Although neither the Doppler probe nor the capnograph are infallible monitors for air embolism they are suitable non-invasive devices for routine use. Central venous catheterisation may present hazards, is troublesome to achieve proper placement, but has distinct advantages in treatment. Swan-Ganz catheterisation is unlikely to find wide acceptance for routine monitoring but will no doubt have its advocates. More sophisticated methods may become available including the use of transoesophageal echocardiography (Furuya *et al* 1983). Prevention of air embolism might include abandoning the sitting posture for posterior fossa surgery.

REFERENCES

Adams R W, Cuccharia R F, Gronert G A, Messick J M Jr, Michenfelder J D 1981 Isoflurane and the cerebrospinal fluid pressure in neurosurgical patients. *Anesthesiology* 54: 97–99

Adams R W, Gronert G A, Sundt T M, Michenfelder J D 1972 Halothane, hypocapnia and cerebrospinal fluid pressure in neurosurgery. *Anesthesiology* 37: 510–517

Adornato D C, Gildenberg P L, Ferrario C M, Smart J, Frost E A M 1978 Pathophysiology of intravenous air embolism in dogs. *Anesthesiology* 49: 120–127

Albin M S, Chang J L, Babinski M, Waterman P, Maivald P, Paulter S 1979 Intracardiac catheters in neurosurgical anesthesia (letter). *Anesthesiology* 50: 67–69

Artru A A 1982 Nitrous oxide plays a direct role in the development of tension pneumocephalus intraoperatively. *Anesthesiology* 57: 59–61

Bedford R F, Marshall W K, Butler A, Welsh J E 1981 Cardiac catheters for diagnosis and treatment of venous air embolism. *Journal of Neurosurgery* 55: 610–614

Bethune R W M, Brechner V L 1968 Detection of venous air embolism by carbon dioxide monitoring. *Anesthesiology* 29: 179

Buckland R W, Manners J M 1976 Venous air embolism during neurosurgery. *Anaesthesia* 31: 633–643

Bunegin L, Albin M S, Helsel P E, Hoffman A, Hung T-K 1981 Positioning the right atrial catheter. *Anesthesiology* 55: 343–348

Campkin T V 1978 Posture and anaesthetic techniques during posterior fossa and cervical surgery. Paper read at the Neurosurgical Anaesthetist's Travelling Club, Wakefield

Campkin T V 1982 Air embolism; placement of central venous catheters. *Anesthesiology* 56: 406–407

Campkin T V 1982 Posterior fossa surgery (letter). *British Journal of Anaesthesia* 54: 574

Christensen M S, Hoedt-Rasmussen K, Lassen N A 1967 Cerebral vasodilatation by halothane anaesthesia in man and its potentiation by hypotension and hypercapnia. *British Journal of Anaesthesia* 39: 927–934

Cuccharia R F, Theye R A, Michenfelder J D 1974 The effects of isoflurane on canine cerebral metabolism and blood flow. *Anesthesiology* 40: 571–574

Eger E 1981 Isoflurane: A review. *Anesthesiology* 55: 559–576

Furuya H, Suzuki T, Okumura F, Kishi Y, Uefuji T 1983 Detection of air ambolism by transesophageal echocardiography. *Anesthesiology* 58: 124–129

Gordon E 1970 The action of drugs on the intracranial contents. In: Boulton T B, Bryce-Smith R, Sykes M K, Gillett G B, Revell A L (eds) *Progress in anaesthesiology.* Excerpta Medica, Amsterdam, p 60

Gronert G A, Messick J M Jr, Cuccharia R F, Michenfelder J D 1979 Paradoxical air embolism from a patent foramen ovale. *Anesthesiology* 50: 548–549

Jackson P L 1978 Intracardiac catheters unnecessary in neurosurgical anesthesia (letter). *Anesthesiology* 48: 154

Jennett W B, Barker J, Fitch W, McDowall D G 1969 Effect of anaesthesia on intracranial pressure in patients with space-occupying lesions. *Lancet* i: 61–64

Johnston R R, Eger E, Wilson C 1976 A comparative interaction of epinphrine with enflurane, isoflurane and halothane in man. *Anesthesia and Analgesia* **55**: 709–712

Lam A M, Gelb A W 1982 Cardiovascular effects and gas exchange during isoflurane-induced hypotension for cerebral aneurysm surgery. *Anesthesia and Analgesia* **61**: 197

Logue V, Hewer A J H 1962 Methods of increasing safety of neuroanaesthesia in the sitting position. *Anaesthesia* **17**: 476–481

McDowall D G 1976 The effects of clinical concentrations of halothane on the blood flow and oxygen uptake of the cerebral cortex. *British Journal of Anaesthesia* **39**: 186–196

MacGillivray R G 1982 Pneumocephalus as a complication of posterior fossa surgery in the sitting position. *Anaesthesia* **37**: 722–725

McKay R D, Sundt T M, Michenfelder J D, Gronert G A, Messick J M, Sharbrough F W, Piepgras D G 1976 Internal carotid artery stump pressure and cerebral blood flow during endarterectomy: modification by halothane, enflurane and Innovar. *Anesthesiology* **45**: 390–399

Martin J T 1970 Neuroanesthesia adjuncts for patients in the sitting position: III Intravascular electrocardiography. *Anesthesiology* **49**: 793–808

Martin R W, Colley P S 1983 Evaluation of transesophageal Doppler detection of air embolism in dogs. *Anesthesiology* **58**: 117–123

Merrill D G, Samuels S I, Silverberg G D 1982 Venous air embolism of uncertain etiology. *Anesthesia and Analgesia* **61**: 65–66

Michenfelder J D, Martin J T, Altenburg B M, Rehder K 1969 Air embolism during neurosurgery: an evaluation of right-atrial catheters for diagnosis and treatment. *Journal of the American Medical Association* **208**: 1353–1358

Michenfelder J D, Miller R H, Gronert G A 1972 Evaluation of an ultrasonic device (Doppler) for the diagnosis of venous air embolism. *Anesthesiology* **36**: 164–167

Michenfelder J D, Cucharia R F 1974 Canine cerebral oxygen consumption during enflurane anesthesia and its modification during induced seizures. *Anesthesiology* **40**: 575–580

Michenfelder J D 1981 Central venous catheters in the management of air embolism: Whether as well as where. *Anesthesiology* **55**: 339–341

Miletich D J, Ivankovich A D, Albrecht R F, Reimann C R, Rosenberg R, McKissic E D 1976 Absence of autoregulation of cerebral blood flow during halothane and enflurane anesthesia. *Anesthesia and Analgesia* **55**: 100–107

Mogos B, Phillips P, Apfelbaum R, Duncalf D 1982 Is right atrial catheterisation always indicated for anesthesia in the sitting position? *Anesthesia and Analgesia* **61**: 205

Morita H, Nemoto E M, Bleyaert A L, Stezoski S W 1977 Brain blood flow, autoregulation and metabolism during halothane anesthesia in monkeys. *American Journal of Physiology* **233**: H670–674

Moss E, Dearden N M, McDowall D G 1983 Effects of 2% enflurane on intracranial pressure and cerebral perfusion pressure. *British Journal of Anaesthesia* **55**: 1083–1087

Munson E S, Paul W L, Perry J C, De Padua C B, Rhoton A L 1975 Early detection of venous air embolism using a Swan-Ganz catheter. *Anesthesiology* **42**: 223–226

Munson E S 1979 Intracardiac catheters in neurosurgical anesthesia (letter). *Anesthesiology* **50**: 67

Murphy F L Jr, Kennell E M, Johnstone R E 1974 The effects of enflurane, isoflurane, and halothane on cerebral blood flow and metabolism in man. Abstracts of Scientific Papers, Annual Meeting of the American Society of Anesthesiologists, p 61–62

Neigh J L, Garman J K, Harp J R 1971 The electroencephalographic pattern during anesthesia with Ethrane: effects of depth of anesthesia, Pa_{CO_2} and nitrous oxide. *Anesthesiology* **35**: 482–487

Rolly G, Van Aken J 1979 Influence of enflurane cerebral blood flow in man. *Acta Anaesthesiologica Scandanavica* **71 (Suppl)**: 59–63

Schettini A, Mahig J 1973 Comparative intracranial dynamic responses in dogs to three halogenated anesthetics. Abstracts of the Scientific Papers, Annual Meeting of the American Society of Anesthesiologists, p 123–124

Shapiro H M, Yoachim J, Marshall L F 1982 Nitrous oxide challenge for the detection of residual intravascular gas following venous air embolism. *Anesthesia and Analgesia* **61**: 304–306

Smith A L, Wollman H 1972 Cerebral blood flow and metabolism. Effects of anesthetic drugs and techniques. *Anesthesiology* **36**: 378–400

Stockard J, Bickford R 1975 The neurophysiology of anaesthesia. In: Gordon E (ed) *A basis and practice of neuroanaesthesia.* Excerpta Medica, Amsterdam, p 3–46

Takasaki M 1974 The effects of enflurane on canine cerebral oxygen consumption and blood flow. *Japanese Journal of Anesthesiology* **23**: 806–808

Thiagarajah S, Frost E A M, Singh T, Shulman K 1982 Cardiac arrest associated with tension pneumocephalus. *Anesthesiology* **56**: 73–75

Tinker J H, Gronert G A, Messick J M Jr, Michenfelder J D 1975 Detection of air embolism, a test for positioning of right atrial catheter and Doppler probe. *Anesthesiology* **43**: 104–105

Walters F, Torrens M J 1982 Posterior fossa surgery (letter). *British Journal of Anaesthesia* **54**: 363

Wollman H, Smith A L, Hoffman J C 1969 Cerebral blood flow and oxygen consumption during electroencephalographic seizure patterns induced by anesthesia with Ethrane. *Federal Proceedings* **28:** 356–358

Zattoni J, Siani C, Rivano C 1974 Effects of enflurane on intracranial pressure. In: Lawin P, Beer R (eds) Ethrane: proceedings of the first European symposium on modern anaesthetic agents, Springer-Verlag, Berlin, p 272

Appraisal of inhalational anaesthetic agents

This chapter describes the virtues of inhalational anaesthesia and the criteria for appraisal of inhalational anaesthetic agents. This is followed by brief notes on agents in current use and the possibility of improving on their characteristics.

Research directed towards the discovery and evaluation of new agents continues to be carried out. The major advantage of inhalational anaesthesia is that the level of control can be readily adjusted by the anaesthetist. When the patient is breathing spontaneously there is a further safeguard in that, with increasing depth of anaesthesia there is respiratory depression which reduces the uptake of agents. Although this feedback mechanism is absent during controlled ventilation, uptake and elimination and consequently partial pressure of the agent at the site of action can still be influenced by the anaesthetist. This includes both the uptake and elimination of the gaseous agent. This situation is preferable to that obtained following intravenous anaesthesia where overdosage or adverse effects cannot readily be terminated: the pattern of elimination is by redistribution metabolism or even excretion.

Additional desirable properties of inhalational anaesthetics are that allergic reactions are virtually unknown and that individual variations in response to such agents is notably less than with intravenous agents. Firm data on this last point is not readily available but an indication may be obtained on analysing information on nine inhalational agents. The difference between MAC, which is an anaesthetising dose 50 (AD_{50}) and the AD_{95} was only 21% for these agents (De Jong & Eger 1975). When this is compared with information collected by Dundee *et al* (1982) on the 'induction' dose of thiopentone, it can be calculated that the comparable range of variation for thiopentone (i.e. twice the standard deviation of the mean dose) was 74%.

A further feature of inhalational agents is that many of their important properties as anaesthetic agents can be accurately predicted from knowledge of their physical properties.

These attributes and the desirable features of an inhalational agent are discussed below.

Non-flammability

It is generally agreed that modern anaesthetic agents must be non-flammable in the range of concentrations and gas mixtures (nitrous oxide and oxygen) used in clinical practice. It was the search for a non-flammable agent which lead finally to the introduction of halothane in 1956. Non-flammability in modern anaesthetics is achieved by halogenation, and in particular by the introduction of fluorine into the molecule. In general this does not greatly change flammability limits but does enormously increase the energy required for ignition and it is this factor which renders these agents non-flammable in clinical use (Larsen 1972). A static spark released within an anaesthetic machine has an energy of a few hundred millijoules whereas to ignite these heavily halogenated compounds, sparks in the range of 10–30 joules are required. Thus the halothane/nitrous oxide/oxygen mixture within the vapourising chamber of a plenum type vaporiser (about 33% halothane at 20°C) is well within the flammable range but could only be ignited by a powerful energy source which could not be present during normal use (Larsen 1972).

Nitrous oxide increases the flammability of organic vapours because it is an endothermic compound whose decomposition results in the evolution of heat together with the production of an oxygen rich (33%) gas mixture. Thus, although the lowest concentration of halothane in oxygen found to be ignitable is around 14%, it has been found that in pure nitrous oxide 2% of halothane is ignitable by an ignition energy as low as 0·3 joules (Brown & Morris 1966).

Compounds showing promise as anaesthetic agents, such as hexafluorobenzene (Garmer & Leigh 1967) have been abandoned because of flammibility. Hexafluorobenzene burns in nitrous oxide at 4%. This should be compared with trichlorethylene, which has had extensive and successful clinical use as a 'non-flammable' agent although it burns in nitrous oxide at 5%. Potential agents of 'borderline' flammability of this order, if they were of sufficient merit, might be rendered non-flammable for clinical purposes by use with quenching gases such as helium or argon. These gases have been shown to reduce the flammability of cyclopropane-oxygen mixtures (Thomas & Jones 1941, Hingson *et al* 1958, Flynn & Young 1966).

Another approach to the problem of flammability which has been suggested is to study compounds of such high boiling point that the concentration at SVP at room temperature is below or close to the level of flammability. Such compounds would require to have very high potency (low MAC) since only low concentrations would be available in clinical practice. Methoxyflurane is an agent in this class. Unfortunately, such a high potency implies slow induction and recovery (eduction)*. This is further discussed below.

Optimum solubility

The importance of agent solubility in regulating the kinetics of inhalation anaesthesia are now well understood. Anaesthetic agents are about twice as soluble in blood as in water (nitrous oxide and diethyl ether are exceptions). The lower the solubility of the agent in blood the less the fall in pulmonary alveolar partial pressure of the agent during the process of induction while the anaesthetising partial pressure of the agent is reached quicker at the site of action in the central nervous system. Low blood solubility is therefore a highly desirable attribute in an inhalational agent.

The potency of the agent, measured by MAC, correlates quite closely with the lipid solubility of the agent. The greater the oil/gas partition coefficient the lower the MAC value. In some discussions of this subject it is suggested that an ideal agent would have low blood solubility and high lipid solubility. Unfortunately it does not appear that oil and water solubility can be discussed as wholly separate entities for anaesthetic agents in current use. This is shown in Fig. 10.1 in which oil solubility is plotted against blood solubility. It can be seen that, in general terms, if an agent is very soluble in blood it is also very soluble in oil and

---

* A case can be made for the use of the word 'eduction' as the inverse of 'induction' in discussions of this nature. It is the obvious antonym, its meaning is clear and it is to be found even in small dictionaries. It is surely preferable to 'recovery' or 'elimination' which are the most commonly used terms in this context although they are not precisely opposite in meaning to induction.

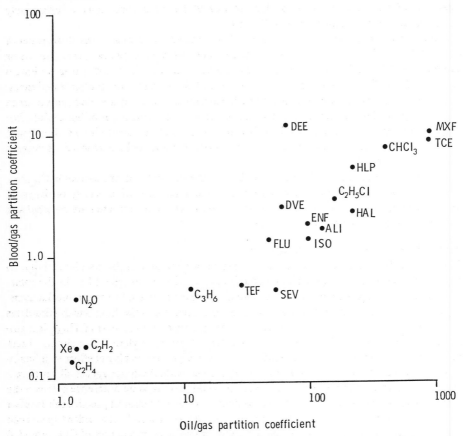

Fig. 10.1 Relationship between oil and blood solubilities for a number of anaesthetic agents. (For abbreviations see Table 10.1.)

vice versa. This means that if the agent is very potent, e.g. methoxyflurane or trichlorethylene, it is also very slow in induction and eduction.

At least one compound, cyclo-octetraene, has been tested for the reason that it has a water solubility less than nitrous oxide and an oil solubility greater than methoxyflurane, but unfortunately it appeared to lack any anaesthetic action (Burns & Bracken 1972).

Stability

The stability of anaesthetics can be considered under two headings: (1) chemical or in vitro, (2) biological or in vivo.

1. *Chemical.* All modern anaesthetics have adequate in vitro stability giving good shelf life under normal conditions but storage in dark bottles and the addition of small amounts of stabilising compounds may be necessary. Stability in the presence of soda lime is also satisfactory except in the case of trichorethylene (and chloroform).

The use of completely closed circuit for prolonged periods imposes a severe test of the chemical stability of an agent because of the continuous passage over the highly alkaline soda lime. The compound CF_2CCLBr, which is toxic to mice in the concentration range 100–5000 p.p.m. has been detected at 5 p.p.m. after 1 hour of closed circuit halothane anaesthesia (Raventos & Lemon 1965, Sharp *et al* 1979). Halothane has been used extensively with soda lime without reports of any ill effect.

2. *Biological.* It has been appreciated since 1964 that metabolic breakdown of anaesthetics occurs and it has become apparent that reactive intermediate compounds, free radicals or inorganic fluoride are the substances chiefly responsible for organic toxicity (liver or kidney) after anaesthesia. The reasons for the introduction of fluorine into the molecules of anaesthetic compounds has already been mentioned. Fluorine is a very unphysiological substance not normally playing any part in the body except as an inert component of bone while free inorganic fluoride in the blood is a relatively toxic substance. In vivo stability is an important feature of modern agents and the percentage of agent metabolised has reached its current nadir of $0 \cdot 2\%$ for isoflurane.

It has become apparent that induction of the cytochome P450 enzyme system in the liver which may result from chronic exposure of the individual to a wide variety of drugs or chemical agents can have a great effect on the extent to which anaesthetics are metabolised and the consequent release of toxic substances.

Minimal depression of vital functions

The two vital functions of principal interest are respiration and cardiovascular activity. In experiments on isolated organs all anaesthetics have a depressant effect but in the intact organisms these depressant effects may be modified or even reversed by various mechanisms.

Thus, diethyl ether exerts a stimulating effect on receptors in the lung which stimulates respiration and opposes depression of the respiratory centre so that a normal Pa_{CO_2} is maintained until deep levels of anaesthesia are reached. Trichlorethylene has a similar direct stimulating effect on the lung which tends to cause a tachypnoea that is not effective in maintaining a normal Pa_{CO_2}. With the exception of nitrous oxide the other agents all produce a concentration dependent depression of respiration and there is some difference between the currently used agents in their tendency to produce this effect. In clinical practice this is offset by the respiratory stimulating effects of surgical stimulus so that all the standard agents can be used in spontaneously breathing patients without undue accumulation of CO_2 provided excessively deep anaesthesia is avoided.

In the case of the cardiovascular system all the agents have a directly depressant action and differences in their overall effect are due to differences in their action on baroreceptor activity and the output of the sympathoadrenal system as reflected in plasma adrenaline and noradrenaline.

On the basis of experimental rather than clinical work (e.g. Skovsted & Price 1972) the inhalation anaesthetics can be divided into two groups. Group 1 agents (ether, cyclopropane, chloroform, trichlorethylene and nitrous oxide) inhibit the baroreceptor response and produce increased sympathetic activity. Group 2 agents (halothane, methoxyflurane, enflurane and isoflurane) preserve or enhance the baroreceptor response and diminish sympathetic activity.

In clinical practice the situation is not simple because direct effects of agents on the cardiovascular system may be opposed by, for instance, sympathetic stimulation resulting from surgical stimulus and the overall change in cardiovascular function as shown by blood pressure, cardiac output or peripheral resistance will depend on the balance between inhibitory and excitatory influences. (See Gothert 1982, Desmonts & Marty 1983.)

Convenient volatility

For agents to be given by an inhalational route, a degree of volatility is essential and this may be expressed by the boiling point or saturated vapour pressure (SVP), at 20°C. Fig. 10.2, in which MAC is plotted against boiling point for a variety of agents, shows that in general the more potent the agent the higher the boiling point. As already mentioned, high potency (low MAC), is accompanied by slow induction and eduction characteristics but it can be argued that such agents are suitable for use with air in draw-over types of anaesthetic apparatus because their presence at low concentration in the inspired air does not depress the inspired oxygen concentration as much as agents of higher volatility and lower potency (but see below under ether). With highly volatile agents, oxygen enrichment of inspired gas becomes more important until in the extreme case of nitrous oxide only 79% of 1 MAC can be administered in the presence of 21% oxygen.

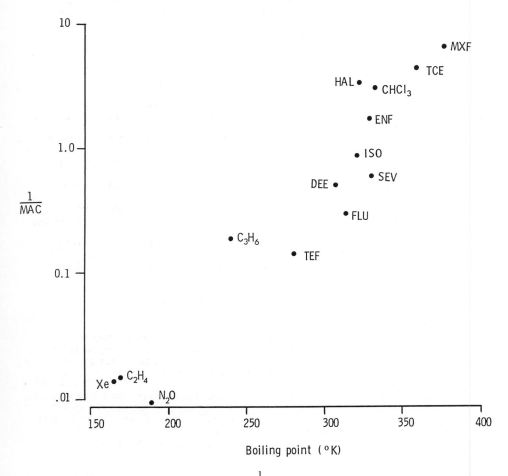

Fig. 10.2 Relationship between boiling point and $\overline{\text{MAC}}$, (For abbreviations see Table 10.1.)

It is generally agreed that for various reasons a minimum inspired oxygen concentration of about 33% is desirable during general anaesthesia and on the assumption that a concentration of 1·3 MAC should be attainable without risk of any degree of hypoxia then the optimum MAC, should be about 50%.

As can be seen from Table 10.1 the boiling points of halothane, enflurane and isoflurane lie within the range 48–58°. Whether this can be considered optimum is discussed later under possibilities for improvement.

Table 10.1 Physical characteristics and MAC values for some anaesthetic agents. ( ) indicates MAC estimated from oil solubility. References from which these data are taken are given below.

Formula		Partition/coefficient			Boiling point	SVP mmHg 20°C	MAC
		H_2O/gas	Blood/gas	Oil/gas			
C_2H_2	Acetylene	0·85	0·88	1·7	103		
	Aliflurane		1·7	124			1·2
$CHCl_3$	Chloroform	4·0	8·0	400	61·2	160	(0·77) dog
C_3H_6	Cyclopropane	0·21	0·55	11·5	−34	4800	9·2
$(C_2H_5)_2O$	Diethyl ether (DEE)	13	12	65	34·6	442	1·92
$(C_2H_3)_2O$	Divinyl ether (DVE)	1·4	2·6	60	283		
$CHClFCF_2OCF_2H$	Enflurane (ENF)	0·78	1·9	98	56·5	180	1·68
C_2H_5Cl	Ethyl chloride (EtCl)	1·2	2·0	169	13·1		
C_2H_4	Ethylene	0·09	0·15	1·3	−103·8		67
$CF_3CH_2OCHCH_2$	Fluroxene	0·85	1·4	48	42·7	286	3·4
$CHF_2CF_2CH_2Br$	Halopropane		5·5	320			
$CHClBrCF_3$	Halothane (HAL)	0·8	2·4	220	50·2	243	0·75
$CF_3CHClOCF_2H$	Isoflurane (ISO)	0·62	1·4	97	48·5	250	1·15
$CHCl_2CF_2OCH_3$	Methoxyflurane (MXF)	4·5	11	950	104·7	23	0·16
N_2O	Nitrous oxide	0·47	0·47	1·4	−89	3900	105
$H_2FCOCH(CF_3)_2$	Sevoflurane (SEV)	0·36	0·6	53	58·5	160	1·7 monkey
CF_3CHBrF	Teflurane (TEF)	0·32	0·60	29	8·66		(7·24)
C_2HCl_3	Trichlorethy-lene (TCE)	1·7	9·0	900	86·7	59	(0·23)
Xe	Xenon	0·085	0·14	1·8	−108		71

Data sheets. May & Baker, Ohio Medical Products

Eger E I II 1974 *Anesthetic uptake and action.* Williams & Wilkins Company, Baltimore, Maryland

Fiserova-Bergerova V 1983 Gases and their solubility: a review of fundamentals. Modeling of inhalation exposure to vapors: uptake, distribution and elimination. CRC Press, Boca Raton, Florida, p 3–28

Halsey M J 1981 Investigations on isoflurane, sevoflurane and other experimental anaesthetics. *British Journal of Anaesthesia* **53:** 43S–47S

Rodgers R C, Hill G E 1978 Equations for vapour pressure versus temperature derivation and use of the Antoine equation on a handheld programmable calculator. *British Journal of Anaesthesia* **50:** 415–424

Steward A, Allott P R, Cowles A L, Mapleson W W 1973 Solubility coefficients for inhaled anaesthetics for water, oil and biological media. *British Journal of Anaesthesia* **45:** 282–293

Secher O 1971 Physical and chemical data and anaesthetics. *Acta Anaesthesiologica Scandinavica, Suppl XLII*

Minimal interaction with other drugs

The most important substances whose actions are affected by anaesthetics are muscle relaxants and circulating catecholamines, particularly adrenaline.

All muscle relaxants are potentiated by inhalational anaesthesia in a dose-dependent manner and since muscle relaxation quite adequate for most forms of surgery can be produced by inhalation agents alone it is reasonable to conclude that at least part of this potentiation is due to the c.n.s. depressant action of the anaesthetic. In addition it has been shown that inhalation agents decrease the sensitivity of the post-junctional membrane of the neuromuscular junction and possibly act at a more distal site such as the muscle membrane (Ngai 1975). There are differences between different anaesthetic agents in the extent to which they potentiate relaxants. For instance, enflurane and isoflurane are considerably more effective in potentiating d-tubocurarine than are halothane or nitrous oxide (Ali & Saverese 1976). The reason for this is quite unknown but it may be considered that it is advantageous for an inhalational agent to potentiate a neuromuscular block since a component of the block can then be removed by eduction of the agent by ventilation of the lungs with a non-rebreathing circuit. This increases flexibility of control as there are then at least two methods of reducing or abolishing the block, neostigmine and ventilation.

The tendency of inhalational agents to sensitise the myocardium to adrenaline, both endogenous and exogenous, has been the subject of much study and one of the few generalisations that can be made about structure-activity relationships in the inhalational agents is that straight chain hydrocarbons tend to sensitise the heart to adrenaline whereas ethers, particularly if fluorinated, do not have this effect. Ethylene is an exception to this generalisation (Burgison et al 1955). The fluorinated ethers in current use confer exceptional myocardial stability to adrenaline and this is a very desirable attribute.

Absence of after effects

Nausea and vomiting and possibly headache are the principal after effects attributable to inhalation anaesthesia. Skvosted & Price (1972), in making their classification considered that group 1 agents (ether, cyclopropane, trichlorethylene and nitrous oxide) 'favoured emesis during recovery'. Clinical experience agrees with this so far as the first three agents named are concerned but there is surprisingly little factual information on the subject. As for nitrous oxide, it is currently used as a component of more than 95% of all inhalational anaesthetic techniques in Britain with the result that there is little control data.

The only conclusion possible is that undesirable after effects will be minimised if the agent remains in the body for as short a time as possible. An agent having low blood solubility is therefore to be favoured.

Good analgesic action

For reasons which are not understood, some inhalation agents produce a considerable degree of analgesia when inhaled at subanaesthetic concentrations (e.g. ether, trichlorethylene, nitrous oxide) whereas others (e.g. halothane) do not (Dundee & Moore 1960). It is tempting to postulate that this effect is caused by the liberation of endorphins (enkephalins) but except in the case of nitrous oxide evidence is conflicting on this subject (Goldstein 1978).

If an agent having a good analgesic action is also of high solubility then eduction will be slow and the agent will provide analgesia in the postoperative period. This is the case with ether (Farman 1981) but as described above other less desirable after effects will also be prolonged and it is probably better to rely on specific analgesic drugs in the postoperative period rather than retention of the anaesthetic agent.

No irritant effects

It is an interesting fact that inhalational anaesthetics all have a smell (Burns & Bracken 1972). If the smell is very pungent then it becomes irritating and this imposes limitations on the use of the agent for inhalational induction. A degree of pungency is one of the few blemishes currently allowed for isoflurane. In the case of diethyl ether, not only is it pungent but it is also very slow in induction and these factors together virtually rule out ether for inhalation induction under normal circumstances.

NOTES ON INHALATIONAL ANAESTHETIC AGENTS

Xenon

Xenon is of considerable theoretical interest but not an agent in current use. It is the only one of the rare gases having adequate lipid solubility to be an anaesthetic agent at pressures of one atmosphere. It has a MAC of 71, and has been shown to be a clinically suitable agent in human subjects although its great cost have limited its use to experimental studies.

One of the features of xenon is that it is biochemically inert and cannot be metabolised in the body. It is therefore of interest to find that exposure of rats to 65% of xenon for 6 days produced 30% leucopenia and also erythropenia. Hopes of being able to render patients unconscious for many days by inhalational agents without causing harm seem unlikely to be realised (Aldrete & Virtue 1967).

Nitrous oxide

Currently the most used inhalational agent in the Western world, nitrous oxide must be assumed to be a very safe agent. Some of its defects have been known for many years. It does not have sufficient potency (MAC 105). It has a diffusing capacity (which is proportional to solubility in blood) 28 times that of nitrogen (Nunn 1977) and consequently tends to enter gas-filled spaces in the body at a higher rate than the nitrogen can diffuse out. If the space is compliant, such as the gut, there is an increase in volume. If the space has a rigid wall, such as the middle ear, there will be a rise in pressure.

It has been known since 1956 that exposure for several days to nitrous oxide at concentrations sufficient for sedation caused bone marrow depression and it is now known that this effect is due to the oxidation of vitamin B_{12}. It is not clear at the present time how long an exposure to nitrous oxide is required to produce clinically significant depression of the bone marrow but it would appear that periods of up to 24 hours are not harmful to patients in normal health. Also it is not clear as to what extent these depressive effects can be reduced or prevented by the administration of folinic acid or activated methionine. Two recent reviews of this important subject are by Brodsky (1983) and Nunn (in press).

Diethyl ether

This was one of the earliest inhalational anaesthetics introduced but its use in the Western world has declined. The chief reason for this is its inflammability and also its great water and blood solubility which, together with its irritant smell, makes for a slow induction and slow recovery associated with a high incidence of vomiting. Nevertheless, ether has always had the highest reputation for safety; it is safe in the presence of adrenaline and, as mentioned previously, does not depress respiration at least in light surgical anaesthesia. It is generally considered a safe agent for the inexperienced anaesthetist because, in addition to being slow in action, it produces a graded series of signs indicating depth of anaesthesia. Cardiac output is well maintained by sympathetic stimulation except at very deep levels of anaesthesia.

Ether does undergo some metabolism but, since it contains no halogens, its intermediate metabolites are such relatively non-toxic substances (ethyl alcohol, acetic acid and acetaldehyde).

Trichlorethylene

Having an oil/gas coefficient of 900, trichlorethylene is at the upper end of the range of feasible agents. Its great merit is that it is non-flammable but it is incompatible with both adrenaline and soda lime. Trichlorethylene is extensively metabolised and is unique in that one of its two principal metabolites, trichlorethanol, is pharmacologically active, having a powerful sedative action which may be very prolonged in enzyme-induced patients.

The kinetics of trichlorethylene and of ether are so different to halothane that those without sufficient experience often have difficulty in using the two older agents with precision.

Cyclopropane

Cyclopropane has solubility characteristics closer to the ideal than the other agents as exemplified by its only use today, which is to produce very rapid induction in children. It is very inflammable and incompatible with adrenaline. The National Halothane Study recorded that the incidence of massive hepatic necrosis following cyclopropane anaesthesia was $1 \cdot 7$ per 10 000 anaesthetics, a higher figure than that recorded after halothane or indeed any other agent. The apparent hepatoxicity of cyclopropane may be due to its sympathetic stimulatory action producing powerfully splanchnic vasoconstriction, but on the other hand, of the 25 cases of postcyclopropane hepatic necrosis reported in the National Halothane Study, 24 patients were in a state of severe shock and the fatal outcome could have been predicted. Despite this cyclopropane was chosen to be the best agent for these very ill patients (Baden & Rice 1981).

It seems likely that trichlorethylene and cyclopropane, as well as methoxyflurane, will all be withdrawn by the manufacturers when anaesthetists can be persuaded to accept their departure.

Halothane

Halothane was introduced into clinical practice in 1956 and, although it was then as expensive as isoflurane is now, it was so greatly superior to existing agents that it soon became universally used. In 1963 the first reports of jaundice and massive hepatic necrosis after halothane anaesthesia appeared. The US National Halothane Study, which reported in 1965, retrospectively surveyed 856 515 anaesthetics of which 30% involved halothane. The true incidence of massive hepatic necrosis associated with halothane in this enormous series was 7 out of 250 000 halothane anaesthetics — about 1 per 35 000 cases (Baden & Rice 1981).

The study of the possible hepatoxicity of halothane has been greatly handicapped by the difficulty of finding an animal model and fairly drastic treatment consisting of enzyme induction by phenobarbitone followed by hypoxic halothane anaesthesia (F_{IO_2} 7–14%) is required to produce centralobular hepatic necrosis. The hypothesis is that when halothane is metabolised by reductive pathways active metabolites are formed which produce hepatocellular damage. If this hypothesis is correct then hypoxia may be a factor leading to halothane hepatotoxicity. There is also some evidence that repeated halothane anaesthetics produce impaired liver function tests. Obesity has also been linked to halothane hepatotoxicity.

The actual incidence of halothane hepatotoxicity remains unknown and widely differing opinions are held. The subject is reviewed by Brown (1982).

Enflurane

Enflurane was introduced clinically in 1958 and is currently the most commonly used agent in North America. Earlier fears about its possibly epileptogenic effects have not been realised. Whereas halothane is about 20% metabolised, this figure is reduced to 2% in the case of enflurane. However, enflurane metabolism unlike that of halothane results in defluorination and serum F^- levels have been shown to reach mildly nephrotoxic levels after 9·6 MAC hours of enflurane anaesthesia (Mazze *et al* 1977). This is not considered likely to present any clinical problems in patients with normal renal function.

As can be seen from its solubility characteristics (Table 10.1) recovery from enflurane should be predictively faster than that from halothane and this has indeed been shown to be the case (Kortilla *et al* 1977, Padfield & Mullins 1980). (See comprehensive review of enflurane anaesthesia by Adams 1981.)

Isoflurane
An isomer of enflurane, isoflurane was introduced into the United Kingdom in 1983. Its physical properties are similar to those of enflurane. Only 0·2% is metabolised. A great deal of experimental work has been carried out in evaluating isoflurane and comprehensive reviews of its pharmacological and clinical properties are by Eger (1981), Wade & Stevens (1981) and Forrest (1983).

Sevoflurane
Sevoflurane is a fluorinated methyl isopropyl ether at present only in the development stage. Its greatest interest lies in its relatively low blood solubility and, in a study using healthy volunteers, the subjects reported being aware of the quite acceptable smell of the agent for only four breaths before losing consciousness (Holaday & Smith 1981). Sevoflurane is reviewed by Holaday (1983).

What is the room for improvement?
It is frequently said that the development of inhalational anaesthetic agents has reached its zenith with isoflurane and that the rapidly mounting costs of basic research and development, together with the increasingly stringent and time-consuming tests demanded by the various governmental drug licensing authorities have finally conspired to make it no longer worthwhile for drug companies to develop new agents. Certainly, it is true to say that there is not much room for improvement in agents having characteristics close to those of the three current leaders in the field, halothane, enflurane and isoflurane. These are all fluorinated hydrocarbons of very similar physical characteristics and it seems likely that research effort has been directed into discovering new agents similar to halothane but marginally better.

However, the considerations set out above (Optimum solubility) strongly suggest that the lowest possible solubility in blood carries the greatest benefit both in speed of induction and eduction and minimisation of after effects. Furthermore, the lowest possible solubility minimises the total quantity of agent required to be taken into the body to produce anaesthesia and this reduces the possibility of damage by harmful metabolites in two ways. Firstly, it minimises their quantity and secondly, it minimises the time available for their production since the agent of low solubility is in the body for the shorter time.

Considered in this light the three current agents are far from optimum and it is worthwhile considering the possibilities of agents of lower solubility. The minimum oxygen requirements mentioned in Convenient volatility (above) limit the reduction in solubility of a prospective agent to one having a MAC of not more than 50% and as can be seen from Fig. 10.2 such an agent would probably be a gas at ambient temperature. It would therefore require to be packed in cyclinders and gas flowmeters, which are quite accurate devices, would give precise control of inspired concentrations. Vaporisers would no longer be necessary.

Deuteration

The substitution of the isotope deuterium ('heavy hydrogen') for one or more of the hydrogen atoms in an anaesthetic molecule increases the resistance of that molecule to metabolic breakdown. This is because deuterium has a larger mass than hydrogen and bonds involving deuterium are stronger than those with simple hydrogen. It has been found that deuteration does not affect the MAC of anaesthetics (Tinker *et al* 1981) and it has been shown to reduce chloroform hepatotoxicity in enzyme-induced rats (Pohl & Krishna 1978).

Deuterisation of halothane decreases oxidative but not reductive metabolism of the molecule — hepatotoxicity may not therefore be decreased. However, deuterisation has been shown to reduce breakdown of methoxyflurane and enflurane (McCarty *et al* 1979) and holds out the possibility of being of value in reducing the metabolism of newer anaesthetics such as sevoflurane (Bentley 1983).

REFERENCES

Adams A P 1981 Enflurane in clinical practice. *British Journal of Anaesthesia* **53:** 27S–41S
Aldrete J A, Virtue R W 1967 Prolonged inhalation of inert gases by rats. *Anesthesia and Analgesia* **46:** 562–565
Baden J M, Rice S A 1981 In: Miller R D (ed) *Metabolism and toxicity of inhaled anaesthetics in anesthesia.* Churchill Livingstone, New York
Bentley J B 1983 Deuterated volatile anesthetics. In: Brown B R (ed) *New pharmacologic vistas in anesthesia.* F A Davis & Co, Philadelphia
Brodsky J B 1983 The toxicity of nitrous oxide. *Clinics in Anesthesiology* **1/2:** 455–462
Brown B R Jr 1982 Current status of hepatoxicity of the halogenated inhalation anaesthetics. In: Peter K & Jesch F (eds) *Inhalation anaesthesia today and tomorrow.* Springer-Verlag, Berlin
Brown T A, Morris G 1966 The ignition risk with mixtures of oxygen and nitrous oxide with halothane. *British Journal of Anaesthesia* **38:** 164–173
Burgison R M, O'Malley W E, Heisse C K, Forrest J W, Krantz J C 1955 Anaesthesia XLVI. Fluorinated ethylenes and cardiac arrhythmias induced by epinephrine. *Journal of Pharmacology and Experimental Therapeutics* **114:** 470–472
Burns T H S, Bracken A 1972 Exploratory and newer compounds. In: Chenoweth M B (ed) *Handbook of experimental pharmacology 30.* Modern inhalation anaesthetics, Springer-Verlag, Berlin, section 7
de Jong R H, Eger E I II 1975 MAC expanded AD_{50} and AD_{95} values of common inhalation anesthetics in man. *Anesthesiology* **42:** 384–389
Desmonts J M, Marty J 1983 Halogenated anesthetics and the sympathetic nervous system. In: Mazze R I (ed) *Clinics in anesthesiology* **1/2:** ch 4
Dundee J W, Hassard T H, McGowan W A W, Henshaw J 1982 The 'induction' dose of thiopentone. *Anaesthesia* **37:** 1176–1184
Dundee J W, Moore J 1960 Alterations in response to somatic pain associated with anaesthesia IV. The effects of sub-anaesthetic concentrations of inhalation agents. *British Journal of Anaesthesia* **32:** 453–459
Eger E I 1981 Isoflurane: a review. *Anesthesiology* **55:** 559–576
Farman J V 1981 Some long established agents — a contemporary view. *British Journal of Anaesthesia* **53:** 3S–9S
Forrest J B 1983 Isoflurane: past, present and future. *Clinics in anesthesiology* **1/2:** 251–274
Göthert M 1982 Influence of inhalation anaesthetics on the autonomic nervous system. In: Peter K & Jesch F (eds) *Inhalation anaesthesia today and tomorrow.* Springer-Verlag, Berlin, p 97–108
Holaday D A 1983 Sevoflurane: an experimental anesthetic. In: Brown B R (ed) *New vistas in anesthesia.* F A Davis & Co, Philadelphia
Larsen E R 1972 The chemistry of modern inhalation anaesthetics. In: Chenoweth M B (ed) *Handbook of experimental pharmacology 30.* Modern inhalation anaesthetics, Springer-Verlag, Berlin, section 2
Mazze R I, Calverley R K, Smith N T 1972 Inorganic fluoride nephrotoxicity. *Anesthesiology* **46:** 265–271
McCarty L P, Malek R S, Larsen E R 1979 The effects of deuteration on the metabolism of halogenated anesthetics in the rat. *Anesthesiology* **51:** 106–110
Ngai S H 1975 Action of general anaesthetics in producing muscle relaxation: interaction of anaesthetics with relaxants. In: Katz R L (ed) *Muscle relaxants.* Excerpta Medica, Amsterdam, p 279–297
Nunn J F 1984 Interaction of nitrous oxide and vitamin B_{12}. *Trends in Pharmacology* **812:** in press
Nunn J F 1977 *Applied respiratory physiology.* Butterworths, London, p 329
Pohl L R, Krishna G 1978 Deuterium isotope effect in bioinactivation and hepatotoxicity of chloroform. *Life Sciences* **23:** 1067–1072

Raventos S, Lemon R G 1965 The impurities in Fluothane. *British Journal of Anaesthesia* **37**: 716–737

Sharp J H, Trudell J R, Cohen E N 1979 Volatile metabolites and decomposition products of halothane in man. *Anesthesiology* **50**: 2–8

Skovsted P, Price H L 1972 The effects of ethrane on arterial pressure, preganglionic sympathetic activity and barostatic reflexes. *Anesthesiology* **36**: 257–262

Summary of the National Halothane Study 1966 *Journal of the American Medical Association* **197**: 775–790

Wade J G, Stevens W C 1981 Isoflurane: an anesthetic for the eighties? *Anesthesia and Analgesia* **60**: 666–682

Gas exchange and anaesthesia

INTRODUCTION

Unpredictable reduction in oxygen delivery to the tissues continues to be a serious complication of general anaesthesia, and is a recurring cause of morbidity and mortality. The two principal causes are (1) arterial hypoxaemia, and (2) impaired cardiac output and regional blood flow. This review is only concerned with the former.

Cyanosis during general anaesthesia is commonly caused by hypoventilation due to obstruction of the airway, but it may occur in apparently normal patients during uncomplicated anaesthesia, where ventilation is uncompromised. The development of techniques for measuring O_2 tension in arterial blood (Pa_{O_2}) has revealed that a reduction in Pa_{O_2} occurs during anaesthesia in the overwhelming majority of patients (Campbell *et al* 1958). While raising the inspired oxygen can often reverse the fall of Pa_{O_2}, this is not always effective. For example, Pa_{O_2} values of $9 \cdot 7$ kPa (72 mmHg) have been reported during anaesthesia in normal patients receiving over 30% oxygen (Nunn *et al* 1965, Hewlett *et al* 1974), as have values as low as $7 \cdot 5$ kPa (56 mmHg) in patients with lung disease receiving over 35% O_2 (Dueck *et al* 1980). This means that it is not acceptable to claim that arterial hypoxaemia is a problem that can simply be overcome by increasing the inspired oxygen tension. Deterioration in gas exchange during anaesthesia therefore remains a practical clinical problem, and clarification of the mechanism would obviously be of value. However, despite intense interest in this subject, the cause of the fall of Pa_{O_2} remains controversial (Nunn 1980, Schmid & Rehder 1981), and there is no single accepted explanation.

To understand this problem, the pathophysiology of pulmonary gas exchange must first be understood, so we shall commence with a review of the basic concepts, and then proceed to the effects of anaesthesia.

FACTORS AFFECTING GAS EXCHANGE: Pa_{O_2} and $PA\text{-}a_{O_2}$

The efficiency of gas exchange is usually assessed by measuring Pa_{O_2} and the alveolar-arterial oxygen tension difference ($PA\text{-}a_{O_2}$). Both these measurements are frequently quoted because although Pa_{O_2} is familiar and is often a good indicator of the degree of abnormality of pulmonary gas exchange, its value takes no account of the alveolar oxygen tension (PA_{O_2}). PA_{O_2} may be reduced by hypoventilation or increased by breathing oxygen, and so the difference between the alveolar and the arterial tensions, $PA\text{-}a_{O_2}$, is often measured, and is a direct indicator of pulmonary gas exchange efficiency.

The factors which influence these values include:

1. Inspired oxygen concentration

2. Ventilation-perfusion ratio
3. Mixed venous oxygen tension
4. Hypoxic pulmonary vasoconstriction
5. Cardiac output
6. Haemoglobin.

1. Inspired oxygen concentration ($F_{I_{O_2}}$)

Raising $F_{I_{O_2}}$ raises $P_{a_{O_2}}$, even when lungs are grossly abnormal. However, it is essential to realise that neither $P_{a_{O_2}}$ nor $P_{A-a_{O_2}}$ is linearly related to $F_{I_{O_2}}$, and the relationship is unpredictable (Lenfant 1963, Harris *et al* 1974). The relationship of $P_{a_{O_2}}$ to $F_{I_{O_2}}$ is illustrated in Figure 11.1, and explained below.

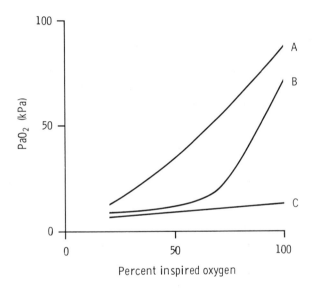

Fig. 11.1   The relationship between % inspired oxygen and $P_{a_{O_2}}$. A: normal lungs. B: low $\dot{V}/\dot{Q}$, without shunt. C: severe shunt.

2. Ventilation-perfusion ratio ($\dot{V}/\dot{Q}$)

The importance of the normal matching of ventilation ($\dot{V}$) to perfusion ($\dot{Q}$) as a determinant of arterial oxygenation cannot be overemphasised. Impairment of normal $\dot{V}-\dot{Q}$ matching represents the major cause of worsening $P_{a_{O_2}}$ following the induction of general anaesthesia, just as it represents the major cause of hypoxaemia resulting from lung disease.

When ventilation is normally matched to perfusion in any lung unit*, then that unit will receive 1 ml of gas for each ml of blood which perfuses it. This unit has a ventilation-perfusion ratio of 1:0. If $\dot{V}/\dot{Q}$ departs from 1:0, the efficiency of gas exchange in the unit will be impaired, and the larger the change of $\dot{V}/\dot{Q}$, the greater the impairment. The nature of the impairment depends upon whether $\dot{V}/\dot{Q}$ is high or low.

*A lung unit is a group of alveoli which share the same $\dot{V}/\dot{Q}$ ratio. The size of a unit may vary from a few alveoli to a few million.

Low $\dot{V}/\dot{Q}$ shunt and the effect of raising inspired oxygen

At one extreme, blood may pass through the lung without coming into contact with alveolar gas at all. The $\dot{V}/\dot{Q}$ ratio is then zero, and this is called a *shunt*. Mixed venous blood passes through the shunt unchanged, and then mingles with the oxygenated blood from other lung units. This reduces the oxygen tension of arterial blood, by an amount dependent on the oxygen content of the mixed venous blood.

When $\dot{V}/\dot{Q}$ is low, but not as low as zero, the effect is in some respects similar to shunt, and in some respects different. For this reason, low $\dot{V}/\dot{Q}$ is sometimes called *virtual shunt*, but to avoid confusion, the term 'shunt' will be reserved for units with a $\dot{V}/\dot{Q}$ of zero. Like shunt, $\dot{V}/\dot{Q}$ units also reduce arterial saturation, by reducing the quantity of oxygen delivered to the alveoli. This is because when $\dot{V}/\dot{Q}$ is low, the amount of oxygen delivered to the alveoli per second is inadequate to saturate the volume of blood flowing through those alveoli per second. The result is blood which has a slightly greater saturation than the blood from a shunt, but still has a lower P_{O_2} than the blood from normal lung units.

However, low $\dot{V}/\dot{Q}$ units differ from shunt in one very important way: increasing the inspired oxygen cannot directly affect the oxygen content of shunted blood but it can improve the oxygenation of blood passing through low $\dot{V}/\dot{Q}$ units. It does this by increasing the delivery of oxygen to these units as shown in Figure 11.2. Thus patients with a low P_{aO_2} resulting from low $\dot{V}/\dot{Q}$ units can be treated by raising inspired oxygen, but this has little

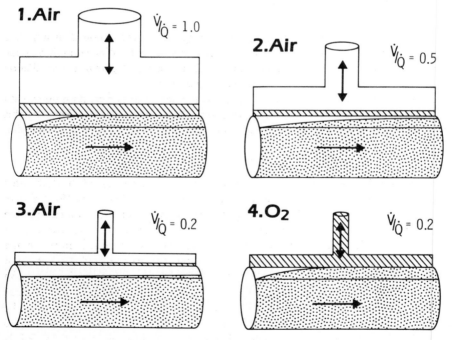

Fig. 11.2 The effect of reduced $\dot{V}/\dot{Q}$, and increased inspired oxygen on saturation of blood leaving a lung unit. Size of upper part of each unit represents ventilation rate, size of lower part perfusion rate. Diagonally striped area represents quantity of O_2 delivered per unit time, stippled area represents % saturated haemoglobin.

1: normal, $\dot{V}/\dot{Q}$ 1·0, O_2 adequate for full saturation of mixed venous blood. 2: $\dot{V}/\dot{Q}$ 0·5, half the quantity of O_2 delivered, nearly adequate for full saturation. 3: $\dot{V}/\dot{Q}$ 0·2, O_2 delivery inadequate, blood leaving unit desaturated. 4: $\dot{V}/\dot{Q}$ still 0·2, O_2 delivery increased by breathing 100% O_2, O_2 delivery once more adequate for full saturation.

effect when the predominant lesion is a shunt. This is why Pa_{O_2} is not linearly related to $F_{I_{O_2}}$, and the different effects of low $\dot{V}/\dot{Q}$ and shunt can often be observed in patients with progressive lung lesions like pneumonia. In the early stages, a patient may have a low Pa_{O_2} while breathing air, but raising $F_{I_{O_2}}$ to $0 \cdot 35$ swiftly restores full oxygen saturation. In these circumstances, the predominant lesion is low $\dot{V}/\dot{Q}$, rather than shunt. As the disease worsens, more low $\dot{V}/\dot{Q}$ units become shunt, and raising $F_{I_{O_2}}$ becomes progressively less effective. Eventually there may be severe desaturation even when $F_{I_{O_2}}$ is $1 \cdot 0$.

Increasing the inspired oxygen is generally beneficial, but may not be entirely so. This is because raising $F_{I_{O_2}}$ may convert a low $\dot{V}/\dot{Q}$ into a shunt by causing absorption atelectasis, the mechanism for which is as follows: if $\dot{V}/\dot{Q}$ in a lung unit is very low, virtually all the oxygen may be taken up from the alveoli. When breathing air this is of little significance, since the remaining nitrogen is very slowly absorbed and holds the alveoli open until the next breath. When breathing oxygen, or when a soluble gas like N_2O is substituted for nitrogen, all the alveolar gas may be absorbed. The alveolus may then collapse, so that the low $\dot{V}/\dot{Q}$ unit has become shunt (Dantzker et al 1975). This effect may play a part in inducing abnormal gas exchange during anaesthesia but it is unlikely to be of great significance since no difference in gas exchange can be detected when N_2/O_2 mixtures are used during anaesthesia rather than N_2O/O_2 (Webb & Nunn 1967, Dueck et al 1980, Heneghan et al 1984).

Breathing oxygen has yet another effect upon the lung, by modifying hypoxic pulmonary vasoconstriction. This is dealt with below.

High $\dot{V}/\dot{Q}$ and dead space

Ventilated but unperfused lung units are called dead space, and ventilation of such units is wasted; these units contribute the alveolar component of dead space. When units have some perfusion, but not enough to match all the ventilation, wasting of part of the ventilation occurs. High $\dot{V}/\dot{Q}$ therefore acts as part of alveolar dead space.

The effect of increased dead space is to divert ventilation from normal lung units, with consequent retention of CO_2. In extreme cases, oxygenation may also be affected by this process, although the usual cause of hypoxia in the presence of high $\dot{V}/\dot{Q}$ is accompanying low $\dot{V}/\dot{Q}$ units.

Physiological $\dot{V}/\dot{Q}$ abnormality

Minor degrees of $\dot{V}/\dot{Q}$ mismatch exist in normal lungs. This is because of the differential effect of gravity on distribution of ventilation and pulmonary blood flow (West 1970). Figure 11.3 illustrates the first of these effects: the dependent parts of the lung are compressed by the weight of the upper parts, so that they are less distended, and are on the lower part of their compliance curve. This means that with inflation, these regions can expand more than the upper regions. There is thus progressively more regional ventilation towards the bottom of the lung. Pulmonary perfusion is also higher at the base of the lung, because the increase in hydrostatic pressure towards the bottom of the lung dilates the dependent pulmonary vessels. This reduces the resistance to flow in the dependent regions, so flow increases towards the lower parts of the lung. However, the rate of change of ventilation and perfusion from top to bottom of the lung are not equal, as shown in Figure 11.4. The result is that $\dot{V}/\dot{Q}$ falls progressively towards the dependent parts of the lung. This spread of $\dot{V}/\dot{Q}$ ratios is responsible for the $PA\text{-}a_{O_2}$ difference (about 1 kPa) observed in normal subjects breathing air.

Closing capacity and $\dot{V}/\dot{Q}$

$\dot{V}/\dot{Q}$ mismatching is also caused by increased closing capacity (CC). Closing capacity is the lung volume at which airway closure begins to occur. If a patient breathes at a lung volume

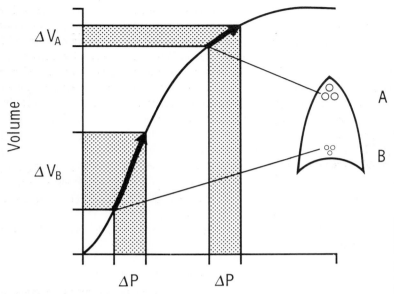

Fig. 11.3 The effect of local pulmonary distension on ventilation distribution. Figure shows a lung compliance curve together with a diagrammatic representation of an upright lung. A: apex, B: base, Δ P: distending pressure of a normal inspiration. ΔV_A & ΔV_B: resultant volume change at apex and base. The lung weight pulls open the apical alveoli, and compresses the basal ones. The apical alveoli are therefore nearer to full distension, and are less expanded by the breath, while the basal ones are lower on the compliance curve and can expand more. Thus ventilation increases progressively towards the bottom of the lung.

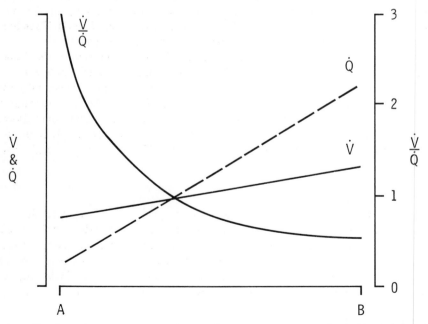

Fig 11.4 Ventilation increases towards the bottom of the lung, and so does perfusion, but perfusion increases more than ventilation, so that $\dot{V}/\dot{Q}$ is higher at the top and lower at the bottom of the lung. (Redrawn from West 1970.)

around closing capacity, then some airways are closed for part of each breath. This reduces ventilation, and hence $\dot{V}/\dot{Q}$, in these units. Thus breathing at or below CC impairs gas exchange. There are two significant consequences of this: firstly, in adult life, closing capacity increases with age, and gas exchange deteriorates. Secondly, there is the effect on changes in lung volume: if a reduction in lung volume increases the amount of airway closure in the tidal range, i.e. if CC impinges more on the tidal volume, then the reduction in lung volume leads to a deterioration in gas exchange. If a reduction in lung volume does not increase airway closure, it does not effect gas exchange (Craig et al 1971).

3. Mixed venous oxygen tension $(P_{\bar{V}O_2})$

A change in $P_{\bar{V}O_2}$ affect Pa_{O_2} in two ways, *directly* or *indirectly*. The *direct* effect is seen in the presence of a shunt or low $\dot{V}/\dot{Q}$ units, when Pa_{O_2} is reduced by venous admixture. The degree of the reduction of Pa_{O_2} is greater the lower the O_2 content of the mixed venous blood, so if $P_{\bar{V}O_2}$ falls Pa_{O_2} also falls, and PA-a_O increases.

The *indirect* effect of $P_{\bar{V}O_2}$ involves an interaction with hypoxic pulmonary vasoconstriction, which is considered next.

4. Hypoxic pulmonary vasoconstriction (HPV)

HPV is a reflex which modifies local pulmonary blood flow in response to local conditions. It constricts pulmonary blood vessels in hypoxic lung units, diverting blood flow to less hypoxic units. Thus blood flow is diverted away from underventilated lung units, improving overall $\dot{V}/\dot{Q}$ matching and thus gas exchange.

Breathing oxygen can profoundly affect this reflex, in two ways: firstly, it increases the P_{O_2} in the gas phase of low $\dot{V}/\dot{Q}$ units, which blocks HPV, and increases blood flow to these units. Secondly, breathing oxygen raises Pa_{O_2}, and thus $P_{\bar{V}O_2}$, increasing the P_{O_2} in blood perfusing shunts. This can inhibit HPV in these units (Pease et al 1982). Thus breathing oxygen can increase blood flow through both low $\dot{V}/\dot{Q}$ units and shunts.

The importance of this effect is that it was once the practice to measure the shunt when breathing air and again when breathing 100% oxygen, and attribute the difference between the two values to the low $\dot{V}/\dot{Q}$ units: this was done because breathing oxygen fully saturates blood perfusing low $\dot{V}/\dot{Q}$ units, and was not thought to affect blood flowing through shunts. This is now no longer done, because breathing oxygen diverts blood flow towards low $\dot{V}/\dot{Q}$ units, but also because of absorption atelectasis. Accurate techniques are now available, using inert gas tracers, to distinguish between shunt and low $\dot{V}/\dot{Q}$ without altering their values (see below).

5. Cardiac output $(\dot{Q})$

Cardiac output may affect Pa_{O_2} and PA-a_{O_2} in two ways: firstly, increasing cardiac outut, by increasing oxygen delivery to the tissues, may increase $P_{\bar{V}O_2}$; and secondly, changes in cardiac output can alter the shunt fraction (Cheney & Colley 1980). This is not usually clinically important, because Q usually increases more than the fall in arterial O_2 content, so oxygen delivery is improved. However, the change in Pa_{O_2} may be sufficiently large to interfere with the interpretation of research data, which is why it is mentioned here.

6. Haemoglobin

This is of considerable clinical importance, although it is usually very easy to keep it constant in the laboratory. This may affect oxygen delivery to the tissues by altering the oxygen combining capacity of the blood. This can influence $P\bar{v}_{O_2}$, and therefore Pa_{O_2} and $PA\text{-}a_{O_2}$, as described above.

These are the factors which may affect pulmonary gas exchange and some of the measurements used to quantify it. Next we shall consider what is known about gas exchange impairment during anaesthesia.

WHY IS GAS EXCHANGE IMPAIRED DURING ANAESTHESIA?

Several theories have been proposed to explain the worsening of pulmonary gas exchange with general anaesthesia. They may loosely be divided into: (a) lung volume-regional ventilation theories, and (b) pulmonary vasculature theories.

Lung volume and regional ventilation

The first explanation for deterioration of gas exchange with induction of anaesthesia was based on the work of Hickey et al (1973) and Hewlett et al (1974). They demonstrated a correlation between the rise in $PA\text{-}a_{O_2}$ occurring on induction of anaesthesia and the fall in functional residual capacity (FRC), and therefore suggested that the fall in lung volume caused the deterioration of gas exchange, the FRC having fallen below CC and thus impaired gas exchange. For this attractively simple theory to be proven, it would have to be shown that when the vast majority of patients were anaesthetised, FRC fell below CC, and that when the lung volume change was reversed, $PA\text{-}a_{O_2}$ returned to pre-anaesthetic value.

The first of these questions, 'does FRC fall below CC in the vast majority of patients when anaesthetised?', was initially investigated by Weenig et al (1973). They measured closing capacity before anaesthesia, and the change of the FRC with induction. They showed that in most patients the fall in FRC would be insufficient to take their tidal range into their CC, as long as CC was not changed by induction of anaesthesia. Juno et al (1978) measured CC both before and during anaesthesia, and showed that although CC did change with induction, in the majority of patients it was still below FRC. Thus the fall in lung volume could not explain the increase in $PA\text{-}a_{O_2}$ in most patients, assuming that, to worsen gas exchange, a fall in lung volume must drop FRC below CC during anaesthesia. This assumes that the lung behaves in the same way during anaesthesia as when awake. This is not necessarily so, as the lung could behave differently during anaesthesia, and *any* reduction in volume could impair gas exchange. This point has now been resolved, and will be returned to later.

The second question, 'does raising lung volume reverse the gas exchange abnormality?', was investigated by Wyche et al (1973). They raised the lung volume of anaesthetised patients with positive end expiratory pressure (PEEP), which produced a trivial improvement in $PA\text{-}a_{O_2}$. This improvement in $PA\text{-}a_{O_2}$ was too small to return it to the awake value, which suggested that the fall of lung volume was **not** the cause of the rise of $PA\text{-}a_{O_2}$. However, two factors made this conclusion less tenable: (a) CC measurements were not made, so it was not known whether FRC actually was raised above CC; and (b) PEEP may reduce cardiac output, which could mask any improvement of $PA\text{-}a_{O_2}$ by reducing $P\bar{v}_{O_2}$ (Colgan et al 1971).

So although these results made it unlikely that the fall in FRC with induction was a major cause of gas exchange impairment, these criticisms introduced some doubt. Recent work has removed this. Bergman & Tien (1983) have measured gas exchange and closing volume during anaesthesia, and identified two groups of patients: one group's FRC was below CC, the other's was above, and gas exchange was initially worse in the first group. They applied just sufficient PEEP to take the first group's FRC just above CC. To the rest they applied PEEP of 5 cmH$_2$O. The first group's gas exchange was much more improved by PEEP than the others, with the result that the mean PA-a$_{O_2}$ *with PEEP on* was the same in both groups. This showed that gas exchange during anaesthesia was affected by CC in exactly the same way as when awake. However, gas exchange with PEEP on was *still worse than when awake*, which confirmed that there was a residual gas exchange abnormality during anaesthesia even when FRC was greater than CC.

Bergman & Tien's study can still be criticised on the grounds that cardiac output changes, which were not measured, could have masked improvement of gas exchange. We have recently (Heneghan *et al* 1984) studied the effect of raising lung volume posturally during anaesthesia, and measured cardiac output changes in the majority of the patients studied. We found no improvement of gas exchange when lung volume increased, and that changes in cardiac output could not explain this, and therefore concluded that the effect of cardiac output was not relevant to the interpretation of the data.

The conclusions at this stage are: (1) Gas exchange is affected by airway closure in exactly the same way during anaesthesia as when awake. (2) The fall in FRC with anaesthesia can only explain part of the increase of PA-a$_{O_2}$, in the unusual case where the fall of FRC increases the amount of airway closure in the tidal range. (3) There is a residual gas exchange abnormality which cannot be explained by this mechanism.

Cause of the residual gas exchange abnormality
One mechanism suggested to explain this residual abnormality is that anaesthesia alters regional distribution of ventilation by altering chest wall motion. This would alter $\dot{V}/\dot{Q}$ in the affected units, increasing PA-a$_{O_2}$.

Froese & Bryan (1974) first reported evidence supporting this: they used lateral radiography to investigate diaphragmatic motion in man, and their results are illustrated in Figure 11.5. There are changes in both end expiratory position and tidal movement during

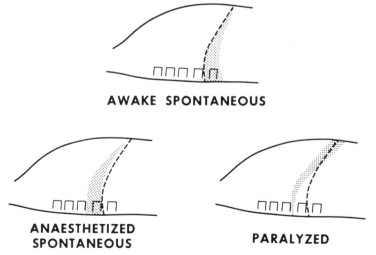

AWAKE SPONTANEOUS

ANAESTHETIZED SPONTANEOUS

PARALYZED

Fig. 11.5   The effect of anaesthesia on diaphragmatic position and motion. Dotted line: resting end-expiratory position awake. Shaded area: tidal movement of diaphragm. End-expiratory position shifts cranially with spontaneously breathing anaesthesia, but motion is little changed; both end-expiratory position and movement are substantially changed during paralysis and ventilation. (From Froese & Bryan 1974 with kind permission of the editors of *Anesthesiology*.)

anaesthesia, movement being particularly affected by mechanical ventilation. This could cause redistribution of ventilation towards the upper, less well perfused, parts of the lung, causing an impairment of gas exchange.

There are two difficulties with this explanation. First, it would be expected that the abnormality of gas exchange would be greater during mechanical ventilation, when the abnormality of diaphragmatic movement was greater, since the abnormality of regional ventilation would then be maximised. This is not so: there is no difference between the efficiency of gas exchange during spontaneous and mechanically ventilated anaesthetised patients (Nunn 1977, Bindslev et al 1981). The second difficulty is that, although changes in the vertical distribution of ventilation can be detected during anaesthesia, they are not sufficient 'to explain the alveolar arterial Po_2 difference usually observed during anaesthesia' (Hulands et al 1970). So, once more, although this appears to be a partial explanation, again it is not a complete solution.

Multiple inert gas technique
Attempts have been made to clarify the causes of the gas exchange abnormality induced by anaesthesia by means of the multiple inert gas technique (Wagner et al 1974). This technique utilises the fact that clearance of a gas by a lung unit depends upon both its solubility and the $\dot{V}/\dot{Q}$ of that unit. The precise method is too complex to be covered here, but it allows lung compartments of 50 different $\dot{V}/\dot{Q}$ values between 0 and infinity to be distinguished with reasonable confidence. This has now been applied to anaesthesia (Dueck et al 1978, 1980, Rehder et al 1979, Bindslev et al 1981), and has confirmed the impression that anaesthesia may increase the proportion of shunt, or low $\dot{V}/\dot{Q}$, or both. It has also shown (Bindslev 1981) that the distribution of $\dot{V}/\dot{Q}$ compartments during the anaesthesia with PEEP is drastically different to that when awake, which confirms the conclusion that the cause of the gas exchange abnormality is not simply the fall in FRC: if it were, then the spread of $\dot{V}/\dot{Q}$ would be the same in both conditions.

However, this technique has little more to offer in the elucidation of this problem, since it suffers from the fault of only measuring ratios of V to Q, and cannot therefore distinguish whether a reduction results from a fall in V, or a rise in Q, or both.

At this stage there are two main conclusions: (a) the fall in lung volume with induction of anaesthesia may cause impairment of gas exchange if FRC falls below CC, but this is uncommon; (b) redistribution of ventilation with a change in chest wall movement can explain part of the gas exchange abnormality. There remains a residue to be explained, and the pulmonary vasculature must now be considered.

Effect of anaesthesia on pulmonary vasculature
The most significant effect of anaesthesia on the pulmonary vasculature is that some anaesthetics have been found to inhibit hypoxic pulmonary vasoconstriction. As described above, HPV diverts blood flow away from hypoxic lung units, improving overall $\dot{V}/\dot{Q}$ matching; impairment on the reflex reverses this, reducing gas exchange efficiency. Several anaesthetic agents have been shown to block HPV, among them halothane, ether and methoxyflurane (Bjertnaes 1977, 1978), and this could contribute to the deterioration of oxygenation occurring with anaesthesia. However, this explanation is also at best a partial one, as intravenous anaesthesia with, for example, ketamine causes a fall in Pa_{O_2} (Zsigmond et al 1976, Rust et al 1978), but ketamine has no direct effect upon HPV (Bjertnaes 1977). Ketamine must therefore be causing the fall in Pa_{O_2} by another mechanism.

Other vascular theories have included the idea that anaesthesia could impair gas exchange by reducing pulmonary arterial pressure and thus adversely affecting the distribution of pulmonary perfusion and hence $\dot{V}/\dot{Q}$ matching. This is not the case: Price et al (1969) showed that halothane anaesthesia in man reduced Pa_{O_2} without altering pulmonary arterial pressure.

Finally, recent reports on the new respiratory stimulant drug Almitrine may require us to revise our thinking on the mechanisms of hypoxic pulmonary vasoconstriction. This has always been thought to be solely a local reflex, but evidence is appearing which suggests that Almitrine enhances HPV (Romaldini et al 1983, Melot et al 1983), and that it does so only when the carotid body is intact (de Backer et al, in press). The respiratory stimulant action of this drug is probably mediated by an increase in the rate of afferent impulses from the carotid body (Labrid, in press) and these facts together suggest that HPV may be modified by alterations in the afferent traffic from the carotid body. The significance of this is that anaesthetics can reduce the afferent traffic from the carotid body (Davies et al 1982), and could be interfering with HPV at a distance from the normally accepted site of action. Therefore the effect of anaesthetics on HPV in, for example, isolated lung may be irrelevant. This, however, is speculation at present.

CONCLUSIONS

A complete understanding of the cause of the deterioration of gas exchange during anaesthesia has not yet been achieved. Contributory factors have been found to include: (1) The fall in lung volume on induction of anaesthesia, if it reduces FRC below CC. (2) An alteration in regional distribution of ventilation, caused by changes in chest wall function. (3) Local inhibition of hypoxic pulmonary vasoconstriction redistributing blood flow to under-ventilated regions. It is not yet clear whether these factors are sufficient in total to explain the observed gas exchange abnormalities. A further possibility has recently arisen, that anaesthesia impairs distant enhancement of HPV via the carotid body.

REFERENCES

Bergman N A, Tien YK 1983 Contribution of the closure of pulmonary units to impaired oxygenation during anaesthesia. *Anesthesiology* **59:** 395–401

Bindslev L, Hedenstierna G, Santesson J, Gottlieb I, Carvallhas A 1981 Ventilation perfusion distribution during inhalational anaesthesia. Effects of spontaneous breathing, mechanical ventilation and positive and expiratory pressure. *Acta Anaesthesiologica Scandanavica* **25:** 360–371

Bjertnaes L J 1977 Hypoxia-induced vasoconstriction in isolated perfused lungs exposed to injectable or inhalational anaesthetics. *Acta Anaesthesiologica Scandanavica* **21:** 133–147

Bjertnaes L J 1978 Hypoxia-induced vasoconstriction in man: inhibition due to diethyl ether and halothane anaesthesia. *Acta Anaesthesiologica Scandanavica* **22:** 570–588

Campbell E J M, Nunn J F, Peckett B W 1958 A comparison of artificial ventilation and spontaneous respiration with particular reference to ventilation-blood flow relationships. *British Journal of Anaesthesia* **30:** 166–175

Cheney F W, Colley P S 1980 The effect of cardiac output on arterial blood oxygenation. *Anesthesiology* **52:** 496–503

Colgan F J, Barrow R E, Fanning G L 1971 Constant positive pressure breathing and cardio-respiratory function. *Anesthesiology* **34:** 145–151

Craig D B, Wahba W M, Don H F, Couture J G, Becklake M R 1971 'Closing volume' and its relationship to gas exchange in seated and supine positions. *Journal of Applied Physiology* **31:** 717–721

Dantzker D R, Wagner P D, West J B 1975 Instability of lung units with low V_A/Q ratios during O_2 breathing. *Journal of Applied Physiology* **38:** 886–895

de Backer W, Bogaert E, van Maele R, Vermeire P (in press) Effect of almitrine bismesylate on arterial blood gases and ventilatory drive in patients with severe chronic airflow obstruction and bilateral carotid body resection. Proceedings of Societas Europa Pneumologica, supplement to *European Journal of Respiratory Diseases*

Davies R O, Edwards McI W, Lahiri S 1982 Halothane depresses the response of carotid body chemoreceptors to hypoxia and hypercapnia in the cat. *Anesthesiology* **57**: 153–159

Dueck R, Rathburn M, Wagner P D 1978 Chromatographic analysis of multiple tracer inert gases in the presence of anesthetic gases. *Anesthesiology* **49**: 31–36

Dueck R, Young I, Clausen J, Wagner P D 1980 Altered distribution of pulmonary ventilation and blood flow following induction of inhalational anesthesia. *Anesthesiology* **52**: 113–125

Froese A B, Bryan A C 1974 Effects of anaesthesia and paralysis on diphragmatic mechanics in man. *Anesthesiology* **41**: 242–255

Harris E A, Kenyon A M, Nisbet H D, Seelye E R, Whitlock R M L 1974 The normal alveolar-arterial oxygen tension gradient in man. *Clinical Science and Molecular Medicine* **46**: 89–104

Heneghan C P H, Bergman N A, Jones J G 1984 Changes in lung volume and $(P_{A_{O_2}} - P_{a_{O_2}})$ during anaesthesia. *British Journal of Anaesthesia* **56**: 437–445

Hewlett A M, Hulands G H, Nunn J F, Milledge J S 1974 Functional residual capacity during anaesthesia. III Artificial ventilation. *British Journal of Anaesthesia* **46**: 495–503

Hickey R F, Visick W D, Fairlie H B, Fourcade H E 1973 Effects of halothane anesthesia on functional residual capacity and alveolar-arterial oxygen tension difference. *Anesthesiology* **38**: 20–24

Hulands G H, Greene R, Iliff L D, Nunn J F 1970 Influence of anaesthesia on the regional distribution of perfusion and ventilation in the lung. *Clinical Science* **38**: 451–460

Juno P, Marsh H M, Knopp T J, Rehder K 1978 Closing capacity in awake and anesthetised-paralysed man. *Journal of Applied Physiology* **44**: 238–244

Labrid C (in press) Almitrine bismesylate: a pharmacological review. Proceedings of Societas Europa Pneumologica, supplement to *European Journal of Respiratory Diseases*

Lenfant C 1963 Measurement of ventilation/perfusion distribution with alveolar-arterial differences. *Journal of Applied Physiology* **18**: 1090–1094

Melot C, Naeije R, Rothschild T, Mertens P, Mols P, Hallemans R 1983 Improvement in ventilation perfusion matching by almitrine in COPD. *Chest* **83**: 528–533

Nunn J F 1977 *Applied respiratory physiology*, 2nd edn. Butterworths, London, p 435

Nunn J F 1980 Anesthesia and the lung. *Anesthesiology* **52**: 1027–1028

Nunn J F, Bergman N A, Coleman A J 1965 Factors influencing the arterial oxygen tension during anaesthesia with artificial ventilation. *British Journal of Anaesthesia* **37**: 898–914

Pease R D, Benumof J L, Trousdale F R 1982 $P_{A_{O_2}}$ and $P\bar{v}_{O_2}$ have both direct and indirect effects on hypoxic pulmonary vasoconstriction. *Anesthesiology* **55**: 380

Price H L, Cooperman L H, Warden J C, Morris J J, Smith T C 1969 Pulmonary hemodynamics during general anesthesia in man. *Anesthesiology* **30**: 629–635

Rehder K, Knopp T J, Sessler A D, Didier E P 1979 Ventilation perfusion relationship in young healthy awake and anesthetised-paralysed man. *Journal of Applied Physiology* **47**: 745–753

Romaldini H, Rodriguez-Roisin R, Wagner P D, West J B 1983 Enhancement of hypoxic pulmonary vasoconstriction by almitrine in the dog. *American Review of Respiratory Diseases* **126**: 288–293

Rust M, Landauer B, Kolb E 1978 Stellenwert von Ketamin in Nottfallsituation. *Anaesthesist* **27**: 205–212

Schmid E E, Rehder K 1981 General anesthesia and the chest wall. *Anesthesiology* **55**: 668–675

Wagner P D, Lavaruso R B, Uhl R R, West J B 1974 Continuous distribution of ventilation perfusion ratios in normal subjects breathing air and 100% O_2. *The Journal of Clinical Investigation* **54**: 54–68

Webb S J S, Nunn J F 1967 A comparison between the effect of nitrous oxide and nitrogen on arterial P_{O_2}. *Anaesthesia* **22**: 69–81

Weenig C S, Pietak S, Hickey R F, Fairley H B 1973 Relationship of preoperative closing volume to functional residual capacity and alveolar arterial-oxygen difference during anesthesia with controlled ventilation. *Anesthesiology* **41**: 3–7

West J B 1970 *Ventilation/blood flow and gas exchange*, 2nd edn. Blackwells, Oxford, p 33

Wyche M Q, Teichner R L, Kallos T, Marshall B E, Smith T C 1973 Effects of continuous positive pressure breathing on functional residual capacity and arterial oxygenation during intra-abdominal operations: studies in man during nitrous oxide and d-tubocurarine anesthesia. *Anesthesiology* **38**: 68–74

Zsigmond E K, Matsuki A, Kothary S P, Jallad M 1976 Arterial hypoxaemia caused by intravenous ketamine. *Anesthesia and Analgesia* **55**: 311–314

Obstetric anaesthesia

Anaesthetists are extending their role in obstetric units, being involved in pain relief in labour and maternal and neonatal intensive care, as well as anaesthesia for operative deliveries. There have been many interesting developments and some of these will be reviewed.

PAIN RELIEF IN LABOUR

Systemic analgesics

Narcotics such as pethidine continue to be used as their administration is simple and accepted for use by unsupervised midwives. They are used particularly in units where regional anaesthetic methods are not always available and for patients unwilling to accept epidural blockade but who require some analgesia, often after relative failure of natural child-birth methods. The pain relief is often poor and side effects such as drowsiness, dysphoria and nausea and vomiting are common. Improved results may be obtained with a patient-controlled intravenous administration system such as the Cardiff palliator rather than conventional intermittent intramuscular injections.

Pethidine may produce depression of the newborn and this is particularly likely to occur if there are obstetric complications or other central depressant drugs are used concurrently. Respiratory depression can be reversed by neonatal naloxone, but subtler effects are more difficult to evaluate. Kuhnert *et al* (1980) have shown that the neonate excretes more unaltered pethidine and less norpethidine than the adult, suggesting that its N-demethylation mechanisms are less effective. The neonate may show lower neuro-behavioural scores for at least 2–3 days after birth. Tomson *et al* (1982) measured maternal plasma levels of pethidine after a dose of $1 \cdot 5$ mg per kg intramuscularly, and showed that they reached a peak concentration of 300–650 ng/ml about 60 minutes after administration. The fetal/maternal ratios varied from $0 \cdot 35$–$1 \cdot 5$ and correlated with the dose delivery interval. Fetal plasma levels of pethidine reached a maximum 1–5 hours after maternal administration, and this is the usual time for neonatal depression to occur. Weiner *et al* (1979) compared bupivacaine epidurals with naloxone-reversed pethidine and showed that the pethidine group had as good neurobehavioural scores. However, all the changes were insignificant as not to be detected by a paediatrician during routine examination.

Inhalational analgesia

Enflurane in concentrations varying from $0 \cdot 25$–$1 \cdot 25\%$ in oxygen has been shown by Abboud *et al* (1981) to produce equivalent analgesia to 40% N_2O. Stefani *et al* (1982) showed that neither 30% N_2O nor $0 \cdot 3$–$0 \cdot 8\%$ enflurane produced any effect on neurobehavioural patterns, and enflurane might have a place as an analgesic for labour pain. Clark *et al* (1979) studied the effects of maternal methoxyflurane on renal function in the neonate and showed significant increases in inorganic fluoride, which decreased more slowly in the neonate than in the mother. However, there were no changes in serum values for urea, creatinine, uric acid, osmolality, sodium, potassium or chloride indicative of gross renal dysfunction. Difficulty is being experienced in obtaining servicing for methoxyflurane Cardiff inhalers and it would appear that this agent, as an obstetric analgesic, is about to take its place in the history books.

Transcutaneous nerve stimulation

A controlled study of transcutaneous nerve stimulation for pain relief in labour, carried out by Nesheim (1981) failed to show any analgesic effect. The same number of patients in each group required other methods of analgesia, and similar pain scores were produced by transcutaneous nerve stimulation or a sham technique. It seems that the more severe nature of the pain explains the differences between the results in labour compared with the treatment of chronic pain.

Epidural analgesia

Epidural technique

Some improvements in epidural technique to raise further the success rate by Evans (1982) who described the Oxford epidural space detector, a polypropylene syringe which is filled with 4 ml of air and has a low-friction piston. A rubber strap applies a fixed pressure of 75 mm Hg, and when the tip of the epidural needle reaches the epidural space the piston advances automatically. It can be used only when the needle tip is in the ligamentum flavum and therefore does not help in the identification of this ligament which is often the most difficult and essential part of the technique.

Debate continues as to whether air or saline is the preferable material for the loss of resistance test. In this context Naulty *et al* (1982) showed that air embolism, detected using a Doppler over the 4th right intercostal space parasternally, occurred during the establishment of epidural catheters in 8 out of 17 patients. In one of the patients the hanging-drop technique was used while in the other 7 the method was loss of resistance to air. Air embolism can occur if there is an open vein and the venous pressure is less than the pressure of the air source. Macdonald (1983) described 4 dural taps in approximately 250 epidurals when air was used (an incidence of 1·6%) and only 15 taps in 5435 epidurals with the saline technique (0·3%). It does appear that saline is safer and more effective than air. The only disadvantage of saline is that confusion may arise occasionally as to whether any fluid issuing from the epidural needle or catheter is cerebrospinal fluid or injected saline.

A useful test to identify false loss of resistance due to cavities in the interspinous ligament or the passage of the needle into the paraspinal tissues has been described by Wilson *et al* (1983). Pressure is applied to the paraspinal muscles; if the epidural needle tip lies superficially to the ligamentum flavum, the resistance to injection will rise, whereas if it lies within the vertebral canal there will not be any change.

Factors affecting spread

Various factors thought to affect the spread of solutions in the epidural space have been evaluated. Crawford & Chester (1949) first suggested that local anaesthetics spread further in the pregnant than the non-pregnant patient and this was confirmed by Bromage (1962). Fagraens *et al* (1983) have shown that local anaesthetics spread further even in early pregnancy than in the non-pregnant state. Using 2% lignocaine with adrenaline they showed that the pregnant patient required 1 ml per segment to be blocked compared to 1·35 ml in the non-pregnant or an average of 20·5 ml for complete spread of analgesia compared to 28·3 ml. Bromage (1961) suggested that epidural injections should not be made during uterine contractions when lumbar epidural pressure rises, as exaggerated spread may occur. However, Sivakumaran et al (1982) have refuted this observation.

The effect of maternal posture on the extent of blockade has also been reviewed. Rickford & Reynolds (1983) using 6–8 ml of 0·5% bupivacaine, could not show any significant differences in onset or duration of blockade, or need for supplements, when injections were made in the lateral or supine positions. Motor block was greater in the lateral position, but this was not felt to be a sufficient disadvantage to counterbalance the adverse circulatory effects of the supine position. An excellent study was published by Thorburn & Moir (1981) who compared 6–8 ml 0·5%, 10–14 ml 0·25% and 6–8 ml 0·25% bupivacaine. Both 6–8 ml 0·5% and 10–14 ml 0·25% produced a higher percentage of complete pain relief in the first stage of labour than 6–8 ml 0·25% (72–74% versus 59%) and the 0·5% produced a higher number of patients with complete pain relief at delivery (64% versus 38–46%). There was no significant difference in the incidence of spontaneous vaginal deliveries between 0·5% (32%) and 10–14 ml of 0·25% (39%), but the low volume of 0·25% produced a higher rate (53%). Motor weakness was initially greater with the 0·5% and the high volume of 0·25%, but by the time the patient had received several 'top ups' there were no significant differences. Postpartum retention of urine was higher in the group receiving 0·5%.

Two studies from Queen Charlotte's Hospital by Morgan et al (1982) and Morgan et al (1982) have looked at the effectiveness of pain relief and maternal satisfaction and have confirmed that epidural analgesia is the best method, although a very low percentage (35%) had complete freedom from pain. However, their scores were made for the entire labour, and not just for the period when analgesia was provided. The mothers not receiving any analgesia had the greater satisfaction, but they probably had the shorter, easier labours, the epidural group often having induction and augmentation of labour and assisted delivery. They confirm that effective analgesia does not necessarily ensure a satisfactory experience. It is apparent that even when epidural analgesia is used, consideration must be given to the surroundings of the mother in labour, the attitudes and compassion of the staff and her partner, and her concepts, desires and expectations for her confinement.

Missed segments
The occasional occurrence of missed segments, particularly pain persisting in the right groin, is a problem. De Campo et al (1980) have suggested that it is due to failure of the local anaesthetic to reach a concentration sufficient to block the particular nerve roots, rather than an anatomical barrier to the spread of the solution. Roberts (1972) postulated that increased afferent input may be caused by stretching of the round ligaments. Thus the treatment of the missed segment is to increase the concentration and volume of local anaesthetic administered, provided always that there is clear evidence that the catheter is within the epidural space. Usubiaga et al (1970) and Doughty (1974) have suggested that only 2–3 cm of epidural catheter should be left in the space to reduce the incidence of unsatisfactory blocks which may result from the catheter tip emerging from an intervertebral foramen or passing round to the anterior part of the space.

Intermittent injections or continuous infusions
There is interest in using continuous infusions of local anaesthetic rather than intermittent

injections into the epidural space. Continuous infusions might reduce the need for 'top ups', and it is hoped that more consistent levels of analgesia could be maintained with greater cardiovascular stability. Davies & Fettes (1981) have used an Intraflo to infuse 5–7 ml $0 \cdot 5\%$ bupivacaine per hour following an initial test dose and 10 ml $0 \cdot 25\%$ bupivacaine. Seventy per cent of the mothers were pain-free for 2–13 hours, 22% required one additional bolus, 8% several additional boluses, and 8% had significant hypotension. Although the results are somewhat better, there remains a need for constant and close supervision of the mother. There will always be a very small risk of the catheter perforating the dura so that the infusion becomes intrathecal, and high spinal anaesthesia might result. If infusions are to be used, it seems safer to use lower concentrations of bupivacaine such as $0 \cdot 1$–$0 \cdot 125\%$ so that earlier warning of spinal block is obtained.

The effect on uterine contractions

Early studies by Tyack *et al* (1973), Lowensohn *et al* (1974) and Raabe & Belfrage (1976) suggested that epidural analgesia was followed by a significant decrease in uterine contractions lasting for about 30 minutes. However, local anaesthetics such as lignocaine or prilocaine had been used often in adrenaline-containing solutions and the importance of avoiding aortocaval compression was not always appreciated. Schellenberg (1977) showed that in the absence of aortocaval compression, bupivacaine epidurals are associated with minimal and insignificant decreases in uterine contractions, the amplitude rather than the frequency being the parameter affected. They confirmed the regularising effect of epidural analgesia on inco-ordinate uterine action, described by Moir & Willocks (1968).

Breech delivery and multiple pregnancy

Studies by Crawford (1974), Donnai & Nicholas (1975), Breeson *et al* (1978), Bowen-Simpkins & Fergusson (1974), Weekes *et al* (1977) and James *et al* (1977) have confirmed the safety and indeed advisability of using lumbar epidural blocks for breech and twin presentations. It allows prompt obstetric intervention, should it become necessary, without the need for hurried and unplanned general anaesthesia with its inherent risks. Although the second stage of labour may be prolonged, there is no increase in the number of assisted deliveries or breech extractions, the condition of the infant, as judged by fetal scalp sampling and Apgar scores, is improved, and perinatal mortality is reduced.

Previous Caesarean sections

Uppington (1983) has reviewed the use of epidural analgesia in patients with previous Caesarean section, and advocates it provided that the scar is transverse in the lower segment and that vaginal delivery is considered safe and possible. Effective analgesia may enable the scar to be palpated more effectively. It is wise to use the weakest concentration of local anaesthetic agent that will produce analgesia, to avoid oxytocic drugs, and to monitor intensively the mother and baby.

Fetal heart rate monitoring

Yeh *et al* (1982) have shown that fetal monitoring leads to a reduction in intrapartum fetal death, but to an increase in Caesarean section rate. This may be due to the monitoring itself, or merely due to the selection of patients being monitored. It has been suggested that all patients having epidural analgesia should have concomitant fetal heart rate monitoring. Maltau (1975) confirmed that bupivacaine epidurals have minimal effect on the fetal heart rate, provided that hypotension is prevented or energetically treated. Colli showed that preloading with 1 litre of Hartmann's solution prior to administration of 10 ml 0·375% bupivacaine reduced fetal heart rate abn 34% to 12%, and the incidence of maternal hypotension from 28% to 2%. Lavin *et al* (1980), have suggested that provided hypotension is avoided, then any fetal heart rate changes should be investigated by the obstetrician in the normal way, and not assumed to be due to the epidural. It is unlikely that local anaesthetic agents in the doses used clinically would produce direct effects on the fetal myocardium, and a much more common reason for fetal heart rate changes is overstimulation of the uterus or obstetric abnormality such as disproportion or placental insufficiency.

The treatment of dural puncture

There will always be a small incidence of dural puncture headaches following attempted epidural anaesthesia, and a larger incidence after spinal anaesthesia. The use of epidural blood patch continues to be debated. Ostheimer *et al* (1974) showed that the use of 10 ml of autologous blood produced over 90% success rate, curing the headache within 1 hour. However, Heyman *et al* (1982) have shown that the larger the volume of blood administered, the greater the incidence of transient symptoms, such as backache, neckache, paraesthesiae in the legs and toes, and cramps in the lower abdomen. Ravindran *et al* (1981) have shown that pushing during the second stage does not influence the incidence of spinal headache. In the present medicolegal climate in relation to forceps delivery, as highlighted by the Whitehouse v Jordan and another case (1980) it seems unwise to alter the obstetric management following a dural puncture. Occasional major neurological complications have followed dural punctures. Newrick & Read (1982) described two cases of intracranial subdural haematoma following spinal anaesthesia. and emphasised the need for constant vigilance, so that persistent or worsening headache is fully investigated. In a similar context, Siegle *et al* (1982) described a patient who had a persistent headache, and developed cerebral infarction following spinal anaesthesia for Caeserean section.

Epidural opioids

Pain relief in labour

Information continues to accumulate about the possible use of spinal opiates in obstetrics. Their site of action appears to be mainly in the posterior horns of the spinal cord and, thus, if injected into the epidural space, they must cross the dura and arachnoid mater or their spinal nerve extensions. The more lipid soluble drugs, such as fentanyl, diamorphine or pethidine appear to cross more readily than morphine. Husemeyer *et al* (1980) studied 2 mg morphine in 8 ml normal saline epidurally, and concluded that it did not provide effective analgesia. Writer *et al* (1981) compared morphine 2 mg–3·5 mg in dextrose with bupivacaine in a double blind trial and found that only 2 out of 8 patients received satisfactory analgesia compared with 100% analgesia with bupivacaine.

Nybell-Lindahl *et al* (1981) gave 4–6 mg morphine in 10 ml normal saline and produced pain relief in only 4 out of 20 patients. Significant blood levels of morphine were achieved, and there could be risks to the fetus if it were delivered rapidly. It seems that epidural morphine alone does not produce adequate analgesia for labour.

Justins *et al* (1982) added either 80 μg fentanyl or saline in a 4 ml volume to bupivacaine epidural solutions. Only 23% of the fentanyl group required supplemental bupivacaine compared with 79% of the saline controls. The fentanyl-bupivacaine patients had a shorter ɹnset time and a longer duration of analgesia than the saline-bupivacaine group, but 23% complained of itching. In another study Justins et al (1983) gave 36 patients a test dose of bupivacaine, and then either epidural or intramuscular fentanyl (100 µg in 2 ml). Sixty-two per cent in the intramuscular group required supplemental bupivacaine in the first hour compared with only 16% in the epidural group. These studies suggest that opiate/local anaesthetic combinations may reduce the amount of bupivacaine required and merit further study. (See chapter by Dr L Kaufman.)

Postoperative analgesia

Several studies have assessed the effects of epidural morphine for postCaesarean section analgesia. Coombs et al (1982) found 2 mg doses to be no better than placebo, while 4.5 mg in 10 ml normal saline gave analgesia for a mean of 26.7 hours. Youngstrom et al (1982) comparing epidural and intramuscular morphine 4 mg, found that the epidural group had a longer onset time, but less pain, a longer duration of analgesia for about 24 hours and lower blood levels (12.5 ng per ml versus 24.8 ng per ml). The addition of adrenaline to epidural morphine did not prolong analgesia. Carmichael et al (1982) confirmed these results, and showed that doubling the epidural morphine dose contributed little extra to the analgesia. Pruritis was again a problem occurring in 90% of the patients and increased in severity with higher doses. It would appear that epidural opiates can produce satisfactory pain relief after Caesarean section. However, pruritis is a common side effect, and there remains the risk of respiratory depression, which may be delayed, so that spinal opioids should only be used when the level of patient supervision is high.

Subarachnoid opioids

Bonnardot et al (1982) studied intrathecal morphine and concluded that, in contrast to epidural morphine, it can produce adequate analgesia for labour, and at a plasma concentration of less than 6 ng per ml. As about 30 ng per ml is required for systemic analgesia, it does seem to confirm a direct spinal action of the drug. However, the disadvantage of dural puncture makes it an unattractive method and it does not seem to offer a reasonable alternative to epidural local anaesthesia.

Epidural analgesia

The effects on the newborn

Thalme et al (1974) stated that epidural anaesthesia causes the least metabolic acidosis, and that provided hypotension is avoided no harmful effects on the baby will result. Lieberman et al (1979) failed to show differences from a control group. However Rosenblatt et al (1981) showed minor neurobehavioural effects following 10–14 ml 0.375% bupivacaine. Corke et al (1982) showed that even 2 minutes of hypotension alters maternal and neonatal acid-base values, but that it needs a longer period to produce neurobehavioural changes.

Treatment of hypotension

Fluid preloading and correct posture to avoid aortocaval compression are used widely to prevent hypotension following spinal and epidural anaesthesia. Ralston et al (1974), studying the pregnant ewe, showed that ephedrine is the vasopressor of choice, as it increases maternal blood pressure by 50% while uterine blood flow remained unaltered. All other vasopressors studied reduced uterine blood flow by 20–62% with detrimental effects on the fetus. Datta et al (1982) have stressed again that hypotension should be treated promptly with ephedrine to improve the neonate and also to reduce the incidence of maternal nausea and vomiting during Caesarean section. Rolbin *et al* (1982) have confirmed that prophylactic intramuscular ephedrine is unnecessary, as it does not reduce the incidence of hypotension, but occasionally produces persistent maternal hypertension and a consequent decrease in umbilical artery pH.

Placental transfer of bupivacaine
Bupivacaine produces a low fetal/maternal ratio of about 0.3. Kuhnert *et al* (1981) have supposed that while this may result from decreased placental transfer due to high protein binding, it may also be due to an increased uptake by fetal tissues. Bupivacaine and its metabolite 2-6 pipedolylxylidine (PPX) persist in neonatal body fluids for several days suggesting considerable uptake by fetal tissues.

Instrumental deliveries
Interest continues on the effect of epidural analgesia on the incidence of instrumental deliveries. Beynon (1957) showed that early pushing does not lead to a shorter second stage. Maresh *et al* (1983) advocates not pushing with epidural analgesia until the head has descended and is visible at the vulva. The second stage can continue as long as there is progress and no evidence of fetal distress. Delaying pushing does not usually cause a deterioration of fetal heart rate, umbilical cord pH or Apgar scores, but is associated with an increase in spontaneous delivery. It is often suggested that epidural blocks should not be 'topped up' for the second stage, as this increases the rate of instrumental deliveries. However, Phillips & Thomas (1983) have shown that the maintenance of selective epidural analgesia throughout the second stage was associated with much less pain, no prolongation of labour, no increase in the total dose of bupivacaine, and that in fact the forceps rate was lower with fewer persistent malrotations. It appears that in most units the use of epidural analgesia is associated with a small increase in the incidence of instrumental deliveries, but that this is due to the beliefs of midwives and obstetricians more than to a true effect of epidural analgesia. The mother may have to choose between a painless second stage and a slightly increased chance of forceps delivery, or a painful second stage with a spontaneous delivery.

Intravenous infusions—glucose administration
Kenepp *et al* (1982) and Mendiola *et al* (1982) have pointed out that excessive administration of glucose to the mother may lead to neonatal hypoglycaemia and hyperbilirubinaemia. Dextrose should be limited to 8 g per hour and crystalloid used in its place whenever possible. Neonatal hypoglycaemia correlated with maternal glucose levels above 120 mg per dl. All the babies that were hypoglycaemic had insulin levels above 40 milliunits per ml. Datta *et al* (1982) agreed that maternal glucose levels should be kept in the range of 90–120 mg per dl, and that dextrose-containing solutions should not be used for volume expansion. Strict control of maternal glucose levels and the avoidance of hypotension should allow neonates of diabetic mothers to be born in optimal condition, with normal acid-base values and no risk of hypoglycaemia.

Epidural anaesthesia for Caesarean section
Epidural anaesthesia for Caesarean section continues to increase in popularity and Morgan *et al* (1983) claim that it is the preferred technique. Craft *et al* (1982) have shown that sensory blockade should extend to the 4th thoracic segment. This will provide the most effective analgesia and adequate abdominal wall relaxation to enable the surgeon to operate gently and

without the need for much retraction or abdominal packs. Crawford (1980) has also stressed the importance of extensive blockade, the added benefit of high oxygen concentrations and the reduction in nausea and vomiting associated with the substitution of syntocinon for ergometrine, all factors known to improve the success rate.

In the United Kingdom the use of supplementary systemic analgesia or sedation is kept to a minimum, as it is accepted that it may remove the essential advantage of the technique, which is the avoidance of the risk of inhalation of gastric contents. Morgan *et al* (1983) showed that following sedation 10% of mothers lost awareness. If this happens at the time of the delivery they will not participate in the birth, a factor which many mothers and fathers believe to be very important. Davis (1982) has suggested that regional anaesthesia could be used for still more Caesarean sections. Patient unwillingness, especially after long, painful labours, must be respected as must other absolute contraindications such as severe haemorrhage or coagulopathy. Technical difficulties and communication problems must also be taken into account, as well as the mother's personality. Time factors are often stressed as a reason for general anaesthesia, but in fact it is fairly unusual for the decision delivery interval to be less than one hour, and if spinal anaesthesia is included as part of the armamentarium then the general anaesthetic rate for Caesarean section could be reduced to about 20%.

Morgan *et al* (1983) carried out an audit of junior anaesthetic staff and showed that more serious difficulties resulted from general anaesthesia than from the use of epidural anaesthesia, including failed intubation, awareness and abnormal reactions to anaesthetic agents. In the epidural group, hypotension and inadequate analgesia and occasional unawareness were the problems. It was concluded that the complications of epidural anaesthesia were more easily managed and therefore that it was safer than general anaesthesia in the hands of trainees.

A recent study by Abboud *et al* (1983) has confirmed a lack of adverse effects of the technique on the newborn.

Local anaesthetic agents

Choice of agent

Interest has continued in the choice of local anaesthetic agents. Bupivacaine remains the most widely used due to excellent sensory analgesia, long duration and low placental transfer. James *et al* (1980) have shown that 3% 2-chloroprocaine produces the most rapid onset of analgesia, but is associated with a three-fold increase in the need for treatment of hypotension and a duration of action of only about 45 minutes. 2-Chloroprocaine, etidocaine and $0 \cdot 75\%$ bupivacaine are not currently available for obstetric anaesthesia in the United Kingdom. One per cent etidocaine has been shown by Datta *et al* (1980) to produce inadequate sensory analgesia and considerable motor block. Bupivacaine $0 \cdot 75\%$, although producing a short onset time, results in excessive motor block and a longer stay in the recovery room, as well as being potentially more cardiotoxic if injected intravenously accidentally.

Neurotoxicity

Further information has become available about the local and systemic toxicity of local anaesthetic agents. Neurological complications have occurred following inadvertent spinal anaesthesia with large volumes of 3% 2-chloroprocaine and have been described by Ravindran *et al* (1980) and reviewed by Covino *et al* (1980). These complications may be due to the acidic pH of $2 \cdot 7$–$4 \cdot 0$. Covino *et al* (1980) have suggested that a large test dose should be used and sufficient time allowed for its real evaluation, that injection of a large single dose be avoided, and that fractional doses through the catheter would be safer. If a dural puncture has occurred, then local anaesthetics with low pH should be avoided. If a full dose is injected intrathecally the subarachnoid space should be irrigated with preservative-free normal saline within 15–20 minutes, after withdrawal of as much cerebrospinal fluid as possible.

Systemic toxicity
Albright (1979) and Marx (1984) have reviewed the potential cardiotoxicity of bupivacaine and etidocaine, which do appear to be more cardiotoxic at high blood levels than other local anaesthetics. De Jong *et al* (1982), using intravenous infusions of long-acting local anaesthetics in animals, have produced nodal and ventricular arrhythmias before or at the onset of seizures, phenomena not seen with lignocaine. It may be that long-acting local anaesthetics have a specific arrythmogenic action. These arrhythmias, and even ventricular fibrillation, can occur even in the absence of hypoxia, hypercarbia or hyperkalaemia, and may be difficult to reverse. Complications can be reduced by fractionation of the dose of local anaesthetic, using 30 mg increments of bupivacaine, waiting 2 minutes, and looking for signs of systemic toxicity before continuing the injection, or by adding adrenaline 5 μg per ml to the test dose to identify intravascular injection. Facilities and equipment for immediate and prolonged resuscitation must be available. It seems proven that bupivacaine is more cardiotoxic than lignocaine, and thus 0·75% bupivacaine is no longer recommended for obstetric patients.

GENERAL ANAESTHETIC TECHNIQUES

Prophylaxis against regurgitation and aspiration
In *Anaesthetic Review 2* there was a detailed discussion on regurgitation and aspiration by Cotton & Smith (1984). Studies by Lahiri *et al* (1973) and Gibbs *et al* (1981) have led to the tendency to replace magnesium trisilicate mixture with 0·3 M sodium citrate. Heaney & Jones (1979) have shown that aspiration of magnesium trisilicate into the lungs may be associated with an acid aspiration syndrome. Gibbs *et al* (1979) suggested that sodium citrate, being non-particulate, was less likely to cause damage if inhaled. Only one dose is required compared to the two-hourly administration recommended for magnesium trisilicate. Holdsworth *et al* (1980) noted a further advantage that sodium citrate mixes better with gastric contents.

Investigations continue into the use of histamine H_2 receptor antagonist drugs to block acid secretion. They do not seem to have any systemic effects on uterine activity or on the fetus, and following detailed study of cimetidine, interest has focused on the newer compound ranitidine. Andrews *et al* (1982) gave 150 mg ranitidine orally the night before and the morning of anaesthesia to surgical patients resulting in gastric volumes less than 25 ml in 90% of patients, and gastric pH greater than 2·5 in all subjects. Studies by Durrant & Strunin (1982), Morison *et al* (1982) and McAuley *et al* (1983) have shown that ranitidine is as effective as cimetidine when given intravenously, but rather more effective when given orally. Daumann *et al* (1982) showed that the effect of ranitidine intravenously comes on in about 4–5 minutes, and lasts for about 6 hours, which seems to give it a longer duration of action than cimetidine.

Induction of anaesthesia
Induction has become rather standardised. A large majority advocate preoxygenation, a sleep

dose of thiopentone, cricoid pressure, paralysis with suxamethonium, and rapid intubation. However, there remain a minority (Green 1978) who feel that it is inappropriate to use suxamethonium, a drug known to raise intragastric pressure, and that it is preferable to intubate following a large dose of non-depolarising relaxant with the patient in a 30-degree head-up tilt.

Inhalational agents and oxygen concentration

It is often stated that halothane has a greater relaxant effect on uterine muscle than other inhalational anaesthetic agents, but a study by Munson & Embro (1977) on isolated human uterine muscle has shown that 0·5 and 1·5 MAC of halothane, enflurane and isoflurane caused an equal decrease in contractility. It is usual practice to supplement nitrous oxide with a low concentration of an inhalational anaesthetic agent, to allow high oxygen concentrations without risking awareness. High oxygen concentrations are desirable for all Caesarean sections and high-risk vaginal deliveries. Rorke et al (1968) stressed the need for an inspired oxygen concentration of about 66% to maximise fetal oxygenation and decrease acidosis in the newborn, and this has been confirmed by Ramanathan et al (1982), who failed to show the plateau and decline in fetal oxygenation previously described with higher oxygen percentages. Hyperventilation should not be used as a means of preventing awareness, as hypocapnoea results in fetal metabolic and respiratory acidosis, probably due to a decrease in placental blood flow, secondary to vasoconstriction or decreased cardiac output. Levinson et al (1974) suggested aiming for normocapnoea, which at term is about 4 kPa (30 mmHg).

Muscle relaxants

The new muscle relaxants have been studied. Flynn et al (1982) gave atracurium 0·3 mg per kg to 12 patients following suxamethonium for intubation. While 9 patients needed increments, only 3 required reversal with neostigmine. Cardiovascular stability was marked and they confirmed that atracurium has insignificant placental transfer, and that the neonates were unaffected. Vecuronium has been administered in doses of 50–80 µg per kg by Demetriou et al (1982) and Baraka et al (1983). There was minimal placental transfer, probably half as much as with pancuronium, the umbilical vein/maternal vein ratio averaging about 11% and uninfluenced by the induction delivery interval. It is possible that the low fetal blood levels reflect extensive fetal uptake.

MATERNAL MORTALITY

The triennial confidential enquiry into maternal deaths in England and Wales for the years 1976–1978 has been published by the DHSS (1982) and reviewed by Hunter & Moir (1983). Thirty deaths were associated directly with anaesthesia, and in 11 patients inhalation of gastric contents was the direct cause of death.

In 16 patients difficulty with intubation was the primary cause. The importance of the pre-anaesthetic assessment of the mother to predict possible difficulties with intubation is well recognised. A failed intubation drill, such as that of Tunstall (1980), must be put into operation as quickly as possible when intubation is impossible, and the anaesthetist should be prepared to abandon a difficult intubation at an early stage. No criticism should be attributed to failure to intubate, but only at persisting unnecessarily. Five deaths were due to inadequate management of blood loss, and there is a need for more intense monitoring of obstetric patients. A severe haemorrhage management policy should be defined, and blood must be available for blood transfusion when required. Although Penney (1982) showed that 86% of blood cross-matched for obstetric patients is not used, it should still be available for all Caesarean sections, for the delivery of multiple pregnancy and abnormal presentations, where antepartum and postpartum bleeding is occurring and in the presence of shock or anaemia. All obstetric patients having anaesthetics should have minimum monitoring of e.c.g. heart rate and blood pressure, and special care should be taken in dark-skinned patients.

Regional anaesthesia is not blameless. Four patients died after extradural blocks, one developing a total spinal in the absence of immediate help; the second appeared to be inadequately supervised in the period following Caesarean section; the third, having a termination of pregnancy, was given an epidural and heavy sedation by an obstetrician; and in the fourth, the use of intravenous ergometrine caused vomiting and severe aspiration. The considerable dangers of major conduction anaesthesia should be well understood by all who practise it, and the patient very carefully and continuously supervised by a doctor or midwife while the blockade is effective.

REFERENCES

Abboud T K et al 1981 Enflurane analgesia in obstetrics. Anesthesia and Analgesia 60: 133–137
Abboud T K et al 1983 Epidural bupivacaine, chloroprocaine or lidocaine for Cesarean section—maternal and neonatal effects. Anesthesia and Analgesia 62: 914–919
Albright G A 1979 Cardiac arrest following regional anesthesia with etidocaine and bupivacaine. Anesthesiology 51: 285–287
Andrews A D, Brock-Utne J G, Downing J W Protection against pulmonary acid aspiration with ranitidine. A new histamine H_2-receptor antagonist. Anaesthesia 37: 22–25
Baraka A, Noueihed R, Sinno H, Wakid N, Agoston S 1983 Succinylcholine-vecuronium (Org NC 45) sequence for Cesarean section. Anesthesia and Analgesia 62: 909–913
Beynon C L 1957 The normal second stage of labour: a plea for reform in its conduct. Journal of Obstetrics and Gynaecology of the British Commonwealth 64: 815–820
Bonnardot J P, Maillet M, Colau J C, Millot F, Deligne P 1982 Maternal and fetal concentration of morphine after intrathecal administration during labour. British Journal of Anaesthesia 54: 487–489
Bowen-Simpkins P, Fergusson I L C 1974 Lumbar epidural block and the breech presentation. British Journal of Anaesthesia 46: 420–424
Breeson A J, Kovacs G T, Pickles B G, Hill J G 1978 Extradural analgesia—the preferred method of analgesia for vaginal breech delivery. British Journal of Anaesthesia 50: 1227–1230
Bromage P R 1961 Continuous lumbar epidural analgesia for obstetrics. Canadian Medical Association Journal 85: 1136–1140
Bromage P R 1962 Spread of analgesic solutions in the epidural space and their site of action: a statistical study. British Journal of Anaesthesia 34: 161–178
Carmichael F J, Rolbin S H, Hew E M 1982 Epidural morphine for analgesia after Caesarean section. Canadian Anaesthetists' Society Journal 29: 359–363
Clark R B, Beard A G, Thompson D S 1979 Renal function in newborns and mothers exposed to methoxyflurane analgesia for labor and delivery. Anesthesiology 51: 464–467
Collins K M, Bevan D R, Beard R W 1978 Fluid loading to reduce abnormalities of foetal heart rate and maternal hypotension during epidural analgesia in labour. British Medical Journal ii: 1460–1461
Coombs D W, Danielson D R, Pageau M G, Rippe E 1982 Epidurally administered morphine for post-Cesarean analgesia. Surgery, Gynecology and Obstetrics 154: 385–388
XCorke B C, Datta S, Ostheimer G W, Weiss J B, Alper M H 1982 Spinal anaesthesia for Caesarean section. The influence of hypotension on neonatal outcome. Anaesthesia 38: 658–662
Cotton B R, Smith G 1984 Regurgitation and aspiration. In: Kaufman L (ed) Anaesthesia review 2. Churchill Livingstone, Edinburgh, ch 12, p 162–176
XCovino B G, Marx G F, Finster M, Zsigmond E K 1980 Prolonged sensory/motor deficits following inadvertent spinal anesthesia. Anesthesia and Analgesia 59: 399–400
Craft J B Jr, Roizen M G, Dao S D, Edwards M, Gilman R 1982 A comparison of T4 and T7 dermatomal levels of analgesia for Caesarean section using the lumbar epidural technique. Canadian Anaesthetists' Society Journal 29: 264–269
Crawford J S 1974 An appraisal of lumbar epidural blockade in patients with a singleton fetus presenting by the breech. Journal of Obstetrics and Gynaecology of the British Commonwealth 81: 867–872

Crawford J S 1980 Experience with lumbar extradural analgesia for Caesarean section. *British Journal of Anaesthesia* **52:** 821–825

Crawford O B, Chester R V 1949 Caudal anesthesia in obstetrics: a combined procaine-pontocaine single injection technic. *Anesthesiology* **10:** 473–478

Damman H G, Muller P, Simon B 1982 Parenteral ranitidine: onset and duration of action. *British Journal of Anaesthesia* **54:** 1235–1236

Datta S, Alper M H, Ostheimer G W, Weiss J B 1982 Method of ephedrine administration and nausea and hypotension during spinal anesthesia for Cesarean section. *Anesthesiology* **56:** 68–70

Datta S, Kitzmiller J L, Naulty S, Ostheimer G W, Weiss J B 1982 Acid-base status of diabetic mothers and their infants following spinal anesthesia for Cesarean section. *Anesthesia and Analgesia* **61:** 662–665

Datta S, Corke B C, Alper M H, Brown W U Jr, Ostheimer G W, Weiss J B 1980 Epidural anesthesia for Cesarean section: a comparison of bupivacaine, chloroprocaine and etidocaine. *Anesthesiology* **52:** 48–51

Davies A O, Fettes I W 1981 A simple safe method for continuous infusion epidural analgesia for obstetrics. *Canadian Anaesthetists' Society Journal* **28:** 484–487

Davis A G 1982 Anaesthesia for Caesarean section. The potention for regional block. *Anaesthesia* **37:** 748–753

De Campo T, Macias-Loza M, Cohen H, Galindo A 1980 Lumbar epidural anaesthesia and sensory profiles in term pregnant patients. *Canadian Anaesthetists' Society Journal* **27:** 274–278

De Jong R H, Ronfeld R A, De Rosa R A 1982 Cardiovascular effects of convulsant and supraconvulsant doses of amide local anaesthetics. *Anesthesia and Analgesia* **61:** 3–9

Demetriou M, Depoix J-P, Diakite B, Fromentin M, Duvaldestin P 1982 Placental transfer of Org NC 45 in women undergoing Caesarean section. *British Journal of Anaesthesia* **54:** 643–645

Donnai P, Nicholas A D G 1975 Epidural analgesia, fetal monitoring and the condition of the baby at birth with breech presentation. *Journal of Obstetrics and Gynaecology of the British Commonwealth* **82:** 360–365

Doughty A 1974 A precise method of cannulating the lumbar epidural space. *Anaesthesia* **29:** 63–65

Durrant J M, Strunin L 1982 Comparative trial of the effect of ranitidine and cimetidine on gastric secretion in fasting patients at induction of anaesthesia. *Canadian Anaesthetists' Society Journal* **29:** 446–451

Evans J M 1982 The Oxford epidural-space detector. *Lancet* **ii:** 1433–1434

Fagraeus L, Urban B J, Bromage P R 1983 Spread of epidural analgesia in early pregnancy. *Anesthesiology* **58:** 184–187

Flynn P J, Frank M, Hughes R 1982 Evaluation of atracurium in Cesarean section using train of four responses. *Anesthesiology* **57:** A286

Gibbs C P, Schwartz D J, Wynne J W, Hood C I, Kuck E J 1979 Antacid pulmonary aspiration in the dog. *Anesthesiology* **51:** 380–385

Gibbs C P, Spohr L, Schmidt D 1981 In vitro and in vivo evaluation of sodium citrate as an antacid. *Anesthesiology* **55:** A311

Green R A 1978 Anaesthesia for Caesarean section *Anaesthesia* **33:** 70

Heaney G A H, Jones H D 1979 Aspiration syndromes in pregnancy. *British Journal of Anaesthesia* **51:** 266–267

Heyman H J, Salem M R, Klimov I 1982 Persistent sixth cranial nerve paresis following blood patch for post-dural puncture headache. *Anesthesia and Analgesia* **61:** 948–949

Holdsworth J D, Johnson K, Mascall G, Gwynne Roulston R, Tomlinson P A 1980 Mixing of antacids with stomach contents. Another approach to the prevention of the acid aspiration (Mendelson's) syndrome. Anaesthesia **35:** 641–650

Hunter A R, Moir D D 1983 Confidential enquiry into maternal deaths. *British Journal of Anaesthesia* **55:** 367–369

Husemeyer R P, O'Connor M C, Davenport H T 1980 Failure of epidural morphine to relieve pain in labour. *Anaesthesia* **35:** 161–163

James F M III, Crawford J S, Davies P, Naiem H 1977 Lumbar epidural analgesia for labor and delivery of twins. *American Journal of Obstetrics and Gynecology* **127:** 176–180

James F M III, *et al* 1980 Chloroprocaine versus bupivacaine for lumbar epidural analgesia for elective Cesarean section. *Anesthesia and Analgesia* **52:** 488–491

Justins D M, Francis D, Houlton P G, Reynolds F 1982 A controlled trial of extradural fentanyl in labour. *British Journal of Anaesthesia* **54:** 409–414

Justins D M, Knott C, Luthman J, Reynolds F 1983 Epidural versus intramuscular fentanyl. Analgesia and pharmacokinetics in labour. *Anaesthesia* **38:** 937–942

Kenepp N B, Kumar S, Shelley W C, Stanley C A, Gabbe S G, Gutsche B B 1982 Fetal and neonatal hazards of maternal hydration with 5% dextrose before Caesarean section. *Lancet* **i:** 1150–1152

Kuhnert B R, Kuhnert P M, Prochaska A L, Sokol R J 1980 Meperidine disposition in mother, neonate and non-pregnant females. *Clinical Pharmacology and Therapeutics* **27:** 486–491

Kuhnert P M, Kuhnert B R, Stitts J M, Gross T L 1981 The use of a selected ion monitoring technique to study the disposition of bupivacaine in mother, fetus and neonate following epidural anesthesia for

Cesarean section. *Anesthesiology* **55:** 611–617

Lahiri S K, Thomas T A, Hodgson R M H 1973 Single-dose antacid therapy for the prevention of Mendelson's syndrome. *British Journal of Anaesthesia* **45:** 1143–1146

Lavin J P, Samuels S V, Misdornik M, Holroyde J, Leon M, Joyce T 1981 The effects of bupivacaine and chloroprocaine as local anesthetics for epidural anesthesia on fetal heart rate monitoring parameters. *American Journal of Obstetrics and Gynecology* **141:** 717–722

Levinson G, Shnider S M, DeLorimier A A, Steffenson J L 1974 Effects of maternal hyperventilation on uterine blood flow and fetal oxygenation and acid-base status. *Anesthesiology* **40:** 340–357

Lieberman B A *et al* 1979 The effects of maternally administered pethidine or epidural bupivacaine on the fetus and newborn. *British Journal of Obstetrics and Gynaecology* **86:** 598–606

Lowensohn R I, Paul R H, Fales S, Yeh S-Y, Hon E H 1974 Intrapartum epidural anesthesia: an evaluation of effects on uterine activity. *Obstetrics and Gynecology* **44:** 388–393

Macdonald R 1983 Dr Doughty's technique for the location of the epidural space. *Anaesthesia* **38:** 71–72

McAuley D M, Moore J, McCaughey W, Donnelly B D, Dundee J W 1983 Ranitidine as an antacid before elective Caesarean section. *Anaesthesia* **38:** 108–114

Maltau J M 1975 The frequency of fetal bradycardia during selective epidural anaesthesia. *Acta Obstetrica et Gynecologica Scandinavia* **54:** 357–361

Maresh M, Choong K-H, Beard R W 1983 Delayed pushing with lumbar epidural analgesia in labour. *British Journal of Obstetrics and Gynaecology* **90:** 623–627

Marx G F 1984 Cardiotoxicity of local anesthetics—the plot thickens. *Anesthesiology* **60:** 3–5

Mendiola J, Grylack L J, Scanlon J W 1982 Effects of intrapartum maternal glucose infusion on the normal fetus and newborn. *Anesthesia and Analgesia* **61:** 32–35

Moir D D, Willcocks J 1968 Epidural analgesia in British obstetrics. *British Journal of Anaesthesia* **40:** 129–138

Morgan B, Bulpitt C J, Clifton P, Lewis P J 1982 Effectiveness of pain relief in labour. Survey of 1000 mothers. *British Medical Journal* **285:** 689–690

Morgan B M, Bulpitt C J, Clifton P, Lewis P J 1982 Analgesia and satisfaction in childbirth (The Queen Charlotte's 1000-mother survey). *Lancet* **ii:** 808–810

Morgan B M, Aulakh J M, Barker J P, Goroszeniuk T, Trojanowski A 1983 Anaesthesia for Caesarean section. A medical audit of junior anaesthetic staff practice. *British Journal of Anaesthesia* **55:** 885–889

Morison D H, Dunn G L, Fargas-Babjak A M, Moudgil G C, Smedstad K G, Woo J 1982 The effectiveness of ranitidine as a prophylaxis against gastric aspiration syndrome. *Canadian Anaesthetists' Society Journal* **29:** 501

Munson E S, Embro W J 1977 Enflurane, isoflurane and halothane and isolated human uterine muscle. *Anesthesiology* **46:** 11–14

Naulty J S, Ostheimer G W, Datta S, Knapp R, Weiss J B 1982 Incidence of venous air embolism during epidural catheter insertion. *Anesthesiology* **57:** 410–412

Nesheim B-I 1981 The use of transcutaneous nerve stimulation for pain relief during labor: a controlled clinical study. *Acta Obstetrica et Gynecologica Scandinavica* **60:** 13–16

Newrick P, Read D 1982 Subdural haematoma as a complication of spinal anaesthetic. *British Medical Journal* **285:** 341–342

Nybell-Lindahl G, Carlsson C, Ingemarsson I, Westgren M, Paalzow L 1981 Maternal and fetal concentrations of morphine after epidural administration in labor. *American Journal of Obstetrics and Gynecology* **139:** 20–21

Ostheimer G W, Palahnuik R J, Shnider S M 1974 Epidural blood patch for postlumbar-puncture headache. *Anesthesiology* **41:** 307–308

Penney G C, Moores H M, Boulton F E, 1982 Development of a rational blood-ordering policy for obstetrics and gynaecology. *British Journal of Obstetrics and Gynaecology* **89:** 100–105

Phillips K C, Thomas T A 1983 Second stage of labour with or without extradural analgesia. *Anaesthesia* **38:** 972–976

Raabe N, Belfrage P 1976 Epidural analgesia in labour. IV: influence on uterine activity and fetal heart rate. *Acta Obstetrica et Gynecologica Scandinavica* **55:** 305–310

Ralston D H, Shnider S M, De Lorimier A A 1974 Effects of equipotent ephedrine, metaraminol, mephentermine and methoxamine on uterine blood flow in the pregnant ewe. *Anesthesiology* **40:** 354–370

Ramanathan S, Gandhi S, Arismendy J, Chalon J, Turndorf H 1982 Oxygen transfer from mother to fetus during Cesarean section under epidural anesthesia. *Anesthesia and Analgesia* **61:** 576–581

Ravindran R S, Bond V K, Tasch M D, Gupta C D, Luerssen T G 1980 Prolonged neural blockade following regional analgesia with 2-chloroprocaine. *Anesthesia and Analgesia* **59:** 447–451

Ravindran R S, Viegas O J, Tasch M D, Cline P J, Deaton R L, Brown T R 1981 Bearing down at the time of delivery and the incidence of spinal headache in parturients. *Anesthesia and Analgesia* **60:** 524–526

Report on confidential enquiries into maternal deaths in England and Wales, 1976–1978. HMSO, London 1982

Rickford W J K, Reynolds F 1983 Epidural analgesia in labour and maternal posture. *Anaesthesia* **38:** 1169–1174

Roberts R B, 1972 The occurrence of unblocked segments during continuous lumbar epidural analgesia for pain relief in labour. *British Journal of Anaesthesia* **44:** 628

Rolbin S H, Cole A F D, Hew E M, Pollard A, Virgint S 1982 Prophylactic intramuscular Ephedrine before epidural anaesthesia for Caesarean section: efficacy and actions on the fetus and newborn. *Canadian Anaesthetists' Society Journal* **29:** 148–153

Rorke M J, Davey D A, Du Toit H J 1968 Fetal oxygenation during Caesarean section. *Anaesthesia* **23:** 585–596

Rosenblatt D B *et al* 1981 The influence of maternal analgesia on neonatal behaviour: II epidural bupivacaine. *British Journal of Obstetrics and Gynaecology* **88:** 407–413

Schellenberg J C 1977 Uterine activity during lumbar epidural analgesia with bupivacaine. *American Journal of Obstetrics and Gynecology* **127:** 26–31

Siegle J H, Dewan D M, James F M III 1982 Cerebral infarction following spinal anesthesia for Cesarean section. *Anesthesia and Analgesia* **61:** 390–392

Sivakumaran C, Ramanathan S, Chalon J, Turndorf H 1982 Uterine contractions and the spread of local anesthetics in the epidural space. *Anesthesia and Analgesia* **61:** 127–129

Stefani S J *et al* 1982 Neonatal neurobehavioural effects of inhalation analgesia for vaginal delivery. *Anesthesiology* **56:** 351–355

Thalme B, Belfrage P, Raabe N 1974 Lumbar epidural analgesia in labour 1. Acid-base balance and clinical condition of the mother, fetus and newborn child. *Acta Obstetrica et Gynecologica Scandinavica* **53:** 27–35

Thorburn J, Moir D D 1981 Extradural analgesia: the influence of volume and concentration of bupivacaine on the mode of delivery, analgesic efficacy, and motor block. *British Journal of Anaesthesia* **53:** 933–939

Tomson G, Garle R I M, Thalme B, Nisell H, Nylund L, Rane A 1982 Maternal kinetics and transplacental passage of pethidine during labour. *British Journal of Clinical Pharmacology* **13:** 653–659

Tunstall M E 1980 Anaesthesia for obstetric operations. In: *Clinics in Obstetrics and Gynaecology,* vol 7, no 3, ch 11, p 665–694

Tyack A J, Parsons R J, Millar D R, Nicholas A D G 1973 Uterine activity and plasma bupivacaine levels after caudal epidural analgesia. *Journal of Obstetrics and Gynaecology of the British Commonwealth* **80:** 896–901

Uppington J 1983 Epidural analgesia and previous Caesarean section. *Anaesthesia* **38:** 336–341

Usubiaga J E, Dos Reis A, Usubiaga L E 1970 Epidural misplacement of catheters and mechanisms of unilateral blockade. *Anesthesiology* **32:** 158–161

Weekes A R L, Cheridjian V E, Mwanje D K 1977 Lumbar epidural analgesia in labour in twin pregnancy. *British Medical Journal* **ii:** 730–732

Weiner P C, Hogg M I, Rosen M 1979 Neonatal respiration, feeding and neurobehavioural state. Effects of intrapartum bupivacaine, pethidine and pethidine reversed by naloxone. *Anaesthesia* **34:** 996–1004

Whitehouse versus Jordan and another 1980 1 All England Law Reports **267:** 650–666

Wilson M A, Swartzman S, Ramamurthy S 1983 A simple test to confirm correct identification of the epidural space. *Regional Anesthesia* **8:** 158–162

Writer W D R, James F M III, Scott Wheeler A 1981 Double-blind comparison of morphine and bupivacaine for continuous epidural analgesia in labour. *Anesthesiology* **54:** 215–219

Yeh S-Y, Diaz F, Paul R H 1982 Ten-year experience of intrapartum fetal monitoring in Los Angeles County/University of Southern California Medical Center. *American Journal of Obstetrics and Gynecology* **143:** 496–500

Youngstrom P C, Cowan R I, Sutheimer C, Eastwood D W, Yu J C M 1982 Pain relief and plasma concentrations from epidural and intramuscular morphine in post-Cesarean patients. *Anesthesiology* **57:** 404–409

Controversies in obstetric practice

FLUID BALANCE

Lind (1983) reviewed many of the factors affecting fluid balance during labour stressing that healthy mothers do not usually develop problems associated with fluid imbalance during the relatively short period of labour. There is an increase in total body water, especially in the extracellular spaces, plasma osmolality decreases during pregnancy and in the last trimester increased fluid intake is not rapidly excreted. The plasma volume increases and there is also an increase in glomerular filtration rate even in early pregnancy. Increased excretion of sodium may be as a result of increased progesterone secretion, but the effect is believed to be lessened by an increase in aldosterone production. Atherton & Green (1983) were unable to conclude whether there were direct hormonal influences on renal function or they were due to an indirect effect resulting from changes in blood volume. Apparently, the mother manages to reset the homeostatic mechanisms, but the changes occur early in pregnancy well before the fetal demands on the mother.

Lind (1983) referred to three situations where fluids were given during labour, despite the fact that there was already an increase of 2 litres of extracellular volume. The indications include:

1. Fluid as a vehicle for oxytocin
2. The management of ketoacidosis
3. During epidural analgesia.

1. Fluid as a vehicle

Spencer *et al* (1981) studied maternal and cord serum sodium levels and the effect of intravenous infusions of glucose during labour. There is a reasonable correlation between maternal and cord sodium and when more than 500 ml of 5% or 10% dextrose was administered the maternal sodium level fell and it decreased further when oxytocin was administered. Similar changes were seen in cord sodium levels. Tarnow-Mordi *et al* (1981) found a high incidence of hyponatraemia in mothers and infants at delivery associated with maternal fluid overload with non-electrolye solution. Some of the infants had cord plasma sodium concentrations of 125 mmol/1 per litre or less. No neonatal neurological damage resulted but there were unexpected large weight losses in the first 48 hours. Mothers given only oral fluids during labour had infants with normal sodium concentrations. There may also be increased levels of antidiuretic hormone (ADH) while there is a possibility that oxytocin may augment this effect. They recommend that not more than 50 ml per hour of 10% dextrose in 0·18% saline should be administered intravenously in labour.

The injection of intravenous glucose may also affect the cardiovascular system. Bocking *et al* (1984) found that 25 g (50% solution or with an equal volume of saline) resulted in a small but significant rise in both maternal and fetal heart rates; this effect was only apparent between a ½ to 1½ hours later.

2. Management of ketoacidosis

Lind (1983) and Foulkes & Dumoulin (1983) questioned the hazards associated with ketosis in normal labour, the latter authors commenting that, although uterine function was reduced in the presence of ketosis, the co-relation was difficult to prove. The fall in pH during labour is often associated with lactate accumulation. Hypertonic carbohydrate solutions may themselves cause lactic acidosis. The common practice of administering 5–10% glucose solutions, apart from causing water intoxication may result in fetal hyperinsulinism and, when the supply of glucose is reduced at birth, fetal hypoglycaemia may ensue. Dumoulin & Foulkes (1984) suggest that intravenous therapy is seldom necessary in the first 24 hours of labour even if there is ketonuria. Intravenous fluid should not exceed 3000 ml per day and consist of alternate solutions of 5% glucose and Hartmann's solution. It is noteworthy that treatment with insulin and glucose has not been advocated in the management of the ketoacidosis during labour.

3. Epidural analgesia

Lind (1983) also presented a critical analysis of fluid given prior to the administration of epidural analgesia. Hypotension developing during epidural analgesia is the result of sympathetic paralysis and perhaps deserves to be treated initially with a vasopressor. The blood volume in late pregnancy is not reduced and the use of Hartmann's solution may be questioned as it failed to remain in the circulation for any length of time. Hypotension may be associated with 'supine hypotension'.

Reluctance to use vasopressors may be due to the fact that, although maternal blood pressure might be restored, there might also be compromise of the fetal blood flow. Hypertension with associated headache has resulted after the injection of vasopressors, especially when intravenous ergometrine has also been given. Ephedrine appears to have been used without obvious major hazard although fetal tachycardia has been reported (James *et al* 1970, Ty Smith & Carbascio 1970). The measurement of umbilical vein blood flow by Doppler ultrasonic apparatus may serve as an early indicator of fetal hypoxia (Jouppila & Kirkinen 1984).

The effects on fetal blood volume by increasing maternal blood volume with intravenous fluids have recently been studied in sheep and it was found that an infusion of an electrolyte solution had little effect on fetal blood volume, whereas use of intravenous dextran caused a moderate expansion of fetal blood volume (Brace 1983). The type of electrolyte solution used for prehydration does not appear to be critical as the administration of normal saline, Ringer's lactate, Ringer's lactate with glucose or plasma-lyte A (containing acetate and gluconate) causes little difference in maternal or neonatal lactate and pyruvate levels (Ramanathan *et al* 1984).

ADRENERGIC MECHANISMS AND OBSTETRICS

Tocolytic therapy—β receptor stimulation

The use of drug therapy to suppress uterine activity in premature labour has introduced further problems. β 2 stimulants, including salbutamol, ritodrine, terbutaline and fenoterol, have been used to relax the uterus in order to delay the onset of premature labour. They are usually given intravenously and may cause maternal tachycardia, tremor, hypertension and even fetal tachycardia. The effects on fetal morbidity and mortality have still to be assessed (Feely *et al* 1984).

Davies & Robertson (1980) reported a case of pulmonary oedema following prolonged intravenous salbutamol infusion. Pulmonary oedema developed two hours postoperatively. Robertson (1982) reviewed many of the factors involved including the concomitant use of steroids to aid fetal maturity and intravenous ergometrine. Ergot derivatives have been known for some time to cause an increase in total peripheral resistance. The ensuing rise in central venous pressure may be maintained for up to 1 hour (Greenhalf & Evans 1970). Johnston (1972) had reservations regarding the use of ergometrine commenting on the possible hazards at the end of the operation when the vasodilator effects of general anaesthesia are removed and the vasoconstrictor action of ergometrine is seen. There are complex actions with intravenous ergotamine including a reduction in renal and hepatic blood flow and a decrease in plasma noradrenaline (Tfelt-Hansen *et al* 1983).

Caritis *et al* (1983) found that the effects on uterine contractions were not closely correlated to the concentration of ritodrine, while in a more detailed study involving echocardiography Hosenpud *et al* (1983) advised caution in its use, especially in patients with cardiovascular disease. However, Benedetti *et al* (1983) reported three cases of pulmonary oedema following treatment with terbutaline: in one patient they were able to measure the pulmonary artery wedge pressure which did not confirm the diagnosis of cardiac failure. It was suggested that the cause of pulmonary oedema was an increase in pulmonary capillary permeability. β 2 receptor stimulation may result in metabolic effects including hypokalaemia, hypoglycaemia and acidosis (Leading article, *Lancet* 1983, Brown *et al* 1983).

Attempts have been made to minimise the cardiovascular actions of β 2 agonists with the use of β 1 antagonists. Metoprolol has been tried by Ross *et al* (1983) to minimise the side effects of terbutaline without success. In fact the serum potassium fell to $2 \cdot 8$ mmol/l within 1 hour. In view of all the hazards of β receptor stimulation (tocolytic therapy) Valenzuela *et al* (1983) defined more closely the indications for treatment, especially for those who were not in true premature labour. Many of their patients responded to sedation and hydration and only in those in whom uterine contractions persisted was tocolytic therapy instituted.

Fetal and maternal catecholamines during labour

Maternal and fetal plasma catecholamine levels have been measured in patients undergoing Caesarean section either under general anaesthesia or epidural analgesia. The highest level was found in patients having normal vaginal delivery and the lowest level was in the group undergoing Caesarean section under epidural analgesia. The neonate delivered vaginally showed the highest level of catecholamines, followed by those delivered by epidural Caesarean section (Irestedt *et al* 1982). In contrast to this study, Shnider *et al* (1983) showed a reduction in maternal catecholamines during normal labour under epidural analgesia. They commented on the beneficial value of reducing maternal pressor amines on the uterine blood flow.

In another study Jouppila *et al* (1984) measured maternal and umbilical plasma cord noradrenaline in patients undergoing normal delivery under epidural analgesia, in normal deliveries without segmental extradural analgesia and in patients undergoing elective Caesarean section under general anaesthesia. The implications of the study are that general anaesthesia and segmental extradural analgesia did not affect catecholamines which are necessary for fetal adaptation, including maintenance of temperature, cardiac output, glucose mobilisation and possibly release of surfactant (Irestedt *et al* 1982).

Jones & Greiss (1982), in a study of maternal and fetal circulating amines, found that the levels were lower in late pregnancy compared with non-pregnant individuals but the levels rose when patients were delivered vaginally. They also found that dopamine levels rose at delivery but were higher if patients were delivered by Caesarean section. Fetal levels were much greater after vaginal delivery compared with those delivered by Caesarean section.

Padbury et al (1982) noted that fetal plasma catecholamines appeared to rise in response to acidosis and hypoxia. This was also observed by Bistoletti et al (1983a), who found that catecholamine levels were significantly raised when the fetal scalp pH was below 7·26 and when there were abnormal fetal heart rate patterns. They also found that maternal analgesia did not influence fetal catecholamine levels. Fetal heart rate variability correlates with fetal noradrenaline levels and may be an early sign of fetal distress even in the fetal pH is normal (Bistoletti et al 1983b).

In the pre-eclamptic patient, Abboud et al (1982a) found higher plasma levels of catecholamines. This could be reduced during labour by the administration of extradural analgesia without any adverse effects on maternal blood pressure, uterine activity or on the fetus. On pregnancy-induced hypertension, there was no evidence of increased sympathetic nervous activity and throughout pregnancy catecholamines were lower than in normotensive patients (Natrajan et al 1982).

Abboud et al (1982b) compared the effects of spinal analgesia in patients having elective Caesarean section with patients having Caesarean who were already in active labour. Plasma catecholamine levels fell in the latter group, but despite adequate analgesia in the elective section group there was no reduction in catecholamine levels.

Ketamine has been recommended for use in obstetric anaesthesia as the blood pressure is maintained and the laryngeal reflex was thought to be protected. Although uterine tone was noted to increase, uterine blood flow was unchanged. Maternal cardiac output increased but these effects could not be correlated with increased plasma catecholamines.

β adrenergic blockade has little effect on fetal heart variability and the fetus seems to have a resting cardioacceleratory drive (Dalton et al 1983). In fetal hypovolemia the β adrenergic system appears to have little influence. β adrenergic agonists may cause a rapid fall in blood pressure during blood loss, but, following blood transfusion, cardiac output recovered more rapidly (Ushioda et al 1983).

Results of these extensive studies may be difficult to correlate but are referred to in detail to alert anaesthetists to the possible dangers of drugs and techniques that alter maternal and fetal catecholamines. They may also complicate the interpretation of the effects of antiarrythmic drug therapy given to the mother during pregnancy (see Rotmensch et al 1983). With advanced technology it is also possible to record fetal cardiovascular dynamics during cardiac dysrhythmias (Wladimiroff et al 1983).

PAIN RELIEF

Epidural analgesia

There have been many claims that epidural analgesia results in healthier infants than those born following the use of systemic analgesics or general anaesthesia. Under epidural analgesia, oxygen consumption and the work of breathing is decreased which may be considered advantageous (Hagerdal et al 1983). Apgar scores were comparable at 1 and 5 minutes whether general anaesthesia or epidural analgesia was employed for Caesarean section (Zagorzycki & Brinkman 1982). Similarly, Fisher *et al* (1983) could not differentiate in the breathing pattern of the neonate following Caesarean section with either epidural or general anaesthesia.

An attempt has been made to compare the effect of various local anaesthetic drugs given epidurally on neonatal behavioural patterns. Although it might be expected that the effects of lignocaine, an amide, would have greater effects than chloroprocaine, an ester, behavioural assessment confirmed that there was a statistical difference which was clinically unimportant (Kuhnert *et al* 1984). Abboud *et al* (1983c) also found that epidural bupivacaine, chloroprocaine or lidocaine had no adverse effect on the neonate as assessed by Apgar score, acid-base status or neurobehaviour. Fetal blood flow has been measured by Lindblad *et al* (1984) using a non-invasive ultrasonic technique. They were able to show that in six patients undergoing Caesarean section under epidural analgesia, using either etidocaine or bupivacaine (both solutions contained adrenaline), there was no alteration in the fetal blood flow at intervals of 15 and 30 minutes following injection of the solution.

There may be an increase in forceps delivery during epidural analgesia and this may be accounted for by the fact that oxytocin levels are reduced compared with a control group (Goodfellow *et al* 1983). Maresh *et al* (1983) found the incidence of forceps delivery could be reduced by instituting 'delayed pushing', which increased the second stage by approximately 100 minutes. Another possible hazard of epidural analgesia is the high incidence of hypotonic bladder in the postpartum period (Weil *et al* 1983).

Endogeous opioids in pregnancy

Interest in endogenous opioids have prompted many studies on the value of epidural or intrathecal opiates in obstetrics. Substance P is believed to be a neurotransmitter in some C afferent fibres and may be involved in the release of gonadotropins and prolactin as well as in the initiation of labour (Skrabanek & Powell 1983; see also Jordan 1983).

In animal studies Craft *et al* (1982) concluded that epidural morphine had no effect on maternal or fetal arterial blood pressure nor on the acid-base status. There was, however, a small decrease in uterine blood flow after 2 hours but this then returned to normal levels.

Newnham *et al* (1983) have shown that there is an increasing level of ACTH, β-lipotrophin and β-endorphin secretion throughout pregnancy although the levels of met-enkephalin are unchanged. Browning *et al* (1983) found that maternal plasma concentrations of β-lipotrophin, β-endorphin and γ-lipotrophin were lower in patients having epidural analgesia, either for normal delivery or Caesarean section, compared with patients who had pethidine and nitrous oxide for normal delivery or general anaesthesia for Caesarean section. This may reflect the effectiveness of epidural analgesia in suppressing painful stimuli. However, segmental epidural analgesia (T 10–12) failed to block the increase in endogenous opioids (Jouppila *et al* 1983). Abboud *et al* (1983d) found that epidural analgesia during labour resulted in a significant decrease in maternal β-endorphin levels.

Following Caesarean section, epidural morphine appears to be successful in relieving post-operative pain for as long as 24 hours and the incidence of nausea, vomiting and urinary retention were not considered significant when compared with the controlled group given intravenous analgesia (Rosen *et al* 1983, Cohen & Woods 1983). The efficacy of pain relief during labour with 'spinal' opioids is debatable. It has been suggested that the drugs are cleared more quickly in labour due to increased blood supply. Niv *et al* (1983) commented on the fact that the visceral afferents involved may be less accessible to the opiate. They obtained reasonable pain relief following Caesarean section, but during labour epidural morphine was augmented with bupivacaine. They also noted that patients were free of perineal pain following episiotomy for 18-24 hours after epidural morphine. In a similar study conducted by Hughes et al (1984) 7·5 mg of epidural morphine provided adequate pain relief for the first stage of labour but was ineffectual during delivery. In contrast, 0·5% bupivacaine gave good results during labour and delivery but was attended by low 1 minute Apgar scores. Epidural morphine produced no evidence of fetal or neonatal distress, the course of labour was unimpaired and maternal venous blood gas tensions were within normal limits. In a personal series of five patients using intrathecal diamorphine, pain-free labour was obtained in two patients while in the others analgesia, while satisfactory, only lasted for 4 hours. There was no cardiovascular or respiratory depression while uterine contractions were not inhibited.

Abboud et al (1983d) reported on the use of intrathecal morphine for pain relief in a patient with severe pulmonary hypertension. During labour there were no significant changes in blood pressure or respiratory depression as confirmed by blood gas analysis. Unfortunately the patient died on the 7th postpartum day and at autopsy was found to have right cardiac hypertrophy and extensive atheroma of the pulmonary arteries. It might be presumptive to claim that the patient with such a degree of disability only survived the hazards of labour because of the intrathecal analgesia.

Hanson et al (1984) conducted an extensive study in 200 patients having epidural analgesia with bupivacaine for Caesarean section. Patients were divided into two equal groups. After delivery of the child the mothers in group one received 3 mg of morphine mixed with 5 ml of 0·25% bupivacaine. In group two the patients received only morphine. They claimed that intraoperative and postoperative analgesia was superior in those patients given both drugs as judged by the need for supplementary analgesia, suggesting some degree of synergism.

It thus seems that the use of epidural and spinal opiates in obstetrics heralds great promise in view of the absence of cardiac and respiratory depression. Although the value in the relief of pain following Caesarean section, the response to pain relief during labour appears variable and short-lived. The explanation may be associated with the increased vascularity in the epidural space or the fact that opiates may exert their action on C fibres rather than on A-δ fibers which mediate acute painful stimuli.

INHALATION OF GASTRIC CONTENTS

Inhalation of gastric contents has been extensively reviewed (Cotton & Smith 1984) and considered by Rubin (see Ch. 11). Johnston et al (1983) reported favourably on the use of oral cimetidine, although 4% of patients requiring emergency anaesthesia had gastric aspirates of approximately 100 ml and a pH less than 2·5. There were no maternal or fetal side effects in this study but drug interactions can occur. Sedman (1984) has reviewed many of the problems showing that cimetidine may affect the absorption of other drugs, the metabolism of oral anticoagulants, the benzodiazepines as well as lignocaine and propranolol. The action of chlormethiozole and morphine were augmented. Renal excretion of drugs may be diminished as creatinine clearance is reduced.

It has also been assumed that the inhalation of acid contents was always deleterious, and efforts should be made to promote an increase in gastric acid pH. However, this results in an alteration in gastric flora: Gram negative organisms appeared to survive in the less acid medium and pulmonary aspiration may result in Gram negative pneumonia (du Moulin 1982).

MISCELLANEOUS

Drugs in pregnancy

In recent years the prescribing of drugs during pregnancy has been thought to be harmful, especially drugs such as aspirin and sulphonamides which affect the fetus. Drug prescribing in pregnancy has been reviewed by McEwan (1982) while Boobis & Lewis (1982) have discussed the problems of altered pharmacokinetics during pregnancy. Ellis & Fidler (1982) have drawn attention to adverse reactions during early pregnancy when congenital malformations may arise and during late pregnancy when drugs may have an adverse effect on the fetus and neonate. Niederhoff & Zahradnik (1983) consider that acetaminophen is the only safe analgesic that may be used during all phases of pregnancy.

Horner's syndrome

Attention has been drawn to Horner's syndrome occurring during lumbar epidural analgesia, suggesting a high level of sympathetic blockade (Schachner & Reynolds 1982). They suggested that the syndrome may be associated with significant maternal hypotension and is an indication for close maternal and fetal monitoring. In a personal and prospective study conducted in association with a neurologist to assess possible neurological hazards of epidural analgesia an incidental finding was the presence of unilateral Horner's syndrome in late pregnancy in 3 patients out of a total of 75.

Phaeochromocytoma

Phaeochromocytoma during pregnancy continues to be misdiagnosed as it often masquerades as pre-eclamptic toxaemia. In the puerperium, Kleiner et al (1982) suggested that undiagnosed fever in association with fluctuating blood pressure levels should suggest the diagnosis of phaechromocytoma and tests should be initiated to locate the tumour.

ADDITIONAL READING

Physiological changes affecting respiration, pulmonary function and gas exchange in pregnancy are reviewed by Weinberger et al (Weinberger S E, Weiss S T, Cohen W R, Weiss J W, Johnson T S (1980). Pregnancy and the Lung. American Review of Respiratory Disease, 121, 559–581).

REFERENCES

Abboud T, Artal R, Sarkis F, Henriksen E H, Kammula R K 1982a Sympthoadrenal activity, maternal, fetal, and neonatal responses after epidural anesthesia in the pre-eclamptic patient. American Journal of Obstetrics and Gynecology 144: 915–918

Abboud T, Artal R, Henriksen E H, Earl S, Kammula R K 1982b Effects of spinal anesthesia on maternal circulating catecholamines. American Journal of Obstetrics and Gynecology 142: 252–254

Abboud T K, Kim K C, Noueihed R et al 1983c Epidural bupivacaine, chloroprocaine, or lidocaine for Cesarean section—maternal and neonatal effects. Anesthesia and Analgesia 62: 914–919

Abboud T K, Sarkis F, Hung T T et al 1983d Effects of epidural anesthesia during labour on maternal plasma β-endorphin levels. Anesthesiology 59: 1–5

Abboud T K, Raya J, Noueihed R, Daniel J 1983d Intrathecal morphine for relief of labour pain in a parturient with severe pulmonary hypertension. Anesthesiology 59: 477–479

Benedetti T J, Hargrove J C, Rosene K A 1982 Maternal pulmonary edema during premature labor inhibition. Obstetrics and Gynecology 59: 339–379

Bistoletti P, Nylund L, Lagercrantz H, Hjemdahl P, Strom H 1983a Fetal scalp catecholamines during labor. American Journal of Obstetrics and Gynecology 147: 785–788

Bistoletti P, Lagercrantz H, Lunell N O 1983b Fetal plasma catecholamine concentrations and fetal heart-rate variability during first stage of labour. British Journal of Obstetrics and Gynaecology 90: 11–15

Bocking A, Adamson L, Carmichael L, Patrick J, Probert C 1984 Effect of intravenous glucose injection on human maternal and fetal heart rate at term. American Journal of Obstetrics and Gynecology 148: 414–419

Boobis A R, Lewis P 1982 Drugs in pregnancy—altered pharmacokinetics. British Journal of Hospital Medicine 28: 566–573

Brace R A 1983 Fetal blood volume responses to intravenous saline solution and dextran. *American Journal of Obstetrics and Gynecology* **147**: 777–781

Brown M J, Brown D C, Murphy M B 1983 Hypokalemia from β 2-receptor stimulation by circulating epinephrine. *New England Journal of Medicine* **309**: 1414–1419

Browning A J F, Butt W R, Lynch S S, Shakespear R A 1983 Maternal and cord plasma concentrations of βlipotrophin, β-endorphin and γ-lipotrophin at delivery; effect of analgesia. *British Journal of Obstetrics and Gynaecology* **90**: 1152–1156

Caritis S N, Lin L S, Toig G, Wong L K 1983 Pharmocodynamics of ritodrine in pregnant women during preterm labor. *American Journal of Obstetrics and Gynecology* **147**: 752–759

Cohen S E, Woods W A 1983 The rôle of epidural morphine in the postcesarean patient: efficacy and effects on bonding. *Anesthesiology* **58**: 500–504

Cotton B R, Smith G 1983 Regurgitation and aspiration. In: Kaufman L (ed) *Anaesthesia review 2.* Churchill Livingstone, Edinburgh, p 162–176

Craft J B, Bolan J C, Coaldrake L A *et al* 1982 The maternal and fetal cardiovascular effects of epidural morphine in the sheep model. *American Journal of Obstetrics and Gynecology* **142**: 835–839

Dalton K J, Phil D, Dawes G S, Patrick J E 1983 The autonomic nervous and fetal heart rate variability. *American Journal of Obstetrics and Gynecology* **146**: 456–462

Davies A E, Robertson M J S 1980 Pulmonary oedema after the administration of intravenous salbutamol and ergometrine. *British Journal of Obstetrics* **87**: 539–541

Dumoulin J G, Foulkes J E B 1984 Ketonuria during labour. *British Journal of Obstetrics and Gynaecology* **91**: 97–98

Dumoulin J G, Paterson D G, Hedley-Whyte J, Lisbon A 1982 Aspiration of gastric bacteria in antacid-treated patients: a frequent cause of postoperative colonisation of the airway. *Lancet* **i**: 242

Ellis C, Fidler J 1982 Drugs in pregnancy—adverse reactions. *British Journal of Hospital Medicine* **28**: 575–584

Feeley J, de Vane P J, Maclean D 1983 β-blockers and sympathomimetics. *British Medical Journal* **286**: 1043–47

Fisher J T, Mortola J P, Smith B, Fox G S, Weeks S K 1983. Neonatal pattern of breathing following Cesarean section: epidural versus general anesthesia. *Anesthesiology* **59**: 385–389

Foulkes J, Dumoulin J G 1983 Ketosis in labour. *British Journal of Hospital Medicine* **30**: 562–564

Goodfellow C F, Hull M G R, Swaab D F, Dogterom J, Buijs R M 1983 Oxytocin deficiency at delivery with epidural analgesia. *British Journal of Obstetrics and Gynaecology* **90**: 214–19

Greenhalf J O, Evans D J E 1970 Effect of ergometrine on the central venous pressure in the third stage of labour. *Journal of Obstetrics and Gynaecology of the British Commonwealth* **77**: 1066–1069

Hagerdal M, Morgan C W, Sumner A E, Gutsche B B 1983 Minute ventilation and oxygen consumption during labor with epidural analgesia. *Anesthesiology* **59**: 425–427

Hanson A L, Hanson B, Matousek M 1984 Epidural anesthesia for Cesarean section. *Acta Obstetricia et Gynecologica Scandinavica* **63**: 134–140

Hosenpud J D, Morton M J, O'Grady J P 1983 Cardiac stimulation during ritodrine hydrochloride tocolytic therapy. *Obstetrics and Gynecology* **62**: 52–58

Hughes S C, Rosen M A, Shnider S M, Abboud T K, Stefani S J, Norton M 1984 Maternal and neonatal effects of epidural morphine for labour and delivery. *Anesthesia and Analgesia* **63**: 319–324

Irestedt L, Lagercrantz H, Hjemdahl P, Hagnevik K, Belfrage P 1982 Fetal and maternal plasma catecholamine levels at elective Cesarean section under general or epidural anesthesia versus vaginal delivery. *American Journal of Obstetrics and Gynecology* **142**: 1004–1010

James F M, Griess F C, Kemp R A 1970 The valuation of vasopressor therapy for maternal hypotension during spinal anaesthesia. *Anesthesiology* **33**: 25–34

Johnson M 1972 The cardiovascular effects of oxytoxic drugs. *British Journal of Anaesthesia* **44**: 826–834

Johnston J R, Moore J, McCaughey *et al* 1983 Use of cimetidine as an oral antacid in obstetric anesthesia. *Anesthesia and Analgesia* **62**: 720–726

Jones C M, Greiss F C 1982 The effect of labor on maternal and fetal circulating catecholamines. *American Journal of Obstetrics and Gynecology* **144**: 149–153

Jordan C C 1983 Anatomical and physiological aspects of pain perception. In: Kaufman L (ed) *Anaesthesia review 2.* Churchill Livingstone, Edinburgh, p 87–107

Jouppila P, Kirkinen P 1984 Umbilical vein blood flow as an indicator or fetal hypoxia. *British Journal of Obstetrics and Gynaecology* **91**: 107–110

Jouppila R, Puolakka J, Kauppila A, Vuori J 1984 Maternal and umbilical cord plasma noradrenaline concentrations during labour with and without extradural analgesia, and during Caesarean section, *British Journal of Anaesthesia* **56**: 251–255

Jouppila R, Jouppila P, Karlqvist K, Kaukoranta P, Leppaluoto J, Vuolteenaho O 1983 Maternal and umbilical venous plasma immunoreactive β-endorphine levels during labor with and without epidural analgesia. *American Journal of Obstetrics and Gynecology* **147**: 799–802

Kleiner G J, Greston W M, Yang P T, Levy J L, Newman A D 1982 Paraganglioma complicating pregnancy and the puerperium. *Obstetrics and Gynaecology* **59**: 29–69

Kuhnert B R, Harrison M J, Linn P L, Kuhnert P M 1984 Effects of maternal epidural anaesthesia on neonatal behaviour. *Anesthesia and Analgesia* **63**: 301–308

Leading article 1983 Adrenaline and potassium: everything in flux. *Lancet* **ii**: 1401–1403

Lind T (1983) Fluid balance during labour: a review. *Journal of the Royal Society of Medicine* **76**: 870–875

Lindblad A, Marsal K, Vernersson E, Renck H 1984 Fetal circulation during epidural analgesia for Caesarean section, 1. *British Medical Journal* **288**: 1329–1340

McEwan H P 1982 Drugs in pregnancy. *British Journal of Hospital Medicine* **28**: 559–565

Maresh M, Choong K H, Beard R W 1983 Delayed pushing with lumbar epidural analgesia in labour. *British Journal of Obstetrics and Gynaecology* **90**: 623–627

Natrajan P G, McGarrigle H H G, Lawrence D M, Lachelin G C L 1982 Plasma noradrenaline and adrenaline levels in normal pregnancy and in pregnancy-induced hypertension. *British Journal of Obstetrics and Gynaecology* **89**: 1041–1045

Niederhoff H, Zahradnik H-P 1983 Analgesics during pregnancy. *American Journal of Medicine* **14 Nov**: 117–119

Newnham J P, Tomlin S, Ratter S J, Bourne G L, Rees L H 1983 Endogenous opioid peptides in pregnancy. *British Journal of Obstetrics and Gynaecology* **90**: 535–538

Niv D, Rudick V, Chayen M S, David M P 1983 Variations in the effect of epidural morphine in gynecological and obstetric patients. *Acta Obstetrica Gynecologica Scandinavica* **62**: 455–459

Padbury F F, Roberman B, Oddie T H, Hobel C J, Fisher D A 1982 Fetal catecholamine release in response to labour and delivery. *Obstetrics and Gynaecology* **60**: 607–611

Ramanathan S, Masih A, Usha A, Arismendy J, Turndorf H 1984 Concentrations of lactate and pyruvate in maternal and neonatal blood with different intravenous fluids used for prehydration before epidural anaesthesia. *Anesthesia and Analgesia* **63**: 69–74

Robertson M J S 1982 Pulmonary oedema: recent developments. In: Kaufman L (ed) *Anaesthesia review 1.* Churchill Livingstone, Edinburgh, p 55–64

Rosen M A, Hughes S C, Shnider S M *et al* 1983 Epidural morphine for the relief of postoperative pain after Caesarean delivery. *Anesthesia and Analgesia* **62**: 666–672

Ross M G Stabblefield P G, Kitzmiller J L 1983 Intravenous terbutaline and simultaneous β 1 blockade for advanced premature labor. *American Journal of Obstetrics and Gynecology* **147**: 897–902

Rotmensch H H, Elkayam U, Frishman W 1983 Antiarrhythmic drug therapy during pregnancy. *Annals of Internal Medicine* **98**: 487–497

Schachner S M, Reynolds A C 1982 Horner syndrome during lumbar epidural analgesia for obstetrics. *Obstetrics and Gynecology* **59**: 318–328

Sedman A J 1984 Cimetidine-drug interactions. *American Journal of Medicine* **76**: 109–114

Shnider S M, Abboud T, Artal R, Henriksen E, Stefani S J, Levinson G 1983 *American Journal of Obstetrics and Gynecology* **147**: 13–15

Skrabanek P, Powell D 1983 Substance P in obstetrics and gynaecology. *Obstetrics and Gynecology* **61**: 641–646

Tfelt-Hansen P, Kanstrup I L, Christensen N J, Winkler K 1983 General and regional haemodynamic effects of intravenous ergotamine in man. *Clinical science* **65**: 599–604

Ty Smith N, Carbascio A N 1970 Use and abuse of pressor agents. *Anesthesiology* **33**: 58–101

Ushioda E, Nuwayhid B, Kleinman G, Tabsh K, Brinkman C R, Assali N S 1983 The contribution of the β-adrenergic system to the cardiovascular response to hypovolemia. *American Journal of Obstetrics and Gynecology* **147**: 423–429

Valenzuela G, Cline S R, Hayashi H 1983 Follow-up of hydration and sedation in the pretherapy of premature labor. *American Journal of Obstetrics and Gynecology* **147**: 396–398

Wladimiroff J W, Struyk P, Stewaet P A, Clusters P, De Villeneuve V H 1983 Fetal cardiovascular dynamics during cardiac dysrhythmia. Case report. *British Journal of Obstetrics and Gynaecology* **90**: 573–577

Weil A, Reyes H, Rottenberg R D, Beguin F, Harrmann W 1983 Effect of lumbar epidural analgesia on lower urinary tract function in the immediate postpartum period. *British Journal of Obstetrics and Gynaecology* **90**: 428–432

Zagorzycki M T, Brinkman C R 1982 The effect of general and epidural anesthesia upon neonatal Apgar scores in repeat Cesarean section. *Surgery, Gynecology and Obstetrics* **155**: 641–645

Recent advances in blood transfusion and blood products (1)

INTRODUCTION

The science and clinical practice of blood transfusion has developed rapidly since 1945. Developments in this field have underlain many of the dramatic advances in surgical and medical treatment during this period. The provision of blood and blood products within the United Kingdom is dependent on the voluntary blood donor, and the role of the Blood Transfusion Service (BTS) is to make optimal use of this finite supply in the face of a continually increasing demand. Recent emphasis has been on more efficient use of these resources at a clinical level by reassessment of prescribing practices. Developments in storage techniques have also improved the efficiency of blood and platelet transfusion. New plasma fractions are being developed as are red cell substitutes. However, transfusion remains a hazardous therapy. A new infective risk has emerged in the form of the acquired immunodeficiency syndrome (AIDS) and 'more established' infective problems have not yet been fully eradicated. In addition unsuspected immunological effects of transfusions have become apparent. In this chapter and the next we will review these recent developments.

ADVANCES IN PRETRANSFUSION TESTING

Tests designed to guarantee normal survival of transfused blood have undergone continual modification since their introduction. Current routine testing involves determination of donor and recipient ABO group and Rhesus D type; a screening test of recipient serum for alloantibodies, and the major crossmatch (recipient serum against donor cells) at room temperature, at 37°C and by indirect (Coombs) antiglobulin reaction.

Overzealous expansion of testing during the 1960s introduced methods designed to detect all antibodies in both recipients and donors. This resulted in the detection of phenomena of little clinical relevance and delayed the release of blood in the clinicians. A recent point of discussion has been the possible safety of abandoning the antiglobulin crossmatch and relying on grouping and antibody screen alone for compatibility testing (Masouredis 1982). The issue is complex and as yet unresolved but such a step would speed up the delivery of blood to patients and be very cost-effective.

The major advance in recent years has been the introduction of low ionic strength solutions (LISS) to enhance the rate of the antibody reaction with the cell surface. Only a slight reduction in ionic strength is possible without inducing non-specific complement fixation (Low & Messeter 1974, Moore & Mollison 1976). The clinical importance of this development is a reduction in the antiglobulin test pre-incubation time from 60 to 5 minutes. Using LISS the time taken to deliver compatible blood to the patient is therefore markedly reduced.

Modifications of the above techniques using very low strength ionic strength saline have been developed with different manoeuvres to inhibit false positive reactions due to complement (Rosenfield et al 1979, Szymanski & Gandhi 1983). These achieve only small further increases in sensitivity but that of Szymanski and Gandhi may be of value in detecting antibodies responsible for delayed transfusion reactions which have eluded routine testing methods.

The LISS technique makes major changes in blood ordering practice possible. Elective surgical lists commit large quantities of blood, technician time and reagents each day to the provision of matched blood, only a small percentage of which is ultimately transfused. Few surgical units have fixed, well thought out criteria for ordering blood. The ratio of cross-matched units to those transfused provides an index of ordering efficiency. High ratios result in increased outdating of units, overworked and error-prone blood bank staff, excessive commitment of units and in increased mean age of units at the time of transfusion (Napier 1983). Groups in the United Kingdom (Smallwood 1983) and United States (Minte et al 1976) have reported how interdisciplinary discussion can devise a crossmatch policy in which blood need not be crossmatched for procedures in which blood is infrequently used, i.e. a mean transfusion rate of 0·5 units or less. These patients are grouped, typed and screened for atypical antibodies. If a requirement for blood develops in these patients, a half-hour crossmatch is immediately available using the LISS technique. In an emergency, group and type specific unmatched blood would be released if a negative antibody screen had been obtained. Patients with a positive antibody screen are fully crossmatched prior to surgery. Boral et al (1979) have provided a useful list on which to base such a policy. Recommendations for common surgical procedures are shown in Table 14.1. The safety of transfusion based on an antibody screen as the only test of compatibility has been proved in this setting (Boral et al 1977).

TRANSFUSION OF RED CELLS

Whole blood or red cell concentrates?

The resolution of this dilemma is the key to efficient use of donated blood. The simple transfer of a unit of blood from the donor to a patient is not only a wasteful use of the contents of that unit but is also needless exposure of that patient to potentially harmful or immunogenic elements. Despite earlier beliefs (Clendening 1933) whole blood does not possess any magical qualities, and transfusions should solely be the replacement of deficient components. Red cell concentrates are therefore the product of choice for nearly all routine transfusions.

There are two strong arguments in favour of transfusion of red cell concentrates rather than whole blood. Firstly, in the majority of situations in which a patient requires a 'blood transfusion', the patient is normovolaemic. Therefore, he requires replacement of oxygen-carrying capacity without volume expansion. Concentrates provide more red cells and oxygen-carrying capacity per unit volume and offer the flexibility of use, either alone, or in combination with electrolyte or colloid solutions. Using concentrates, the risk of congestive cardiac failure is reduced. When both oxygen-carrying capacity and volume expansion are required, it is clearly less convenient and more expensive to infuse red cells in conjunction with plasma protein fraction (PPF). In such circumstances, as in continuing massive haemorrhage, whole blood is the product of choice (Schmidt 1978). The indications for the use of whole blood have become very few and the contraindications more numerous (McCullough & Crosby 1980). Red cell concentrates are as effective in the management of

Table 14.1 Transfusion guidelines for elective surgery

General surgery	
Cholecystectomy	Type and screen
Exploratory laparotomy	Type and screen
Hiatal hernia repair	Type and screen
Colectomy and hemicolectomy	2 units
Splenectomy	2 units
Breast biopsy	Type and screen
Radical mastectomy	1 unit
Simple mastectomy	1 unit
Gastrectomy	2 units
Antrectomy and vagotomy	2 units
Inguinal herniorrhaphy	Type and screen
Vein stripping	Type and screen
Cardiovascular surgery	
Saphenous vein bypass	8 units
Congenital open heart surgery	8 units
Valve replacement	8 units
Aortobifemoral bypass	8 units
Thoracotomy	3 units
Closed mediastinal exploration	Type and screen
Resection abdominal aortic aneurysm	8 units
Carotid endarterectomy	2 units
Obstetric-gynaecologic surgery	
Total abdominal hysterectomy	Type and screen
Exploratory laparotomy	Type and screen
Total vaginal hysterectomy	Type and screen
Laparoscopy	Type and screen
Repeat Caesarean section	Type and screen
Labour and delivery requests	Type and screen
Plastic surgery	
Mammoplasty	Type and screen
Thoracoabdominal flap	Type and screen
Orthopaedic surgery	
Open reduction	2 units
Arthroplasty	Type and screen
Shoulder reconstruction	Type and screen
Total hip replacement	2–3 units
Total knee replacement	Type and screen
Genitourinary surgery	
Transurethral resection of prostate	Type and screen
Radical nephrectomy	1 unit
Renal transplantation	1 unit
Prostatectomy	2 units

Reproduced with kind permission of the author and editor from *American Journal of Clinical Pathology (1979)* **71**: 680–684.

haemorrhage of the order of 1000 ml (Robertson & Polk 1975) and in less severe haemorrhage, volume expansion alone may be sufficient in a previously fit person. In these situations transfusion of blood products may expose patients to unnecessary risks without discernible benefits (Simon 1980).

The second argument in favour of an increased use of red cell concentrates is a more general one. The availability of fresh frozen plasma and plasma fractions depends on the removal of plasma from freshly donated blood. The use of component therapy in red cell transfusion liberates un-needed components for use in other patients. In addition, any shortfall in the supply of high demand products, such as factor VIII concentrate and albumin must be met from commercial sources. As well as the attendant increase in cost, there is an increased risk of infection from these products as they are frequently prepared from blood collected among high risk communities. Their importation into the United Kingdom is therefore to be discouraged on both economic and public health grounds.

A widely available red cell concentrate, 'plasma depleted red cells' is prepared by removal of 180 ml of plasma per unit following centrifugation. It has a haematocrit of 60–65% and is a satisfactory product for use in slow continuous haemorrhage, pre- and postoperatively, intraoperatively and in liver disease and symptomatic anaemia (Mitchell 1976). Although variable amounts of potentially harmful ammonia, citrate, titratable acidity, free haemoglobin and microaggregates are removed (Chaplin 1969, Grindon 1974) inadequate numbers of platelets and leucocytes are removed to prevent allosensitisation or reaction to their antigens.

Autologous blood transfusion

Autologous blood transfusion has the major advantages of absolute compatibility and of absent risk of disease transmission or allosensitisation. Despite this, it is an uncommon practice in this country, but has been more extensively used in the United States where it is used to conserve blood bank stocks of homologous blood. Autologous blood transfusion takes two forms: (1) collection and storage for later elective use; (2) salvage of red cells during active bleeding.

Blood can be collected and stored in either the liquid or frozen state and then reinfused into patients during elective surgical procedures. Major obstacles to this practice have been: (1) lack of facilities, (2) anxiety about the patients' fitness to donate blood, (3) the unpredictability of requirements. Clearly the advantages of this form of transfusion are lost if extra blood is required. In recent years a number of centres in the USA have provided facilities for the collection and storage of autologous blood (Silvergleid 1979) and collections have been carried out in potentially high risk subjects without adverse effects (Mann et al 1983). Milles et al (1971) have suggested that any patient fit enough to undergo elective surgery is medically fit to donate blood preoperatively. Clearly the procedure has an application in the rare patient for whom there is unusual difficulty in obtaining blood for an elective operation.

Salvage of blood shed into the peritoneal cavity after rupture of an ectopic pregnancy or of the spleen has a long history. However, this blood is frequently unsuitable because of haemolysis or coagulation (Pathak 1970). Recent technological advances have dramatically improved the safety of blood salvage.

Blood shed at an operative site can be retrieved by suction by the Haemonetics 'Cell Saver' (Haemonetics Corporation, Braintree, MA, USA) heparinised, filtered, washed with saline, packed and concentrated to a haematocrit above 50%. These washed packed cells are then removed into a transfer pack and may be transfused immediately or up to 24 hours later. They are devoid of free haemoglobin, myoglobin, bone particles, fat, heparin, activated coagulation factors and cellular debris. One large study reported this system to be safe and efficient and blood-bank blood requirements were reduced by over 50% (Kelling et al 1983) It is, however, expensive, both in capital cost, and in software and provision of trained personnel, particularly on a 24-hour basis.

Less sophisticated machines without a washing-cycle can produce a product indistinguishable from that infused during total cardiopulmonary bypass, and which compared favourably with stored blood at 14 days (Glober & Broadie 1982). These authors provide a review of this technique and an account of its application as an emergency service.

Leucocyte poor red cells

Patients repeatedly transfused frequently develop antileucocyte antibodies and non-haemolytic febrile transfusion reactions. The severity of these reactions appears to be related to the titre and type of antibody and to the number of leucocytes in the transfused blood (Payne 1957, Brittingham & Chaplin 1957, Perkins et al 1966). A number of techniques have been developed to produce a leucocyte poor red cell product for use in sensitised patients and to prevent sensitisation in those commencing multiple-transfusion programmes. These techniques may be used either individually or in combination: (1) serial centrifugation and washing, (2) red cell sedimentation with macromolecular polymers (dextran, gelatin or hydroxyethyl starch), (3) freezing-thawing and washing, (4) filtration through cotton wool, nylon or cellulose acetate filters. Hughes & Brozovic (1982) have reviewed these methods in detail.

The extent of leucocyte depletion achieved varies according to the method employed, as does the removal of platelets and plasma, concomitant red cell loss, preparation time and cost. Leucocyte depletion of at least 80% is the desired target as transfusion of less than 5×10^8 leucocytes appears to prevent non-haemolytic febrile transfusion reactions in the majority of sensitised patients (Perkins et al 1966). However leucocyte depletion of greater than 95% does not necessarily render blood non-immunogenic (Crowley & Valeri 1974) and antibodies to leucocytes, platelets and HLA antigens can develop after transfusion of frozen-washed cells (Minchinton et al 1980). All leucocyte-poor red cell products have a shelf life of only 24 hours due to the risk of bacterial contamination. Saline-washed or frozen-washed red cells are the products of choice in the rare cases of sensitivity to IgA in IgA deficient individuals (Pineda & Toswell 1975, Vyas et al 1975).

A recent controlled trial in sensitised thalassaemic patients revealed that methyl-cellulose filtered cells were as efficient at reducing reactions as frozen-thawed red cells and that there was no difference in transfusion requirement between the groups (Marcus et al 1984). The preparation of frozen-washed cells is cumbersome, costly and time consuming and there is a relatively high red cell loss (Chaplin 1982). For these reasons, filtered or unfrozen washed cells are more widely used.

A 95% reduction in non-haemolytic febrile transfusion reactions among previously sensitised individuals has been reported by Wenz et al (1980) by transfusing stored blood through ordinary microaggregate filters. Only 40% leucocyte and platelet depletion was obtained. The therapeutic effect is thought to be due to more efficient removal of granulocytes, as these cells are the most immunogenic component of blood. This method clearly has advantages of simplicity and economy and should probably be used in the first instance before resorting to one of the more complicated and time consuming depletion techniques.

Neocyte transfusion ('young red cells')

It is possible to exploit age related changes in size and density of erythrocytes to obtain from a donor a population of younger than average red cells (neocytes) using a cell separator (Propper et al 1980, Corash et al 1981). The half-life of these cells after transfusions is longer than that of unfractionated frozen cells using ^{51}Cr (Corash et al 1981). A technique to obtain neocytes from fresh or frozen units of blood using a cell processor has also been described and they too have improved in vivo survival (Graziano et al 1982). This method is said to be more cost effective.

Long-term administration of neocytes was suggested as a manoeuvre to improve the management of chronically transfused patients. It was hoped that a decreased frequency of transfusion requirements would result and that the rate of iron accumulation would thereby be reduced. Propper et al (1980) reported an increase in transfusion intervals in thalassaemic children using neocytes but this is not universal experience (Marcus et al 1984) and the methods of preparation are expensive. Neocytes have been successfully used for intrauterine transfusion to prevent haemolytic disease of the newborn.

Advances in liquid storage of red cells

For 20 years from its development in 1943, acid-citrate-dextrose (ACD) was the standard anticoagulant-preservative for red cells (Loutit et al 1943). A 24-hour cell survival of 70% was deemed the minimal acceptable viability after transfusion and established a 21-day shelf life for ACD stored blood (Ross et al 1947). The introduction of citrate-phosphate-dextrose (CPD) reduced acidosis and improved ATP synthesis (Gibson et al 1957), and was later found to improve red cell function by better preservation of 2,3 diphosphoglycerate (2,3 DPG) in the first week of storage (Sohmer & Dawson 1979). Recently this anticoagulant has been further modified by the addition of 25% more dextrose and of $0 \cdot 25$ mM adenine. This new anticoagulant-preservative has rapidly attained wide usage due to an increase in the shelf life of red cell products to 35 days (Zuck et al 1977). This solution has been named CPDA–1 and further modifications with more dextrose and adenine designated CPDA–2 and CPDA–3 have been examined to further improve viability at 35 days (Valeri et al 1982).

These new CPD solutions with added adenine all preserve viability better through maintenance of ATP levels during storage, but at the expense of a fall in 2,3 DPG concentrations. An accelarated deterioration in 2,3 DPG levels is found with all these solutions in the first week of storage compared with CPD solutions. Very low levels are reached by 10–14 days (Akerblom et al 1967, Valeri et al 1982).

The shift to the left in the oxygen dissociation curve of stored blood has been known since 1954 (Valtis & Kennedy 1954), and the role of 2,3 DPG depletion was deduced by Akerblom et al in 1968. However, it has proved difficult to demonstrate a deterimental effect from the use of 2,3 DPG depleted red blood cells and the clinical relevance of low 2,3 DPG has not been established (Mollison 1983, Collins 1983).

Recent animal studies suggest that 2,3 DPG depletion of transfused blood may affect survival if other impairment of oxygen delivery coexists (reviewed by Collins 1983).

Prolongation of shelf life by 14 days will result in a reduction of blood shortages and a decrease in the number of units reaching the expiration date unused (Kreuger et al 1975, Dawson 1983).

Other additives and rejuvenation of expired blood

A number of other additives have been developed to supply nutrients to red cells prior to storage. These permit maximal plasma removal from the unit by lowering the viscosity of the residual red cells. Saline-adenine-glucose (SAG) and SAG–M, a similar solution with added mannitol are used in this way to resuspend packed red cells to a haematocrit of around 60% (reviewed by Dawson 1983). More widespread use of these solutions would increase the yield of plasma for fractionation and help reduce the deficit in factor VIII and albumin production.

Red cell concentrates resuspended and preserved in SAG have been shown to contain considerably fewer microaggregates than whole blood and to have excellent post-transfusion survival after 35 days storage (Högman et al 1978). The viscosity of these preparations is comparable to that of whole blood (Dawson 1983).

Healing of intestinal anastomoses after surgery (Tagart 1981) and of distal amputation stumps in diabetics (Bailey et al 1979) appears to be compromised by increased blood viscosity. Red cell concentrates resuspended in these solutions may be the most appropriate preparation for the intraoperative transfusion of such patients. Red cells resuspended in SAG–M will be more widely available in the very near future.

2,3 DPG levels can be restored to normal or even supra-normal levels in stored blood by incubation with inosine, phosphate and pyruvate. Maintenance of 2,3 DPG levels near normal for two weeks has been attained after addition of ascorbates (Dawson 1983). A recently introduced product designated FRES (frozen rejuvenation of erythrocytes for storage) allows even outdated red cells to be rejuvenated for frozen storage with normal or supranormal concentrations of 2,3 DPG and ATP (Dawson 1983). The introduction of these techniques into clinical use will depend on demonstration of the importance of a normal oxygen dissociation curve in the transfused red cells.

RED CELL SUBSTITUTES

A number of solutions are currently undergoing development as red cell substitutes. Some of these have been dubbed 'artificial blood' but this term is erroneous as only oxygen transport and volume expansion of the multitude of functions of blood, are provided. None of the solutions developed to date meets the ideal criteria for safety, efficiency, convenience of storage and ease of use.

Perfluorocarbon emulsions

Perfluorocarbons are intermediate length, branched or cyclic carbon skeletons in which all the hydrogen atoms are replaced by fluorine (Tye 1982). They have the property of dissolving oxygen, carbon dioxide and carbon monoxide in proportion to the partial pressure of the gas (Henry's law). In addition they are extremely inert and unreactive with body tissues and are excreted unchanged, primarily by expiration and perspiration (Yokoyama et al 1975). However, they are immiscible in aqueous solution and maintenance of a stable emulsion has proved a major development problem. Micellar size is critical and increased toxicity and reduced intravascular half-life are associated with increasing particle size.

Many perfluorocarbons have been examined as potential red cell substitutes and a mixture of two of these compounds produced by the Green Cross Corporation of Japan has been marketed as 'Fluosol-DA'. A 20% emulsion of Fluosol-DA has undergone preliminary clinical trials. The emulsion has an average particle size of $0.1\ \mu$m (Tye 1982) and an intravascular half-life of about 7 hours (Mitsuno et al 1982). There are several problems with this solution. It is unstable at room temperature and must be reconstituted with electrolytes, hydroxyethyl starch and bicarbonate, prior to infusion (Yokoyama 1975). A further disadvantage is an oxygen solubility only three times that of plasma alone with a linear relationship between oxygen content and tension (Collins 1983). In order to deliver adequate volumes to the tissues, the patient must inspire air with an F_{O_2} of $0 \cdot 75$ or greater (Naito & Yokoyama 1978, Tye 1983).

Early clinical trials in Japan revealed few adverse effects (Mitsuno et al 1982, Suyama et al 1981). However, transient hypotension associated with pulmonary infiltrates was noted in the first USA clinical studies. Activation of complement was subsequently demonstrated in in vitro studies by the same group (Vercelloti et al 1982). These investigators found that steroid administration diminished the pulmonary effects in the patient and in experimental animals. A test dose of $0 \cdot 5$ ml is required by the USA clinical protocol prior to infusion of

Fluosol-DA 20% (Tye 1982) and transient hypotension in response to this, has also been reported (Tremper *et al* 1982).

The long-term effects of Fluosol-DA infusion have not yet been established. It is clear that prolonged retention of the compound occurs in reticuloendothelial system (Naito & Yokoyama 1978). At autopsy of a patient who died of renal failure following a severe haemolytic transfusion reaction and received 67 ml/kg of Fluosol-DA 20%, over a 4-day period, foamy histocytes containing perfluorocarbon were found throughout the body (Ohnishi & Kitazawa 1980).

Though perfluorocarbons are the solutions at the most advanced stage of development, the requirement for hyperbaric oxygen pressures, test doses and the complexities of storage and reconstitution will limit their application. They may have a role in patients with religious objections to blood transfusions, in acute hypovolaemic shock and in the prevention of ischaemic damage where red cells are excluded by blocked or partially obstructed blood vessels.

Modified haemoglobin solutions

The realisation that haemoglobin itself has practically no toxicity and that the coagulant and renal effects associated with its infusion or with intravascular haemolysis are caused entirely by other red cell components has led to examination of this compound as a possible red cell substitute. Haemoglobin solutions can be prepared such that most of these other elements and their effects can be eliminated (Rabiner *et al* 1967). However, these simple stroma-free haemoglobin solutions are rapidly excreted in the urine, are not very effective in delivering oxygen and are oxidised in the circulation to non-functioning methaemoglobin (De Venuto *et al* 1979).

The haemoglobin molecule can be modified in a number of ways to overcome some of these problems. Near normal oxygen-affinity and augmented oxygen-delivering properties can be produced (Greenburg *et al* 1977). Further modifications of the molecule and intermolecular crosslinkages have been examined in an attempt to increase intravascular retention (Sehgal *et al* 1983, De Venuto 1983). An alternative approach has been to link the haemoglobin chemically to other macromolecules such as hydroxyethyl starch (Cerny *et al* 1982).

Modified haemoglobin solutions have many advantages. The solutions are compatible with aqueous solutions and no crossmatch is required as the antigens are removed with the stroma (Zuck *et al* 1978). A 7% solution is oncotically active, less viscous than whole blood (Usami *et al* 1971) and can achieve greater delivery of oxygen at normal gas tensions than Fluosol-DA 20%. Storage is easy and lyophilised preparations ensure prolonged storage at room temperature. In addition, the danger of transmitting hepatitis has been removed.

These solutions appear to be viable candidates as a useful red cell substitute. In addition a readily available source exists in the form of time-expired red cell preparations. Their effects on the immune, coagulation and fibrinolytic mechanisms await study before they can be considered for clinical trials.

No red cell substitutes are licensed for use in the United Kingdom at the time of writing. The perfluorocarbons have already attained limited clinical use overseas and seem likely to be available here in the near future. However, their associated disadvantages suggest that they will be swiftly superseded and modified haemoglobin solutions appear to have a far greater potential. Another approach has been the development of synthetic oxygen-binding chelators with the property of reversible oxygen-binding. These have not yet been studied in a biological setting.

PLATELET TRANSFUSION

Platelet concentrates containing about 5×10^{10} platelets in 50–70 ml of plasma can be prepared from freshly donated units of whole blood by a double centrifugation procedure. This represents 70–80% of the platelets in the original unit of whole blood but in addition it contains about 10% of the lymphocytes and a small quantity of red cells.

The aim of therapy with platelet concentrates is to provide sufficient circulating platelets to terminate haemorrhage and 6 units of platelet concentrate are usually required, thereby raising the platelet count by 40–$60 \times 10^9/l$. Failure to obtain an increment 1 hour after transfusion is usually due to antiplatelet antibodies or to splenomegaly: the platelet count 24 hours after transfusion is affected by the presence of infection, inflammation, fever or coagulopathy (Daly et al 1980).

Platelet concentrates are stored best at 22°C with constant agitation (Filip & Aster 1978, Holme et al 1978). Until recently the shelf life of platelet concentrates has been restricted to 72 hours due to a marked fall in pH and viability (Murphy et al 1970). Three-day-old concentrates result in smaller increments than fresher platelets (Lazarus et al 1982).

A container constructed of polyolefin (Fenwal PL 732, Travenol Laboratories Inc, Deerfield, Il., USA) with increased permeability to oxygen and carbon dioxide has recently been marketed. This prevents the hypoxic conditions which resulted in increased lactic acid production with the earlier PVC containers (Murphy & Gardner 1975, Murphy et al 1982) and permits a shelf life of 5 days. In vivo studies have confirmed the therapeutic value of these 5-day-old concentrates (Murphy et al 1982, Gunson et al 1983). Another permeable storage container made of PVC using a new plasticiser (trade mark CLX, Cutter Laboratories Inc, Berkley, CA, USA) can maintain the pH at an acceptable pH for 5–7 days storage at 22°C (Archer et al 1982).

Although platelets carry blood group A and B antigens and HLA-A and HLA-B antigens, platelet transfusions do not require a crossmatch. These antigens may be absorbed on to the platelets from the plasma (Kelton et al 1982, Blumberg et al 1984). Platelets do not carry rhesus antigens, but most concentrates are contaminated by sufficient red cells to sensitise an Rh-negative recipient. Concentrates from an ABO-compatible donor are preferable and Rh-negative donor platelets should be obtained for Rh-negative recipients if possible. However, although decreased recovery following ABO incompatible platelet transfusions has been described (Duquesnoy et al 1979), a haemostatic response is usually obtained (Menitove & Aster 1983). Platelet concentrates should be infused through a standard blood bank filter (170 μ).

Chill-fever reactions following platelet transfusions suggests the presence of alloimmunisation and this can be confirmed by a 1 hour post-transfusion platelet count where an increment of less than $10 \times 10^9/l$ is usually associated with cytotoxic antibody (Daly et al 1980). This is most commonly seen in multiply transfused patients or multiparous women and is usually a result of sensitisation to HLA antigens and rarely to specific platelet antigens. Such patients become refractory to random donor platelet transfusions. Experimental evidence suggests that alloimmunisation after platelet transfusion is usually due to contaminating leucocytes (Claas et al 1981). Leucocyte poor platelet concentrates eliminate the chill fever reaction in these patients, but do not improve the incremental response (Eernisse & Brand 1981). These patients may respond to HLA-matched platelet concentrates from a relative or unrelated donor though up to 39% of HLA matched platelet transfusions fail (Schiffer 1980) and this may be due to antibodies to specific platelet antigens. Single donor platelet concentrates are obtained using a cell separator and contain at least $3 \cdot 5 \times 10^{11}$

platelets in about 250 ml plasma. Autotransfusion of cryopreserved platelet concentrates harvested during remission have been used for allosensitised adult leukaemic patients (Schiffer *et al* 1982). As immunisation appears to be dose-dependent (Pegels *et al* 1982), the use of single donor platelet transfusions may delay alloimmunisation by limiting the number of antigens to which the recipient is exposed. A recent randomised trial in acute leukaemia suggests that this is the case (Gmür *et al* 1983).

Platelet transfusions should be given to any patient with major bleeding who has a quantitative or qualitative platelet defect. Menitove & Aster (1983) recommend 1 unit of platelet concentrate for each 10 kg of body weight as a reasonable initial dose, though this may need to be doubled in patients with splenomegaly, fever, infections or DIC. The likelihood of controlling haemorrhage is directly related to the increment in the post-transfusion platelet count (Slichter & Harker 1978). Patients with alloantibodies, sepsis, splenomegaly or DIC may not have a post-transfusion increment. Nevertheless, they should receive platelet concentrates if they have thrombocytopenic bleeding.

The value of prophylactic platelet transfusion has been clearly demonstrated in leukaemic patients (Higby *et al* 1974). Most haematologists attempt to maintain platelet counts in these patients above $20 \times 10^9/l$. Patients with counts slightly above this will require prophylactic platelets if blood is transfused as the dilutional effect of stored blood further aggravates pre-existing thrombocytopenia. The administration of prophylactic platelets to patients with acute self-limiting thrombocytopenia due to infections, drugs or other causes would also seem prudent when the count falls to these levels. There is, however, no absolute level at which haemorrhage will occur or be prevented.

GRANULOCYTE TRANSFUSION

When the technology for delivering granulocyte transfusions became available in the 1960s there was considerable optimism about the potential of this therapy for treating and preventing serious opportunistic infection. Despite early clinical studies indicating that transfused granulocytes influence the outcome in infected neutropenic patients, larger better controlled studies have shown no significant difference in outcome and survival (Winston *et al* 1982). Therapeutic granulocyte transfusions remain controversial.

The main problem of granulocyte transfusion appears to be numerical. A maximum of $2 \cdot 5 \times 10^{10}$ leucocytes can be obtained by leucapheresis with the aid of macromolecule infusion and glucocorticoid pretreatment of a normal donor. This is roughly equal to the circulating granulocyte pool of an adult but represents only 5% of the daily granulocyte production and $0 \cdot 5\%$ of the total body stores of granulocytes (McCullough & Quie 1981). In the early days of granulocyte transfusion up to $1-5 \times 10^{11}$ cells were transfused from patients with chronic granulocytic leukaemia (CGL). There are no controlled trials of granulocyte transfusions obtained from CGL patients, although interest in the use of CGL donors has recently revived (Benbunan 1980, Schiffer 1983).

There is no place for prophylactic granulocyte transfusions. The high incidence of hypersensitivity reactions, alloimmunisation (Schiffer *et al* 1979) and the risk of cytomegalovirus (CMV) transmission (Winston *et al* 1980) for no clear benefit, make this practice unacceptable. Therapeutic granulocyte transfusions should be considered, if adequate doses are assured, for specific infective indications as an adjunct to established anti-infective therapy in neutropenic patients in whom there is a chance of controlling the underlying disease (Higby

& Burnett 1980). They may also have a place in the management of the septicaemic neonate (Laurenti *et al* 1981) but should be irradiated prior to infusion to avoid the risk of graft versus host disease.

REFERENCES
See end of chapter 15.

Recent advances in blood transfusion and blood products (2)

PLASMA COMPONENTS AND FRACTIONS

A range of plasma products, components separable by physical means and fractions obtained by chemical processes are available from the Blood Transfusion Service (BTS). Refinements in processing and handling have been introduced in an attempt to provide sufficiency of potent products free from adverse effects. However, national self-sufficiency in some high demand products such as factor VIII concentrate and salt-poor human albumin has not yet been attained.

The products currently obtainable from the BTS and their indications for use are detailed in Table 15.1. In addition a number of immunoglobulin preparations for subcutaneous or intramuscular administration are available. These are prepared either from unselected healthy donors (human normal immunoglobulin:HNI) or from individuals with high titres of antibodies of particular specificity (specific immunoglobulin preparations). A detailed review is provided by Crawford & Mitchell (1983). The specific immunoglobulins are scarce and should be used with discretion. An immunoglobulin product for intravenous use has recently become available and a number of other plasma proteins are being evaluated for clinical use.

Intravenous immunoglobulin

Imbach *et al* (1981) first reported the beneficial effect of intravenous infusion of human normal immunoglobulin in children with refractory chronic idiopathic thrombocytopenia purpura (ITP). Elevation of the platelet count by intravenous immunoglobin was subsequently confirmed in adults with acute and chronic ITP (Fehr *et al* 1982). A beneficial effect on the neutrophil count is seen in immune neutropenia (Pollack *et al* 1982).

The elevation of the platelet count or neutrophil count may be transient or prolonged. Following an initial 2 g/kg over 5 days, boosters of 400 mg/kg may be required to maintain the desired platelet count. Few adverse reactions have been reported. The elevation of the circulating platelet count appears to be a result of reticuloendothelial blockade rather than suppression of autoantibody production (Fehr *et al* 1982). Increments in excess of 200 000 platelets/μl have been obtained (Imbach *et al* 1981) and almost all patients will have an increment lasting at least 2 weeks (Bussel & Hilgartner 1984). Intravenous immunoglobulin has been used to prepare thrombocytopenic patients for surgery, either alone or in combination with steroid therapy (Bussel & Hilgartner 1984).

Antithrombin III (ATIII)

This circulating α-2 globulin is the major inhibitor of thrombin in blood. It also inhibits the

Table 15.1 Characteristics of blood products available in the United Kingdom

Product	Unit volume (ml)	Protein content (g/100 ml)	Sodium content (mmol/g protein)	Clotting factors	Non-icterogenic	Storage (°C)	Indications
Plasma protein fraction (PPF/SPPS)	400	4·5	3·1	No	Yes	2–25	Oligaemic shock, burns, plasma exchange
Salt-poor albumin	100	20	0·65	No	Yes	2–25	Hypoproteinaemia of liver disease, nephrotic syndrome
Fresh frozen plasma	200	—	—	All	No	−30	Acquired haemostatic disorders, Von Willebrand's disease, haemophilia B, plasma exchange
Cryoprecipitate	30	—	—	FVIII fibrinogen fibronectin	No	−30	Haemophilia A, acquired haemostatic disorders
Factor VIII concentrate	15	—	—	FVIII	No	+4	Haemophilia A
Factor IX concentrate	20	—	—	II, IX, X	No	+4	Haemophilia B, reversal of warfarinisation

action of activated factors IX, X, XI and XII and thus plays a key role in inhibiting intravascular coagulation. This effect is markedly enhanced by even low concentrations of heparin (Biggs et al 1970).

Familial deficiency of ATIII is associated with a tendency to venous thromboses often in uncommon sites like the mesenteric veins. This deficiency may occur in as many as 1 in 2000 and is therefore more common than haemophilia. Inheritance is generally autosomal dominant and the defect may be qualitative or quantitative. Thrombotic events in these individuals usually occur in response to a challenge such as trauma, pregnancy or surgery. Acquired deficiency of ATIII may occur in women on the oral contraceptive pill, post-operatively, in thrombotic states and in severe liver disease (Winter et al 1982).

Several ATIII concentrates are available. They clearly have a role as replacement therapy for patients with familial ATIII deficiency during a thrombotic episode (Winter et al 1982) and prophylactically in these individuals during surgery or labour (Mannucci et al 1982, Samson et al 1984). ATIII concentrate has been used in patients with shock and DIC; 5 out of 6 patients so treated survived compared to 5 deaths out of 5 historical controls treated with heparin alone (Blauhut et al 1982). It has been reported to improve the coagulopathy of hepatic cirrhosis (Schipper & Ten Cate 1982) and acute hepatic failure (Braude et al 1981).

The precise indications for ATIII concentrate in non-familial deficiency await clarification. Controlled trials are urgently required. However the evidence to date suggests that it is worth consideration in acute hepatic dysfunction or cirrhotic patients undergoing surgery. In addition it may be of value in disseminated intravascular coagulation, particularly if heparin is contraindicated because of bleeding sites.

Fibronectin

The fibronectins are a family of immunologically related proteins which occur in a soluble circulating form or as a less soluble form on cell surfaces and basement membranes. The circulating form is an α-2 glycoprotein with adhesive properties for fibrin, actin, collagen, *Staphlococcus aureus* and heparin (Sherman 1984). It is thought by some to have opsonic properties for reticuloendothelial phagocytes (Saba & Jaffee 1980) though it may not be a true opsonin (Bevilacqua et al 1981).

Several reports exist of reduced plasma fibronectin levels in patients with intravascular coagulation (Mosher & Williams 1978), shock and trauma (Saba et al 1978) and infection (Boughton & Simpson 1982). Improved fibronectin levels have been correlated with response to antibiotic therapy (Boughton & Simpson 1982). Lower levels of fibronectin have been associated with increased mortality (Mosher & Williams 1978).

The relationship between low fibronectin levels and reticuloendothelial dysfunction in clinical sepsis has not been established. Accumulation of harmful particulate matter normally eliminated by the reticuloendothelial system has been postulated to result from decreased circulating fibronectin. Damage to the microcirculation and vital organs was a suggested consequence (Editorial, *Lancet* 1983).

Infusion of cryoprecipitate can restore circulating fibronectin concentrations for several hours (Saba et al 1978). Improved circulating fibronectin levels has been followed by improved pulmonary function in critically ill patients (Scovill et al 1979, Saba & Jaffee 1980). However, clinical reports to date have dealt with only small numbers of patients and an early report of a controlled trial does not confirm any beneficial effect from cryoprecipitate infusion (Mosher & Grossman 1983). The variability in cryoprecipitate content makes interpretation of reports from different centres difficult and further study is clearly necessary.

However, it seems unlikely that fibronectin infusion will prove a panacea for critically ill patients and there is, at present, no strong evidence to support its use.

C1 esterase inhibitor

Autosomal dominant hereditary deficiency of this protein results in the syndrome of angioneurotic oedema. This may lead to asphyxiation from oedema in the upper respiratory tract. Fresh frozen plasma has been found to be effective in acute episodes but its use results in the infusion of further complement components which may, in theory, be harmful. A crude preparation of C1 esterase inhibitor has been prepared and is of value in acute attacks and to cover surgery in affected individuals (Gadek et al 1980).

Alpha–1–antitrypsin

Deficiency of this protein is associated with severe progressive pulmonary emphysema. A concentrate has been prepared and encouraging results have been reported in an early clinical trial (Gadek et al 1983). Long-term maintenance therapy may be required in affected individuals in view of the chronic nature of the condition. This concentrate may have a use in adult respiratory distress syndrome.

SYNTHETIC PLASMA SUBSTITUTES

Colloidal solutions of macromolecules can provide effective plasma volume expansion for varying periods after infusion according to the molecular weight of the macromolecule infused. Ideally these substances should be non-toxic, non-allergenic and should not persist in the body for prolonged periods. A large number of macromolecules have been examined: naturally occurring polysaccharides (pectin); chemically modified polysaccharides (hydroxyethyl starch); bacterial polysaccharides (dextran); natural or chemically modified proteins (gelatin, modified fluid gelatin, urea-bridged gelatin); plastics (polyvinyl pyrrolidone) (Mischler 1984).

Volume expansion

Dextran, modified gelatins and hydroxyethyl starch solutions all augment blood volume and maintain colloid osmotic pressure in patients who have sustained blood loss (Gruber 1969, Lundsgaard-Hansen et al 1969, Mischler 1982).

Augmentation of plasma volume by macromolecule infusion may be transient or prolonged according to the size of molecule infused. Small molecules (dextran 40, chemically modified gelatins and hydroxyethyl starch 240/0·43) are potent osmotic agents and may increase blood volume to an amount greater than the volume of solution infused. They are, however, rapidly eliminated from the vascular compartment and only a small amount of the infused dose remains at 24 hours (Mischler 1984). Larger molecules (dextran 70, hydroxyethyl starch 450/0·70) are less potent osmotic agents and have less effect on plasma volume in relation to the volume of colloid infused, but up to 38% of the infused dose persists at 24 hours and the therapeutic effect is more prolonged. The biophysicochemical characteristics of these solutions are summarised in Table 15.2.

Clearly synthetic plasma substitutes have a potential role in the acute management of hypovolaemic shock. It has been suggested that maintenance of colloid osmotic pressure by these solutions may lessen the risk of peripheral or pulmonary oedema following large volumes of lost blood (Mischler 1984). However, the colloid: crystalloid debate is complex and unresolved.

Table 15.2 Biophysicochemical characteristics of macromolecules*

Macromolecule	Proprietary preparation	Concentration	$Mn^{\dagger}$	T½ (hours)	Overall survival in blood	Frequency of reactions
Modified fluid gelatin		3–4%	22 600	2·5	168 hours	0.066
Urea linked gelatin	Haemaccel (Hoechst)	3–4%	24 500	2.5	168 hours	0·146
Dextran 70	Macrodex (Pharmacia)	6%	35 – 40 000	25·5	4–6 weeks	0·016
Dextran 40	Rheomacrodex (Pharmacia)	10%	25 000	2·5	144 hours	0·008
HES 450/0·70	Hespan (USA)	6%	71 000	25·5	17–26 weeks	0·007
HES 264/0·43		10%	63 000	2·5	96 hours	—

*Modified from Gruber (1969), Mischler (1982), Collins (1981) amd Mischler (1984).
†Mn = number average molecular weight: the best measure of the variable molecular size and configuration of a polydisperse colloid.

American experience in Vietnam favoured crystalloid: blood combinations over colloid: blood combinations. The subject is reviewed in detail by Collins (1981). Synthetic plasma substitutes have no advantage over plasma, other than cost of production and availability, and are useful alternatives to plasma in the management of hypovolaemic shock, while compatible blood is being obtained. In smaller haemorrhages (<1000 ml) electrolyte solutions are adequate replacement therapy.

These solutions only provide the volume expansion and osmotic effect of plasma and will be superseded in this field when an effective red cell substitute also providing oxygen-transport becomes available. In addition, infusion of plasma substitutes results in dilution of coagulation factors and will fail to correct any pre-existing haemostatic deficit. When large volumes are infused, fresh frozen plasma should also be administered. They should be avoided in situations where a haemostatic defect is suspected (see adverse effects below).

The use of dextran 40 is contraindicated in the treatment of hypovolaemic shock as it may obstruct the renal tubes (Rush 1974) and precipitate renal failure (Feast 1976). This preparation is used to improve blood flow in conditions with peripheral circulatory problems. Dextran 70 infusions should not exceed 20 ml/kg body weight in 24 hours. Up to 10 litres of modified gelatin may be infused in 24 hours by replacing a 1500–4000 ml blood loss with equal volumes of blood and gelatin and greater losses in a ratio of 2 volumes of blood to 1 volume gelatin. Hydroxyethyl starch is not yet licensed for use as a plasma volume expander in the United Kingdom, but has been widely used in the United States and Europe to a maximum dose of 20 ml/kg/day. The haematocrit should not be permitted to fall below 25% when infusing plasma substitutes.

A sample of the recipients blood must be drawn for grouping and compatibility testing before infusion of plasma substitutes as macromolecules may promote rouleaux formation and interfere with interpretation of these tests.

Adverse effects

Anaphylactoid reactions may occur following infusion of any of the plasma substitutes. These range from mild skin reactions to severe life threatening shock and cardiorespiratory arrest (Ring & Messmer 1977). Most reactions are mild and may be related to histamine release. Reactions are most common after gelatin and least common after hydroxyethyl starch infusions (Mischler 1984).

Infusion of plasma substitutes produces a haemostatic defect through dilution of factors and enhanced conversion of fibrinogen to fibrin (reviewed by Mischler 1984). This effect is most marked with dextran and a lesser effect is seen with the other macromolecules in large dosage (Strauss 1981). The dextrans also have a specific inhibitory effect on factor VIII, thereby reducing platelet aggregability and thrombus stability and making them useful agents for the prophylaxis of deep venous thrombosis and pulmonary embolism (Bergentz 1978, Borgqvist 1982). Artificial plasma substitutes are therefore best avoided in patients with suspected coagulopathies.

IMMUNOLOGICAL EFFECTS OF TRANSFUSION THERAPY

The catastrophic effect of transfusion of incompatible blood has been recognised since the early part of this century. Manipulation of the immune response to incompatible red cells has been successfully practised for many years by the administration of anti Rh (D) immuno-globulin. This may soon be routinely obtained from a monoclonal cell line (Crawford et al

1983). Despite the familiarity of these immunological effects, unsuspected and as yet unexplained immunological effects of transfusion therapy have become apparent.

Blood transfusion and allograft survival

For many years only leucocyte-poor frozen-thawed red cells were administered to prospective renal transplant recipients to restrict their exposure to HLA-antigens and reduce their risk of allosensitisation. Many patients received no blood transfusions to avoid the risk entirely. In 1973, Opelz et al reported improved allograft survival in patients who had received previous blood transfusion. The beneficial effects of blood transfusion on allograft survival have since been widely confirmed and the leucocyte component appears to be critical in providing benefit. Blood from donors HLA identical for class I antigens with the recipient and for both class I and II antigens with the donor will improve graft survival (reviewed in Woodruff & Van Rood 1983). The kidney donor himself may therefore provide blood prior to the transplant. Multiple transfusions appear better than a single transfusion (Opelz & Terasaki 1978) and pretransplant transfusions are more effective than those given at the time of surgery (Terasaki 1984).

The precise mechanism of this effect has not yet been defined, though there is evidence of a role for T-lymphocyte suppression and anti-idiotype antibodies (Woodruff & Van Rood 1983). Terasaki (1984) has suggested that transfusions may act as a primary immune stimulus, resulting in a vigorous secondary response to the renal graft which may then be readily immunosuppressed.

In marked contrast, patients with aplastic anaemia who have received red cell, granulocyte or platelet transfusions prior to a bone marrow transplant have a significantly increased incidence of graft rejection (Storb et al 1977). Clearly the response of these two groups of patients to blood transfusions results in a radically different outcome and further research in this field is necessary.

Impaired cellular immunity in haemophilia

As a result of more intensive study of the immune system in haemophiliac patients (see AIDS below), T-lymphocyte abnormalities have been identified in a large number of these patients (Goldsmith et al 1983, Lederman et al 1983, Luban et al 1983, Menitove et al 1983). The majority of reports consist of disturbances of circulating T-lymphocyte subpopulations similar to those seen in homosexual men, Haitians and drug addicts (i.e. reduction in 'helper T-cells' and reduced 'helper:suppressor ratio'). These abnormalities have been found in the presence or absence of opportunistic infection among haemophiliacs with no history of homosexuality or drug abuse.

It has been suggested that these abnormalities may be due to repeated exposure to commercial lyophilised factor VIII concentrate with possible transfer of undefined blood-borne agents (Lederman et al 1983, Menitove et al 1983). Similar T-lymphocyte subpopulation abnormalities have been found in patients repeatedly exposed to other blood products for von Willebrand's disease and sickle cell anaemia (Kessler et al 1983). Thus repeated exposure to many blood products appears to be associated with the development of T-lymphocyte subpopulation disturbances in the peripheral blood. It is not yet clear whether this effect is produced by an infective agent (such as the AIDS virus) contaminating the transfusions or by repeated exposure to alloantigens in the blood products themselves. In addition, the long-term effect of these lymphocyte disturbances on otherwise healthy haemophiliacs remains to be seen.

INFECTIVE PROBLEMS OF TRANSFUSION THERAPY

Non-A, non-B hepatitis

This diagnosis of exclusion, emerged as an important cause of post-transfusion hepatitis when hepatitis B surface antigen positive donor blood was eliminated (Prince *et al* 1974). It is not exclusively a transfusion-associated infection, for the majority of cases do not follow blood transfusion. Most of the patients do not become jaundiced. Aach *et al* (1981) used two serial alanine aminotransferase (ALT) elevations as the diagnostic criteria. They found the incidence post-transfusion to range from 4%, with middle-class donors and recipients to 18% with donors and recipients of lower socioeconomic background. Non-transfused hospital controls had an incidence of 2.2% by the same criteria. If elevated transaminases reliably reflects non-A, non-B hepatitis it is clearly a common infection. Non A, non-B post-transfusion hepatitis appears to progress to chronic liver disease in some patients (Realdi *et al* 1982).

Blood donors with elevated serum ALT levels appear to have an increased likelihood of transmitting non-A, non-B hepatitis (Aach *et al* 1981) and this study concluded that 40% of non-A, non-B hepatitis could have been prevented by discarding units with an ALT of 45 IU or above. Confirmatory observations have been reported (Alter *et al* 1981).

The pros and cons of routine ALT screening of donors have been extensively discussed (Holland *et al* 1981, Barker & Hässig 1983). A major objection is the observation that not all units with an elevated ALT are infective while transfusion of many units with normal ALT levels is followed by infection (Holland *et al* 1981). There are many causes of an elevated ALT, including mild to moderate use of alcohol. In addition it is neither clear what a donor rejected on these grounds should be told, nor whether he should be rejected permanently. The majority of transfusion centres worldwide do not use ALT screening.

Cytomegalovirus (CMV) infection

Post-transfusion CMV infection may occur in both immunocompetent or immunocompromised recipients. Subclinical infections occurs in about 16% of immunocompetent transfusion-recipients. It is more common in seronegative individuals and the risk of infection is directly related to the quantity of blood transfused (reviewed in Bayer *et al* 1984). Clinically apparent infections only occurred in 1·6% of 1410 patients reviewed. Studies of infants have demonstrated that post-transfusion CMV infections are associated with transfusion from seropositive donors (Monif *et al* 1976, Yeager *et al* 1981, Adler *et al* 1983) and in bone marrow transplant patients CMV infection is most frequent among those receiving granulocyte transfusions (Winston *et al* 1980, Hersman *et al* 1982).

Immunocompromised patients have an increased incidence of morbidity and mortality from CMV infection (Ho 1982). Heart, renal and bone marrow transplant recipients, children with leukaemia and premature infants are all at risk groups. The source of infection in these patients may occasionally be endogenous reactivation of latent CMV in seropositive individuals. Alternatively, CMV infection in recipients of transplants from seropositive donors may originate from the graft itself (Bayer *et al* 1984).

Clinically apparent CMV infection commonly takes the form of heterophile-antibody-negative mononucleosis with fever, lymphadenopathy and hepatosplenomegaly. In immunocompromised patients interstitial pneumonitis, hepatitis and retinitis may occur and neonates may develop haemolytic anaemia and thrombocytopenia. Among bone marrow transplant recipients, CMV infection occurs in about 50% (Hersman *et al* 1982) and CMV interstitial pneumonitis has a mortality of up to 90% (Meyers *et al* 1982). CMV infection may itself have immunosuppressive effects on previously immunocompetent individuals (Carrey *et al* 1983).

Diagnosis is often difficult, particularly in immunocompromised individuals. Virus isolation is the most reliable diagnostic test. No specific therapy is yet available.

A number of centres have established panels of seronegative blood donors for immunocompromised patients and neonates. The prevalence of CMV antibody in blood donors varies directly with age and with sex and social class (reviewed in Bayer *et al* 1984). The lowest frequency of antibodies is found in males under 23 years of age and females have a higher frequency at all ages. There is a steady rate of seroconversion among all donors and such panels require continual review. In view of the low incidence and mild nature of clinically apparent CMV infection in immunocompetent individuals, such screening fortunately need not be introduced generally.

Alternate manoeuvres under investigation to reduce the risk of CMV infection are (1) the use of frozen or washed blood, (2) the use of blood stored for more than 48 hours and (3) the use of irradiated blood. Immunoprophylaxis of seronegative bone marrow transplant recipients with CMV-immune globulin reduces the overall infection rate (Meyers *et al* 1983).

Acquired immunodeficiency syndrome (AIDS)

AIDS has attained worldwide publicity and speedy notoriety. It is defined by the Centers for Disease Control (1982) as the occurrence of either life-threatening opportunistic infection (most commonly *Pneumocystis carinii* pneumonia) or the development of Kaposi's sarcoma in a person under 60 years of age who has not received immunosuppressive therapy. The syndrome has occurred most frequently among sexually active homosexual or bisexual men with multiple partners, Haitians, past or present intravenous drug abusers and the sexual partners of these groups. It has also occurred in haemophiliacs receiving factor VIII concentrate from commercial sources. Two of these cases have occurred in the United Kingdom. A characteristic finding in AIDS patients has been a marked reduction in total lymphocyte count and 'T-helper:T-suppressor ratio' due to reduced 'T-helper' cells but these changes are not pathognomonic.

Recently two centres have independently identified human retroviruses in AIDS patients. The two viruses: lymphadenopathy associated virus (LAV:Barre-Sinoussi *et al* 1983, Vilmer *et al* 1984) and human T-cell leukaemia-lymphoma virus type III (HTLV-III:Gallo *et al* 1984) may be identical and may prove to be the infective agent. Antibody to HTLV-III is virtually absent in the general population, but is found in 79% of patients with prodromal AIDS and 88% of those with fully developed disease (Sarngadharan *et al* 1984).

The pattern of disease occurrence suggests that person-to-person transmission through blood products can occur. The long incubation period (2–22 months) has prompted fears that a carrier state may exist during which apparently healthy people could donate infective blood. In January 1984, Curran *et al* reported 18 adult cases of AIDS who were not in any high-risk group but had received blood transfusions in the preceding 5 years. These patients had received blood from 2 to 48 donors (median 14), some of whom were high-risk donors. The only reported case of AIDS in a donor and recipient is that of a newborn infant who received blood products from 18 donors, one of whom subsequently died of AIDS. The infant developed AIDS-like symptoms at 6 months (Ammann *et al* 1983). Acceleration in the reports of transfusion-associated AIDS in haemophiliacs in the early part of 1984 parallels the original explosion of cases in high-risk groups and may confirm fears of transfusion-associated spread. Nevertheless, approximately 12 million people have been transfused in the

USA since AIDS was first recognised (Bayer *et al* 1984). Although Curran's data suggest that it is a possible complication of transfusion, the risk of contracting AIDS from blood transfusion is clearly extremely low.

The incidence in haemophiliacs is higher (29 cases reported in the USA at the time of writing; an incidence of about 1 in 500) and may be related to the preparation of factor VIII concentrate from plasma pooled from several thousand donations. However, many other haemophiliacs have received the same batches of concentrate without developing AIDS. It appears likely that pre-existing susceptibility in the recipient, perhaps an anomalous immune response to the virus, may predispose him to develop AIDS following transfusion of blood products containing the infective agent. Alternatively, infectivity may be low, as suggested by the absence of reports of AIDS in health workers or laboratory personnel exposed to AIDS patients or samples, or in casual contacts of patients.

At present, blood donors are discreetly requested to voluntarily refrain from donation if they feel that they may belong to a high-risk group. Unfortunately a number of these groups have been a regular source of commercially prepared blood products and it appears prudent to limit patient exposure to these preparations. Cryoprecipitate rather than factor VIII concentrate is being administered to newly diagnosed haemophiliacs, children under 4 years and those requiring infrequent treatment. Identification of a putative infective agent raises the prospect of a screening test for donors as well as prophylactic immunisation for at-risk individuals. In the meantime, transfusion recipients may be added to the at-risk group. This new risk underlines the importance of considering the benefits, hazards and alternative measures before the administration of blood and blood products.

FUTURE DEVELOPMENTS

Recombinant DNA technology offers great promise to blood transfusion. The prospect of ample supplies of blood products free of risk of transmissible infection, though not at low cost, has stimulated much interest in this field. Human albumin has been produced from bacteria (Lawn *et al* 1981) and a functional factor VIII molecule has already been produced from a mammalian cell line (Tuddenham 1984). Despite pressure for rapid development, particularly of factor VIII, clinical application may still be distant. 'Scaling up' production is not always a minor problem and purification of the 'soup' needs careful evaluation so that we do not replace known human pathogens with those harboured by cell lines.

Clearly blood and blood product transfusion remain important, indeed often life-saving, therapeutic modalities. Nevertheless, as with many other therapeutic options, they are not without risk and should be seen to offer clear benefit to the patient before administration.

REFERENCES

Aach R D, Szmuness W, Mosley J W *et al* 1981 Serum alanine aminotransferase of donors in relation to the risk of non-A and non-B hepatitis in recipients. TTV study. *New England Journal of Medicine* **304:** 989–994

Adler S P, Chandrika T, Lawrence L, Baggett J 1983 Cytomegalovirus infections in neonates acquired by blood transfusions. *Paediatric Infectious Diseases* **2:** 114–118

Akerblom O, De Verdier C H, Finlayson M *et al* 1967 Further studies on the effect of adenine in blood preservation. *Transfusion* **7:** 1–9

Akerblom O, De Verdier C H, Garby L, Hogman C 1968 Restoration of defective oxygen transport function of stored red blood cells by addition of inosine. *Scandinavian Journal of Clinical Laboratory Investigation* **21:** 245–248

Alter H J, Purcell R H, Holland P V, Alling D W, Koziol D E 1981 Donor transaminase and recipient hepatitis. Impact on blood transfusion services. *Journal of the American Medical Association* **246:** 630–634

Ammann A J, Cowan M J, Wara D W, Weintrub P, Dritz S, Goldman H, Perkins H A 1983 Acquired immunodeficiency in an infant: possible transmission by means of blood products. *Lancet* i: 956–958

Archer G T, Grimsley P G, Jindra J et al 1982 Survival of transfused platelets collecting into new formulation plastic packs. *Vox Sanguinis* 43: 223–230

Barre-Sinoussi F, Chermann J C, Rey F et al 1983 Isolation of a T-lymphotrophic retrovirus from a patient at risk for acquired immune deficiency syndrome (AIDS). *Science* 220: 868–870

Barker L F, Hässig A (eds) 1983 International forum on ALT screening of blood donors to reduce the incidence of non-A, non-B post-transfusion hepatitis. *Vox Sanguinis* 44: 48–64

Bayer W L, Tegtmeier G E, Barbara J A J 1984 The significance of non-A, non-B hepatitis, cytomegalovirus and the acquired immune deficiency syndrome in transfusion practice. *Clinics in Haematology* 13: 253–269

Benbunan M 1980 Granulocyte transfusions—an established or still an experimental therapeutic procedure? *Vox Sanguinis* 38: 40–44

Bergentz S E 1978 Dextran in the prophylaxis of pulmonary embolism. *World Journal of Surgery* 2: 19–25

Bergqvist D 1982 Dextran and haemostasis: a review. *Acta Chirurgica Scandinavica* 148: 633–640

Bevilacqua M P, Amroni D, Mosesson M W, Bianco C 1981 Receptors for cold insoluble globulin (plasma fibronectin) on human monocytes. *Journal of Experimental Medicine* 153: 42–60

Biggs R, Denson K, Akman N, Borrett R, Hadden M 1970 Antithrombin III, antifactor Xa and heparin. *British Journal of Haematology* 19: 283–305

Blauhut B, Necek S, Vinazzer H, Bergmann H 1982 Substitution therapy with an antithrombin III concentrate in shock and DIC. *Thrombosis Research* 27: 271–278

Blumberg N, Masel D, Mayer T, Horan P, Heal J 1984 Removal of HLA-A, B antigens from platelets. *Blood* 63: 448–450

Boral L I, Dannemiller F J, Stanford W, Hill S S, Cornell T A 1979 A guideline for anticipated blood usage during elective surgical procedures. *American Journal of Clinical Pathology* 71: 680–684

Boral L I, Henry J B 1977 The type and screen. A safe alternative and supplement in selected surgical procedures. *Transfusion* 17: 163–168

Boughton B J, Simpson A 1982 Plasma fibronectin in acute leukaemia. *British Journal of Haematology* 51: 487–491

Bowman R J 1983 Red blood cell substitutes and artificial blood. *Human Pathology* 14: 218–220

Braude S, Arias J, Hughes R et al 1981 Antithrombin III infusion during fulminant hepatic failure. *Thrombosis and Haemostasis* 46: 369 (abstract)

Bussel J B, Hilgartner M W 1984 The use and mechanism of action of intravenous immunoglobulin in the treatment of immune haemolytic disease. *British Journal of Haematology* 56: 1–7

Carney W P, Iacoviello V, Hirsch M S 1983 Functional properties of T-lymphocytes and their subsets in cytomegalovirus mononucleosis. *Journal of Immunology* 130: 390–393

Centers for Disease Control 1982 Update on acquired immune deficiency syndrome (AIDS)—United States. Morbidity and Mortality Weekly Report 31: 507–514

Cerny L C, Stasiw D M, Cerny E L 1982 Biophysical properties of resuscitation fluids. *Critical Care Medicine* 10: 254–260

Chaplin H 1969 Current concepts: packed red blood cells. *New England Journal of Medicine* 281: 364–367

Claas F H J, Smeenk R J T, Schmidt R et al 1981 Alloimmunisation against the MHC antigen after platelet transfusions is due to contaminating leukocytes in the platelet suspension. *Experimental Haematology* 9: 84–89

Clendening L 1933 *The romance of medicine.* Garden City Publishing Company, New York

Collins J A 1981 Haemorrhage, shock and burns: pathophysiology and treatment. In: Petz L D, Swisher S N (eds) *Clinical practice of blood transfusion,* Churchill Livingstone, New York, p 425–453

Collins J A 1983 Pertinent recent developments in blood banking. *Surgical Clinics of North America* 63: 483–495

Corash L, Klein H, Deisseroth A et al 1981 Selective isolation of young erythrocytes for transfusion support of thalassaemia major patients. *Blood* 57: 599–606

Crawford D H, Barlow M J, Harrison J F, Winger L, Huehns E R 1983 Production of human monoclonal antibody to Rhesus D antigen. *Lancet* i: 386–388

Crawford R, Mitchell R 1983 Use and supply of human immunoglobulin preparations. *Scottish Medical Journal* 28: 306–310

Curran J W, Lawrence D N, Jaffe H et al 1984 Acquired immunodeficiency syndrome (AIDS) associated with transfusions. *New England Journal of Medicine* 310: 70–75

Daly P A, Schiffer C A, Aisner J, Wiernik P H 1980 Platelet transfusion therapy: one hour post-transfusion increments are valuable in predicting the need for HLA-matched preparation. *Journal of the American Medical Association* 243: 435–438

Dawson R B 1983 Preservation of red blood cells for transfusion. *Human Pathology* 14: 213–217

De Venuto F 1983 Modified haemoglobin solution as a resuscitation fluid. *Vox Sanguinis* 44: 129–142

De Venuto F, Friedman H I, Neville J R, Peck C C 1979 Appraisal of haemoglobin solution as a blood substitute. *Surgery, Gyneacology and Obstetrics* **149:** 417–436

Duquesnoy R J, Anderson A J, Tomasulo P A, Aster R H 1979 ABO compatibility and platelet transfusions of alloimmunised thrombocytopenic patients. *Blood* **54:** 595–599

Editorial 1983 Fibronectin and infection. *Lancet* **i:** 106–107

Eernisse J G, Brand A 1981 Prevention of platelet refractoriness due to HLA antibodies by administration of leukocyte-poor blood components. *Experimental Haematology* **9:** 77–83

Feest T G 1976 Low molecular weight dextran: a continuing cause of acute renal failure. *British Medical Journal* **ii:** 1275

Fehr J, Hoffman V, Kappeler V 1982 Transient reversal of thrombocytopenia in idiopathic thrombocytopenic purpura by high dose intravenous immunoglobulin. *New England Journal of Medicine* **356:** 1254–1258

Filip D J, Aster R H 1978 Relative haemostatic effectiveness of human platelets stored at 4°C and 22°C. *Journal of Laboratory and Clinical Medicine* **91:** 618–624

Gadek J E, Crystal R G 1983 Experience with replacement therapy in the destructive lung disease associated with severe alpha-1-antitrypsin deficiency. *American Review of Respiratory Diseases* **127:** 545–546

Gadek J E, Hosea S W, Gelfand J A 1980 Replacement therapy in hereditary angioedema. Successful treatment of acute episodes of angioedema with partly purified C1-inhibitor. *New England Journal of Medicine* **302:** 542–546

Gallo R C, Salahuddin S Z, Popovic M *et al* 1984 Frequent detection and isolation of cytopathic retroviruses (HTLV-III) from patients with AIDS and at risk from AIDS. *Science* **224:** 500-502

Gibson J G, Reese S B, McManus T J, Scheitlin W A 1957 A citrate phosphate dextrose solution for the preservation of human blood. *American Journal of Clinical Pathology* **28:** 569–578

Glover J L, Broadie T A 1982 Intraoperative autotransfusion. In: Collins J A Murawski K, Shafer A W (eds) *Massive transfusion in surgery and trauma.* Alan R Liss Incorporated, New York. p 151–170

Gmür J, Von Felton A, Osterwalder B *et al* 1983 Delayed alloimmunisation using random single donor platelet transfusions.

Goldsmith J C, Moseley P L, Monick M, Brady M, Hunninghake G W 1983 T-lymphocyte subpopulation abnormalities in apparently healthy patients with haemophilia. *Annals of Internal Medicine* **98:** 294–296

Graziano J H, Piomelli S, Seaman C *et al* 1982 A simple technique for preparation of young red cells for transfusion from ordinary blood units. *Blood* **59:** 865–868

Greenburg A G, Schooley M, Peskin G W 1977 Improved retention of stroma-free haemoglobin solution by chemical modification. *Journal of Trauma* **17:** 501–504

Grindon A J 1974 Whole blood transfusions for volume expansion. *New England Journal of Medicine* **291:** 50

Gruber U F 1969 Blood replacement, Springer-Verlag, Berlin

Gunson H H, Merry A H, Thomson E E, Carter A C 1983 Five-day storage of platelet concentrate. II in-vivo studies. *Clinical and Laboratory Haematology* **5:** 287–294

Hersman J, Meyers J D, Thomas E D, Buckner C D, Clift R 1982 The effects of granulocyte transfusions upon the incidence of cytomegalovirus infection after allogeneic bone marrow transplantation. *Annals of Internal Medicine* **96:** 149–152

Higby D J, Burnett D 1980 Granulocyte transfusions: current status. *Blood* **55:** 2–8

Higby D J, Cohen E, Holland J F, Sinks L 1974 The prophylactic treatment of thrombocytopenic leukaemia patients with platelets: a double-blind study. *Transfusion* **14:** 440–446

Ho M 1982 Cytomegalovirus. *Biology and infection,* Plenum, New York

Holland P V, Bancroft W, Zimmerman H 1981 Post transfusion viral hepatitis and the TTVS. *New England Journal of Medicine* **304:** 1033–1035

Holme S, Vaidja K, Murphy S 1978 Platelet storage at 22°C: effect of type of agitation on morphology, viability and function in vitro. *Blood* **52:** 425–435

Hughes A S B, Brozovic B 1982 Leucocyte depleted blood: an appraisal of available techniques. *British Journal of Haematology* **50:** 381–386

Imbach P, D'Apuzzo V, Hirt A *et al* 1981 High dose intravenous immunoglobulin for idiopathic thrombocypotenic purpura. *Lancet* **i:** 1228–1231

Keeling M M, Gray L A, Brink M A, Hillerich V K, Bland K I 1983 Intraoperative autotransfusion: experience in 725 consecutive cases. *Annals of Surgery* **197:** 536–540

Kelton J G, Hamid C, Aker S, Blajchman M A 1982 The amount of blood group A substance on platelets is proportional to the amount in the plasma. *Blood* **59:** 980–985

Kessler C M, Schulof R S, Goldstein A C *et al* 1983 T-lymphocyte subpopulations associated with transfusions of blood-derived products. *Lancet* **i:** 991–992

Kreuger A, Akerblom O, Hogman C F 1975 A clinical evaluation of citrate-phosphate-dextrose-adenine blood. *Vox Sanguinis* **29:** 81-89

Laurenti F, Ferro R, Isacchi G et al 1981 Polymorphonuclear leukocyte transfusions for the treatment of sepsis in the newborn infant. *Journal of Paediatrics* **98:** 118–123

Lawn R M, Adelman J, Bock S C et al 1981 The sequence of human serum albumin and its expression in *E. Coli.* Nucleic Acids Research **9:** 6103–6114

Lazarus H M, Herzig R H, Warm S E, Fishman D J 1982 Transfusion experience with platelet concentrates stored for 24 to 72 hours at 22°C. *Transfusion* **22:** 39–43

Lederman M M, Ratnoff O D, Scillian J J, Jones P K, Schacter B 1983 Impaired cell mediated immunity in patients with classic haemophilia. *New England Journal of Medicine* **308:** 79–83

Loutit J F, Mollison P L, Young M 1943 Citric acid-sodium citrate-glucose mixtures for blood storage. *Quarterly Journal of Experimental Physiology* **32:** 183–193

Low B, Messeter L 1974 Antiglobulin test in low ionic strength salt solution for rapid antibody screening and crossmatching. *Vox Sanguinis* **26:** 53–61

Luban N L C, Kelleher J F, Reaman G H 1983 Altered distribution of T-lymphocyte sub-populations in children and adolescents with haemophilia. *Lancet* **i:** 503–505

Lundsgaard-Hansen P, Haessig A, Nitschmann H 1969 Modified gelatins as plasma substitutes. *Bibliotheca Haematologica* **33**

Mann M, Sacks H J, Goldfinger D 1983 Safety of autologous blood donation prior to elective surgery for a variety of potentially 'high-risk' patients. *Transfusion* **23:** 229–232

Mannucci P M, Boyer C, Wolf M, Tripodi A, Larrieu M J 1982 Treatment of congenital antithrombin III deficiency with concentrates. *British Journal of Haematology* **50:** 531–535

Marcus R E, Wonke B, Bantock H M et al 1984 A prospective trial of young red cells in 48 patients with transfusion dependent thalassaemia. (In preparation)

Masouredis S P 1982 Pretransfusion tests and compatibility: questions of safety and efficiency. *Blood* **59:** 873–875

McCullough J, Crosby W H 1980 Contempo '80: haematology. *Journal of the American Medical Association* **243:** 2188–2190

McCullough J, Quie P G 1981 Granulocyte transfusion: a current appraisal. In: Allen J C (ed) *Infection in the compromised host,* 2nd edn. Williams and Wilkins, Baltimore

Menitove J E, Aster R H 1983 Transfusion of platelets and plasma products. *Clinics in Haematology* **12:** 239–266

Menitove J E, Aster R H, Casper J T et al 1983 T-lymphocyte subpopulations in patients with chronic haemophilia treated with cryoprecipitate and lyophilised concentrates. *New England Journal of Medicine* **308:** 83–86

Meyers J D, Fluornoy N, Thomas E D 1982 Non bacterial pneumonia after allogeneic marrow transplantation: a review of ten years' experience. *Review of Infectious Diseases* **4:** 1119–1132

Meyers J D, Leszcynski J, Zaia J A et al 1983 Prevention of cytomegalovirus infection by cytomegalovirus immune globulin after marrow transplantation. *Annals of Internal Medicine* **98:** 442–446

Milles G, Langston H T, Dalessandro W 1971 Autologous transfusion. Charles C Thomas, Springfield

Minchinton R M, Waters A H, Baker L R I, Cattell W R 1980 Platelet, granulocyte and HLA antibodies in renal dialysis patients transfused with frozen blood. *British Medical Journal* **281:** 113–114

Mintz P D, Nordine R B, Henry J, Webb W R 1976 Expected haemotherapy in elective surgery. *New York State Journal of Medicine* **76:** 532–537

Mischler J M 1982 Pharmacology of hydroxyethyl starch. Use in therapy and blood banking. Oxford University Press, Oxford

Mischler J M 1984 Synthetic plasma volume expansers—their pharmacology, safety and clinical efficiency. *Clinics in Haematology* **13:** 75–92

Mitchell R 1976 Red cell transfusion. *Clinics in Haematology* **5:** 33–51

Mitsuno T, Ohyanagi H, Naito R 1982 Clinical studies of a perfluorochemical whole blood substitute (Fluosol-DA). *Annals of Surgery* **195:** 60–69

Mollison P L 1983 Blood transfusion in clinical medicine, Blackwell Scientific Publications, Oxford

Monif G R G, Daicoff G I, Flory L L 1976 Blood as a potential vehicle for the cytomegaloviruses. *American Journal of Obstetrics and Gynecology* **126:** 445–448

Moore H C, Mollison P L 1976 Use of low ionic strength medium in manual tests for antibody detection. *Transfusion* **16:** 291–296

Mosher D F, Grossman J E 1983 Clinical use of fibronectin (potential applications). Ricerca in *Clinica e in Laboratorio* **13:** 43–54

Mosher D F, Williams E M 1978 Fibronectin concentration is decreased in plasma of severely ill patients with disseminated intravascvular coagulation. *Journal of Laboratory and Clinical Medicine* **91:** 729–735

Murphy S, Gardner F H 1975 Platelet storage at 22°C: role of gas transport across plastic containers in maintenance of viability. *Blood* **46:** 209–218

Murphy S, Kahn R A, Holme S et al 1982 Improved storage of platelets for transfusion in a new container. *Blood* **60:** 194–200

Murphy S, Sayar S N, Gardner F H 1970 Storage of platelet concentrates at 22°C. *Blood* **35:** 549–557
Naito R, Yokoyama K 1978 Perfluorochemiocal blood substitutes: Fluosol-43, Fluosol-DA 20% and 35%. *Technical Information. Series 5,* Green Cross Corporation, Osaka, Japan
Napier J A F 1983 Use of blood in general surgery. *British Medical Journal* **286:** 1142 (letter)
Ohnishi Y, Kitazawa M 1980 Application of perfluorochemicals in human beings: a morphological report of a human autopsy case with some experimental studies using rabbit. *Acta Pathologica, Japan* **30:** 489–504
Opelz G, Sengar D D S, Michey M R, Terasaki P I 1973 Effect of blood transfusion on subsequent kidney transplants. *Transplantation Proceedings* **5:** 253–259
Opelz G, Terasaki P I 1978 Improvement of kidney graft survival with increased numbers of blood transfusions. *New England Journal of Medicine* **299:** 799–803
Pathak U N, Stewart D B 1970 Autotransfusion in ruptured ectopic pregnancy. *Lancet* **i:** 961–964
Pegels J G, Bruynes E C E, Engelriet C P, Vondem Borne A E, 1982 Serological studies in patients on platelet and granulocyte substitution therapy. *British Journal of Haematology* **52:** 59–68
Perkins H A, Payne R, Ferguson J, Wood M 1966 Non-haemolytic febrile transfusion reactions. Quantitative effects of blood components with emphasis on isoantigenic incompatibility of leukocytes. *Vox Sanguinis* **11:** 578–600
Pineda A A, Taswell H A 1975 Transfusion reactions associated with anti IgA antibodies: report of four cases and review of the literature. *Transfusion* **15:** 10–15
Pollak S, Cunningham-Rundles C, Smithwick E M, Barandun S, Good R A 1982 High dose intravenous gammaglobulin for autoimmune neutropenia. *New England Journal of Medicine* **307:** 253
Prince A M, Brotman B, Grady G F *et al* 1974 Long incubation post-transfusion hepatitis without serological evidence of exposure to hepatitis-B virus. *Lancet* **ii:** 241–246
Propper R D, Button L N, Nathan D G 1980 New approaches to the transfusion management of thalassaemia. *Blood* **55:** 55–60
Rabiner S F, Helbert J R, Lopas H, Friedman L H 1967 Evaluation of stroma-free haemoglobin solution for use as a plasma expander. *Journal of Experimental Medicine* **126:** 1127–1142
Realdi G, Alberti A, Rugge M *et al* 1982 Long term follow-up of acute and chronic non-A non-B post-transfusion hepatitis: evidence of progression to liver cirrhosis. *Gut* **23:** 270–275
Regional Transfusion Directors 1984 Notes on transfusion. HMSO, London
Renck H, Ljungstrom K G, Hedin H, Richter W 1983 Prevention of dextran induced anaphylactic reactions by hapten inhibition: a Scandinavian multicentre study on the effect of 20 ml Dextran 1, 15% administered before dextran 70 or dextran 40. *Acta Chirurgica Scandinavica* **149:** 355–360
Ring J, Messmer K 1977 Incidence and severity of anaphylactoid reactions to colloid volume substitutes. *Lancet* **i:** 466–469
Robertson H D, Polk H C 1975 Blood transfusions in elective operations. *Annals of Surgery* **181:** 778–783
Rosenberg R 1975 Action and interaction of antithrombin and heparin. *New England Journal of Medicine* **292:** 146–151
Rosenfield R E, Shaikh S H, Innella F, Kaczera Z, Kochwa S 1979 Augmentation of haemagglutination by low ionic conditions. *Transfision* **19:** 499–510
Ross J F, Finch C A, Peacock W C, Sammons E 1947 The in vivo preservation and post-transfusion survival of stored blood. *Journal of Clinical Investigation* **26:** 687–703
Rush B F 1974 Volume replacement: when, what and how much? In: Schumer W, Nyhus L M (eds) *Treatment of shock: principles and practice.* Lee and Febiger, Philadelphia
Saba T N, Blumenstock F A, Scovill W A, Bernard H 1978 Cryoprecipitate reversal of opsonic alpha-2 surface binding glycoprotein deficiency in septic surgical and trauma patients. *Science* **201:** 622–624
Saba T M, Jaffee E 1980 Plasma fibronectin (opsonic glycoprotein): its synthesis by vascular endothelial cells and role in cardiopulmonary integrity after trauma as related to reticuloendothelial function. *American Journal of Medicine* **68:** 577–594
Samson D, Stirling Y, Woolf L, Howarth D, Seghatchian M J, De Chazal R 1984 Management of planned pregnancy in a patient with congenital antithrombin III deficiency. *British Journal of Haematology* **56:** 243–249
Sarngadharan M G, Popovic M, Bruch L, Schupbach J, Gallo R C 1984 Antibodies reactive with human T-lymphotrophic retrovirus (HTLV-III) in the serum of patients with AIDS. *Science* **224:** 506–508
Schiffer C A 1980 Clinical importance of antiplatelet antibody testing for the blood bank. In: Bell C A (ed) *A seminar on antigens on blood cells and body fluids.* American Association of Blood Banks, Washington DC, p 189–208
Schiffer C A 1983 Granulocyte transfusion therapy. *Cancer Treatment Reports* **67:** 113–119
Schiffer C A, Aisner A J, Daly P A, Schimpff S C, Wiernik P H 1979 Alloimmunisation following prophylactic granulocyte transfusion. *Blood* **54:** 766–774
Schiffer C A, Aisner A J, Dutcher J P *et al* 1982 A clinical program of platelet cryopreservation. *Progress in Clinical Biological Research* **88:** 165–180
Schipper H G, Tencate J W 1982 Antithrombin III transfusion in patients with hepatic cirrhosis. *British*

Journal of Haematology **52:** 25–33

Scovill W A, Annest S, Saba T M *et al* 1979 Cardiovascular haemodialysis after opsonic alpha 25B glyoprotein therapy in injured patients. *Surgery* **86:** 284–293

Sehgal L R, Rosen A L, Gould S A, Sehgal H L, Moss G L 1983 Preparation and in vitro characteristics of polymerised pyridoxylated haemoglobin. *Transfusion* **23:** 158–162

Sherman L A 1984 New plasma components. *Clinics in Haematology* **13:** 17–38

Silvergleid A J 1979 Autologous transfusions: experience in a community centre. *Journal of the American Medical Association* **241:** 2724–2725

Simon E R 1980 Whole blood and red cells. In: Mayer K (ed) *Guidlines to transfusion practices.* American Association of Blood Banks, Washington DC, p 25–39

Slichter S J, Harker L A 1978 Thrombocytopenia: mechanisms and management of defects in platelet production. *Clinics in Haematology* **7:** 523–539

Smallwood J A 1983 Use of blood in elective general surgery: an area of wasted resources. *British Medical Journal* **286:** 868–870

Sohmer P R, Dawson R B 1979 The significance of 2,3 DPG in red blood cell transfusion. *Critical Reviews of Clinical Laboratory Science* **11:** 107–174

Storb R, Prentice R L, Thomas E D 1977 Marrow transplantation for the treatment of aplastic anaemia. An analysis of factors associated with graft rejection. *New England Journal of Medicine* **296:** 61–66

Strauss R G 1981 Review of the effects of hydroxyethyl starch on the blood coagulation system. *Transfusion* **21:** 299–302

Suyama T, Yokoyama K, Naito R 1981 Development of perfluorochemical whole blood substitute (Fluosol-DA 20%): an overview of clinical studies with 185 patients. *Progress in Clinical and Biological Research* **55:** 609–628

Szymanski I O, Gandhi J G 1983 A new low ionic strength test for assessment of pretransfusion compatibility. Studies in vitro and in volvo. *American Journal of Clinical Pathology* **80:** 37–42

Terasaki P I 1984 The beneficial effect on kidney graft survival attributed to clonal deletion. *Transplantation* **37:** 119–125

Tremper K K, Friedman A E, Levine E, Lapin R, Camarillo D 1982 The preoperative treatment of severely anaemic patients with a perfluorochemical oxygen-transport fluid, fluosol-DA. *New England Journal of Medicine* **307:** 277–283

Tuddenham E G D 1984 Personal communication

Tye R W 1982 Blood substitutes as therapy in massive surgery and trauma. In: Murawski K (ed) *Massive transfusion in surgery and trauma.* Alan R Liss, New York, p 79–90

Usami S, Chien S, Gregerson M I 1971 Haemoglobin solution as a plasma expander: effects on blood viscosity. *Proceedings of the Society of Experimental Biology and Medicine* **136:** 1232–1235

Valeri C R, Valeri D A, Gray A, Melaragno A, Dennis R C, Emerson C P 1982 Viability and function of red blood cell concentrate stored at 4°C for 35 days in CPDA-1, CPDA-2 and CPDA-3. *Transfusion* **22:** 210–216

Valtis D J, Kennedy A C 1954 Defective gas transport function of stored red blood cells. *Lancet* **i:** 119–124

Vercellotti G, Hammerschmidt D E, Craddock P R, Jacobs H S 1982 Activation of plasma complement by perfluorocarbon artificial blood: probable mechanism of adverse pulmonary reactions in treated patients and rationale for corticosteroid prophylaxis. *Blood* **59:** 1299–1304

Vilmer E, Barre-Sinoussi F, Rouzioux C *et al* 1984 Isolation of a new lymphotrophic retrovirus from two siblings with haemophilia B, one with AIDS. *Lancet* **i:** 753–757

Vyas G N, Perkins H A, Yang Y M, Basatani G K 1975 Healthy blood donors with selective absence of immunoglobulin A: prevention of anaphylactic transfusion reactions caused by antibodies to IgA. *Journal of Laboratory and Clinical Medicine* **85:** 838–842

Winter J H, Fenech A, Mackie M, Bennett B, Douglas A S 1982 Treatment of venous thrombosis in antithrombin III deficient patients with concentrates of antithrombin III. *Clinical and Laboratory Haematology* **4:** 101–108

Winter J H, Fenech A, Ridley W *et al* 1982 Familial antithrombin III deficiency. *Quarterly Journal of Medicine* **204:** 373–395

Winston D J, Ho W G, Gale R P 1982 Therapeutic granulocyte transfusions for documented infections. A controlled trial of 95 granulocytopenic episodes. *Annals of Internal Medicine* **97:** 509–515

Winston D J, Ho W G, Howell C L *et al* 1980 Cytomegalovirus associated with leukocyte transfusions. *Annals of Internal Medicine* **93:** 671–675

Woodruff M F A, Van Rood J J 1983 Possible implications of the effect of blood transfusion on allograft survival. *Lancet* **i:** 1201–1203

Yeager A S, Grumet F C, Hafleigh E B, Arvin A M, Bradley J S, Prober C G 1981 Prevention of transfusion acquired cytomegalovirus infection in newborn infants. *Journal of Paediatrics* **98:** 281–287

Yokoyama K, Yamanouchi K, Watanabe M *et al* 1975 Preparation of perfluorodecalin emulsion, an approach to the red cell substitute. *Federation Proceedings* **34:** 1478–1483

Zuck T F, Bensinger T A, Peck C C *et al* 1977 The in vivo survival of red blood cells stored in modified CPD with adenine: report of a multi-institutional co-operative effort. *Transfusion* **17**: 374–382

Zuck T F, De Venuto F, Neville J R, Friedman H I 1978 Oncotic and oxygen transport effects of haemoglobin solutions. *Progress in Clinical and Biological Research* **19**: 111–147

Additional references

Bailey M J, Johnston C L W, Yates C J P, Somerville P G, Dormandy J A 1979 Preoperative haemoglobin as a predictor of outcome of diabetic amputations. *Lancet* **ii**: 168–170

Högman C F, Hedlund K, Zetterström H 1978 Clinical usefulnes of red cells preserved in protein-poor mediums. *New England Journal of Medicine* **299**: 1377–1382

Tagart R E B 1981 Colorectal anastamosis: factors influencing success. *Journal of the Royal Society of Medicine* **74**: 111–118

AIDS UPDATE

HTLV-III and LAV have been shown to be identical and the evidence for a role in the pathogenesis of AIDS is compelling. A reliable assay for serum antibody to HTLV-III has been developed and is being commercialised. Transmission of HTLV-III by blood transfusion has been conclusively demonstrated by serological studies of a small number of donor-recipient pairs, both in the USA and in this country. Screening of donors for antibody to HTLV-III may reduce the number of potentially infective units transfused but HTLV-III has been isolated from a small number of seronegative individuals (Salahuddin *et al* 1984) and other assays for viral antigens must be developed. The risk from blood transfusion remains very low — estimated at 1 per 100 000 transfusions on American experience over the past 3 years. However, the risk for haemophiliacs is much higher (now 52 cases of AIDS in the USA and 3 in the UK) and a recent report by Melbye *et al* (1984) suggests that European haemophiliacs have acquired the virus mainly via commercial American concentrates. Efforts to achieve national self sufficiency in blood products and studies of methods of rendering concentrates non-infective whilst maintaining potency must continue.

References

Editorial 1984 Blood transfusion, haemophilia and AIDS. *Lancet* **ii**: 1433–1435

Salahuddin S Z, Groopman J E, Marikham P D *et al* 1984 HTLV-III in symptom-free seronegative persons. *Lancet* **ii**: 1418–1420

Melbye M, Froebel K S, Madhok R *et al* 1984 HTLV-III seropositivity in European haemophiliacs exposed to factor VIII concentrate imported from the USA. *Lancet* **ii**: 1444–1446

Burns and the inhalation injury

The mortality rate of patients admitted to specialised burn units is approximately 14% (Feller *et al* 1978). Constant improvements in management are reducing this and overall mortality rates of 10% have now been reported (Venus *et al* 1981). In the USA this amounts to about 5000 fatalities a year (2:100 000) from house fires (Mierley & Baker 1983). A similar picture exists in the UK where in 1979 there were approximately 1000 fatalities from fires (United Kingdom Fire Statistics).

Mortality rises with increasing size of burn and with increasing age. Significant and even dramatic increases in mortality occur when the cutaneous burn is associated with respiratory damage from inhalation of smoke, hot gases or chemicals (Table 16.1).

MECHANISMS OF INHALATIONAL INJURY

How does the inhalation of smoke and hot gases produce pulmonary damage? Firstly by thermal injury, mainly confined to the upper respiratory tract. Secondly by systemic carbon monoxide poisoning. Thirdly by chemicals present in the smoke and, lastly, by sepsis. Iatrogenic injury, for example by trauma during attempted intubation adds to the overall damage.

Thermal injury

This causes oedema of the pharynx and larynx. Further injury is prevented by the efficient cooling mechanism afforded by the tissues of the upper airway acting as a heat sump. In support of this is the rapid cord closure which occurs in the face of hot air inhalation. With the exception of steam, hot gases possess a low specific heat which restricts the extension of thermal injury down the bronchial tree.

Smoke inhalation

Smoke analysis (Zawacki *et al* 1977) demonstrates the following contents:

O_2 17·70%± 0·39
CO_2 0·94%± 0·24
CO   0·19%± 0·03

In addition other workers (Zikria *et al* 1972, Chi-shing Chu 1981) have demonstrated aldehydes 0·11% and acrolein (50 ppm) as well as significant quantities of arsenic and cyanide.

The source of these chemicals has been showed by Genovesi *et al* (1977) (Table 16.2) to

Table 16.1 Distribution of patients by extent of total body surface burns and percentage mortality*

	Percentage burn									
	<10	11–20	21–30	31–40	41–50	51–60	61–70	71–80	81–90	91–100
Percentage Mortality										
Patients with inhalational injury	15·6	11·0	31·8	58·0	78·0	100	100	100	100	100
Patients without inhalational injury	0·9	4·0	14·2	33·0	46·0	50·0	65·0	100	100	100

* Data from 914 patients with acute thermal injuries and demonstrates the higher mortality of patients who receive cutaneous burns as well as an inhalational injury when compared with patients receiving skin burns only. (From Venus et al 1981 with kind permission of the editor of *Critical Care Medicine* and The Williams & Wilkins Co., Baltimore.)

Table 16.2 Sources of pulmonary irritants (P) in smoke

Material	Use	Major toxic chemical products of combustion
PVC	Wall and floor covering Telephone cable insulation	Hydrogen Chloride (P) Phosgene (P) Carbon Monoxide
Polyurethane	Upholstery	Isocyanates (P) Hydrogen cyanide
Lacquered wood Veneer Wallpaper	Wall covering	Acetaldehyde (P) Formaldehyde (P) Oxides of Nitrogen (P) Acetic acid
Acrylic	Light diffusers	Acrolein (P)
Nylon	Carpet	Hydrogen cyanide
Acrilan	Carpet	Hydrogen cyanide
Polystyrene	Miscellaneous	Styrene Carbon Monoxide

From Genovesi *et al* 1977 with kind permission of the editor of *Chest*.

arise predominantly from the plastics now widely used in building materials. PVC in particular is capable of producing highly toxic fumes when heated to temperatures above 225°C. This chloroethylene polymer is manufactured at a rate of over 8·3 billion kg per annum (Dyer & Esch 1976) and has found widespread use as a rubber substitute covering electric cables, telephone wires, 'non-inflammable' upholstery, seatcovers in aircrafts and cars as well as many other household uses.

As a result, although buildings may be constructed of fire-resistant elements, their contents (over which there is no control) may constitute a huge fuel load.

Notable pulmonary irritants amongst the chemicals present in smoke are hydrogen chloride, phosgene and acrolein. These substances are carried into the small airways in vapour form or absorbed on to small soot particles. There they adhere to the mucous membrane and in the presence of water form corrosive acids. Ulcers develop in the mucosal lining which may slough. Interstitial oedema, congestion and haemorrhages are also described as well as effects on surfactant production (Nieman *et al* 1980). Not only is there local tissue damage but systemic poisoning may occur from the absorption of lethal quantities of arsenic (Chu 1981) and cyanide.

Carbon monoxide poisoning

Carbon monoxide combines avidly with haemoglobin and in as low a concentration as 0·1% in room air will produce equal concentrations of oxyhaemoglobin and carboxyhaemoglobin. The result is a 50% reduction in oxygen carrying capacity. Allied with a leftward shift of the dissociation curve there is a significant reduction in the tissue availability of oxygen and cellular hypoxia results (Fein 1980).

Iatrogenic damage

The injured lung now presents a very vulnerable surface and sepsis is easily introduced. Instrumentation, intubation, or tracheal suction of the bronchial tree may lacerate the sloughing mucosal layer. Immunological deficiency has been described (Miller & Trunkey 1977, Fick et al 1980) and 'in association with the mechanical alterations significantly predisposes the thermally injured patient with inhalational injury to the development of infection in general and specifically to the development of pneumonia' (Tranbaugh et al 1983).

Either as a result of sepsis, the cutaneous burn, or chemical inhalation, there may be increases in the permeability of the pulmonary capillaries leading to interstitial pulmonary oedema. Several workers have investigated the extravascular lung water (EVLW) content after burns. The consensus opinion is that early increases (first 24 hours) in EVLW are uncommon. When it does occur it is usually the result of inhaling noxious fumes. At a later stage, however, there is evidence that increases in EVLW (Tranbaugh et al 1983) do occur in association with skin or pulmonary sepsis. At this point overenthusiastic and inaccurate fluid replacement may increase the oedema. Fluid transudation however may occur even in the absence of raised venous pressure and the question of colloid versus crystalloid resuscitation then becomes relevant and controversial.

Proponents of the Starling principle assert that administration of crystalloid will increase interstitial oedema by lowering colloid osmotic pressure (COP). However, Brigham (1979) states that pulmonary lymphatic flow is capable of increasing many fold and removing extra-interstitial fluid. Furthermore, as Brown (1982) points out, any movement of crystalloid solution into the pulmonary interstitial space will lower the COP there and tend to reverse the osmotic pressure gradient towards normal.

Clearly the mechanism of interstitial pulmonary oedema is complex. It seems sensible, however, to monitor atrial pressure in these circumstances so that excessive hydrostatic forces can be avoided.

DIAGNOSIS

History
Inhalation injury (see Fig. 16.1) should be suspected in the presence of:

1. A history of burn in an enclosed space
2. Facial burns or singed nasal hair
3. Hoarseness and wheezing
4. Carbonaceous sputum
5. High carboxyhaemoglobin levels.

Blood Tests
Carboxyhaemoglobin and blood gases
Measurement of carboxyhaemoglobin is a useful test if the patient is seen within several hours of the burn. Elevated levels (above 15%) indicate a strong likelihood of smoke inhalation. Because the partial pressure of dissolved oxygen (Pa_{O_2}) is not affected by carbon monoxide poisoning, this parameter may be normal. On the other hand the arterial oxygen saturation (Sa_{O_2}) will be low in the presence of carboxyhaemoglobin and this combination of a normal Pa_{O_2} and low Sa_{O_2} should arouse suspicion. When haematological techniques are used which derive Sa_{O_2} from Pa_{O_2} a false picture will result.

As far as the clinical appearance of the patient is concerned, the presence of carboxy-haemoglobin below levels of 40% is unlikely to cause the classical cherry red colouration of the skin. Cyanosis is more likely. Furthermore, because the carotid body responds to

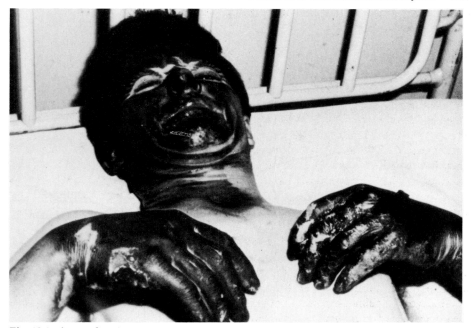

Fig. 16.1   A case of smoke inhalation. By kind permission of Mr B Morgan, FRCS.

changes in Pa_{O_2} and not Sa_{O_2} there may be no increase in minute volume. The failure of oxygen delivery to the tissues as a result of this intoxication leads to lactic acid production and a metabolic acidosis.

Respiratory function tests
Several workers describe the usefulness of simple respiratory function tests (Whitener *et al* 1980, Haponik *et al* 1984) in the diagnosis of respiratory injury. Using spirometric techniques (FEV_1 and FVC) Whitener *et al* (1980) described severe airway obstruction soon after burn injury and confirmed that the incidence of respiratory complication is related to the severity of surface burn and the presence or absence of smoke inhalation. Specifically, they noted that in patients without cutaneous burn, abnormal spirometry supported the diagnosis of smoke inhalation whereas normal spirometry excluded significant exposure. Haponik *et al* (1984) measured flow volume curves and found good correlation between abnormal curves and the severity of anatomic injury in the upper airway visualised at fiberoptic endoscopies. In particular they described good correlation between abnormal curves and the eventual need for endotracheal intubation. Both groups of workers recognised however that patients with severe facial injuries did not always make good candidates for this type of study.

Radiological investigations
All workers are agreed that chest X-ray is of little value in the early diagnosis of inhalational injury. Xenon washout scans (Moylan *et al* 1972) are more helpful. An intravenous injection of 6–10 μCi of xenon 133 is given and lung scans obtained at intervals over the next 2–3 minutes. Normally the isotope is completely cleared within 90 seconds. Significant delays in

clearance or segmental retention of the isotope suggest lung injury. False negative and positive results occur.

Instrumentation

Fiberoptic bronchoscopy is a useful aid to diagnosis and will demonstrate both the level and severity of the injury. In the absence of an expert bronchoscopist, indirect laryngoscopy with light and mirror can provide invaluable information about the condition of the larynx and pharynx.

TREATMENT

Oxygen

In the presence of carbon monoxide poisoning oxygen in high concentration should be given at once, remembering that concentrations of more than 60% are difficult to achieve with a face mask.

The administration of 100% oxygen increases the elimination half time of carbon monoxide from 250 minutes when breathing air to 40–50 minutes (Fein *et al* 1980). Should severe intoxication be suspected on the basis of coma or severe confusion (carboxy-haemoglobin more than 60%), then intubation and ventilation with 100% oxygen should be instituted. The inspired oxygen concentration can be reduced to 60% after 4 hours and 40% at 8 hours.

The ability to measure cyanide levels quickly, at least in the UK, seems limited, although American writers (Crapo 1981) refer to the importance of this test. Where cyanide poisoning is suspected, in the presence of a severe metabolic acidosis without much evidence of carbon monoxide intoxication, treatment may be initiated using sodium nitrite (300 mg over 2–4 minutes) to produce methaemoglobin. This unites with cyanide to form cyanmethaemoglobin. A slow (10-minute) infusion of 12.5 g of aqueous sodium thiosulphate will then change cyanide to thiocyanate which is less toxic and is excreted in the urine (Berlin 1977).

Airway obstruction

This is an early development in patients with inhalational injuries and one which may progress rapidly and insidiously (see Fig. 16.2). Delay in securing the airway by intubation can result in major difficulties with oedema of pharynx and larynx preventing visualisation of the cords. Bartlett (1976), in a review of 740 patients with acute burns recommended specific indications for intubation:

1. Stridor
2. Facial burns and c.n.s. depression
3. Full thickness burns of nose and lips
4. Facial burns and circumferential full thickness burns on the neck
5. Visible oedema of pharynx.

Although tracheostomy has been implicated as a potent cause of pulmonary sepsis it is noteworthy that Bartlett (1976) reported no association between mortality and the method of upper airway control. Most clinicians will, however, prefer to use nasotracheal intubation introducing a nasogastric tube at the same time. Extubation should be delayed until the facial oedema subsides and a leak can be demonstrated around the tube with the open end occluded and the cuff deflated.

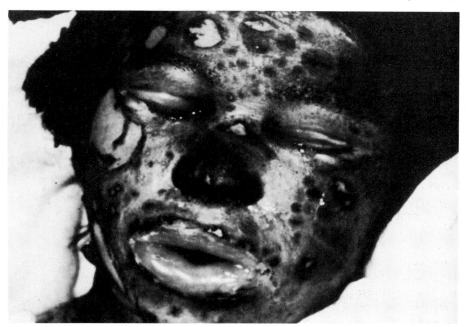

Fig. 16.2   Facial burns and oedema. By kind permission of Mr B Morgan, FRCS.

Steroids

Until 1977, steroids were used routinely in the early management of smoke inhalation injury. A common regime was to administer methyl prednisolone 30 mg/kg a day for 2 days. In 1978, however, Moylan and Alexander demonstrated steroid coverage to be of no benefit and even detrimental. This study has been supported by Robinson *et al* (1982) in a study of the victims of the MGM Grand and Hilton hotel fires in Las Vegas. At present the consensus opinion is that steroids are not indicated. The use of antibiotics is more controversial and will depend on local practice. Certainly several authors recommend penicillin routinely during the first 5 days after injury.

Fluids

Fluid resuscitation is the cornerstone of burn treatment and is usually instituted when burns exceed 15% in adults and 10% in children. Because of the pulmonary complications associated with burns, fluid replacement should be accurately monitored either by central venous pressure measurement or in the more complicated case by left atrial pressure measurement. In either case the best opportunity to insert these lines is early in the course of management before oedema, bandages and burn ointments render the task more difficult. Good anchorage of these lines is absolutely essential.

Various fluid regimes exist, examples of which can be simplified as follows:

Mount Vernon: 2·5 ml colloid/percentage burn/kg body weight/24 hours and 2500 ml 5% dextrose.

Evans: 1 ml colloid and 1 ml electrolyte solution/kg body weight/percentage burn and 5% dextrose 2000 ml to cover evaporative water losses . . . in first 24 hours.

Brooke: 0·5 ml colloid and 1.5 ml electrolyte solution/kg body weight/percentage burn and 2000 ml of 5% dextrose . . . in first 24 hours.

Parkland: 4 ml Hartmanns/kg body weight/percentage burn in first 24 hours.

Clearly a variety of techniques work although controversy exists regarding types of fluid, salt content and the timing of colloid administration. Whichever formula is decided upon, careful attention must be given to the vital signs, packed cell volume, electrolytes and urine output (Table 16.3). Pruitt (1978) recommends urinary outputs of 30–50 ml/hour, although

Table 16.3 Clinical guide to adequacy of fluid therapy in burns

1. Urine volume 50–100 ml/hour
2. Sensorium clear and lucid
3. Pulse < 120 beats/min
4. Blood pressure normal or high
5. CVP > 5 cmH$_2$O
6. Lack of nausea or ileus
7. Serum bicarbonate > 18 mmol/litre
8. Sodium excretion > 30 mmol/litre

From Gilbertson A A 1984 *Intravenous technique and therapy.* William Heinemann, London.

higher hourly volumes (50–100 ml) have been suggested by workers in the UK (Brown & Ward 1984). Generally speaking, it is agreed that patients with inhalational injury have increased fluid needs but Scheulen & Munster (1982) suggest that meeting this need may predispose patients with inhalational injury to pulmonary fluid overload thus prolonging their dependence on IPPV. In their opinion lower urine volumes (20–35 ml/hour) are more appropriate. They also recommend increased use of left atrial monitoring.

Respiratory care

Deterioration in pulmonary function may occur during the first day or two post-burn even without smoke inhalation. Brown (1982) points out that the earliest signs are usually auscultatory but elevation of respiratory rate and worsening arterial blood gases provide good objective evidence.

Once respiratory disorder is recognised, standard procedures of humidified oxygen administration, chest physiotherapy and bronchodilator therapy should be instituted. Escharotomy may be necessary to prevent splinting of the chest wall and regular cultures of burn wound, sputum, blood and urine organised.

During the first 24 hours after inhalation injury Robinson *et al* (1981) demonstrated that large areas of lung had low ventilation perfusion ratios consistent with small airway oedema and closure. Efforts to maintain small airway patency have led some workers to advocate early prophylactic intubation (Venus 1981) with constant positive airway pressure (CPAP). Others oppose this regime on the basis of increased likelihood of pulmonary sepsis and pulmonary oedema.

Respiratory Failure

Should respiratory deterioration develop intermittent positive pressure ventilation should be started using the following criteria:

Respiratory rate   >35/min
Vital capacity   <10-15 ml/kg
Shunt fraction   >15–20%
Pa_{O_2} ($Fi_{O_2}·4$)   <11·0 kPa
Dead space/tidal volume   >0·55–0·6

As usual in these therapeutic circumstances efforts should be made to keep the F_{IO_2} as low as possible compatible with a Pa_{O_2} of above $8 \cdot 0$ kPa. High airway pressures should be avoided to minimise pulmonary barotrauma. Although IMV has received enthusiastic support, recent reviews (Weisman et al 1983) point out that, as yet, none of the putative advantages have been proved.

Nutrition

The value of early attention to nutrition cannot be overemphasised, taking into account the marked increase in whole body protein synthesis and breakdown which occurs in proportion to the size of the burn. A simple formula (Curreri et al 1974) such as the one recommended by Munster et al (1980) can be used:

$$\text{calories per day} = 25 \text{ cal/kg body weight} + 40 \text{ cal/percentage burn}$$

Ideally these calories should be administered enterally by fine-bore nasogastric tube using one of the iso-osmolar ready to use preparations containing the complete nutritional requirements of the patient. Measurement of nitrogen and electrolyte losses in urine will facilitate accurate replacement. Finally, increasing ambient temperatures will prevent to some extent evaporative water losses from the burn and thus reduce calorie expenditure.

Long-term effects of smoke inhalation

Reports of chronic lung damage after smoke inhalation are uncommon. However, some authors have described bronchiectasis and obliterative bronchiolitis in these circumstances.

A recent report from this unit (Cooke 1982) suggests that severe but asymptomatic airflow obstruction can persist for as long as 15 months after the exposure to smoke. In this patient, who initially suffered a severe smoke inhalation episode without cutaneous burn, serial flow volume loops demonstrated preservation of maximum flow rates but severe reduction in flow rates at 50% and 25% of vital capacity. Lung volumes were normal (Table 16.4). These findings, which persisted until his failure to attend follow-up at 15 months, were not improved by steroids and were consistent with widespread damage to small airways.

Table 16.4 Serial pulmonary function tests in a patient who received smoke inhalation (percentage of predicted value in parenthesis)

| | Number of days postinjury | | | | | | | | |
	10	15	20	27	45	59	86	103	470
FEV_1 litres	2·00	2·12	2·29	2·48	2·36	2·11	2·30	2·20	2·86
	(43)	(46)	(49)	(53)	(51)	(45)	(50)	(47)	(62)
FVC litres	3·69	4·23	4·27	3·90	4·16	4·18	4·40	4·10	5·53
	(63)	(73)	(73)	(67)	(71)	(72)	(75)	(70)	(96)
FEV_1/FVC %	54	50	53	63	56	50	52	53	51
V_{max} litres/second		4·62	8·42	9·21	9·82	9·07	8·81	9·20	9·51
		(54)	(98)	(108)	(115)	(106)	(103)	(107)	(111)
$V_{max\,50}$ litres/second		0·92	1·00	1·36	1·25	0·86	1·00	1·03	1·33
		(17)	(19)	(26)	(23)	(16)	(19)	(25)	(24)
$V_{max\,25}$ litres/second		0·33	0·46	0·57	0·48	0·33	0·46	0·46	0·52
		(14)	(20)	(27)	(21)	(14)	(20)	(19)	(23)
DLCO mmol/min/kPa		6·76	7·56	7·82	8·06	7·98	8·72		8·60
		(53)	(60)	(62)	(64)	(63)	(69)		(68)
KCO mmol/min/kPa/litre		1·28	1·31	1·37	1·40	1·42	1·56		1·62
		(66)	(68)	(71)	(72)	(73)	(80)		(84)

From Cooke et al 1982 with kind permission of the editor of *Anaesthesia* and The Association of Anaesthetists of Great Britain and Ireland.

REFERENCES

Bartlett R H, Niccole M, Travis M J, Allyn P A, Furnas D W 1976 Acute management of the upper airway in facial burns and smoke inhalation. *Archives of Surgery* **3:** 744–749

Berlin C 1977 Cyanide poisoning: a challenge. *Archives of Internal Medicine* **137:** 993–994

Brigham K L 1979 Pulmonary oedema: cardiac and non-cardiac. *American Journal of Surgery* **138:** 361–367

Brown J, Ward D 1984 Immediate management of burns in casualty. *British Journal of Hospital Medicine* **31:** 360–368

Brown J 1982 Management of injury due to smoke inhalation. *Journal of the Royal Society of Medicine Supplement no 1* **75:** 45–50

Chi-Shing Chu 1981 New concepts of pulmonary burn injury. *Journal of Trauma* **21:** 958–961

Crapo R O 1981 Smoke inhalation injuries. *Journal of the American Medical Association* **246:** 1694–1696

Cooke N T, Cobley A J, Armstrong R F 1982 Airflow obstruction after smoke inhalation. *Anaesthesia* **37:** 830–832

Curreri P W, Richmond D, Marvin D, Marvin J A, Baxter C R 1974 Dietary requirements of patients with major burns. *Journal of the American Dietary Association* **65:** 415–417

Dyer R F, Esch V H 1976 PVC toxicity in fires. *Journal of the American Medical Association* **235:** 393–397

Feller I, Richards K E, Pierson C L, Flanders S J 1978 Causes of death in burned patients. 5th International Congress on Burn Injuries, Stockholm

Fein A, Leff A, Hopewell P C 1980 Pathophysiology and management of the complications resulting from fire and the inhaled products of combustion. *Critical Care Medicine* **8:** 94–98

Fick R B, Paul E, Reynolds H Y *et al* 1980. Impaired phagocytic and bacteriocidal functions of smoke exposed rabbits' alveolar macrophages. *Chest* **78:** 516–518

Genovesi M G, Tashkin D P, Chopra S 1977 Transient hypoxaemia in firemen following inhalation of smoke. *Chest* **71:** 441–444

Haponik E F, Munster A M, Wise R A *et al* 1984 Upper airway function in burn patients. *American Review of Respiratory Disease* **129:** 251–257

Mierley M C, Baker S P 1983 Fatal house fires in an urban population. *Journal of the American Medical Association* **249:** 1466–1468

Miller C L, Trunkey D D 1977 Thermal injury: defects in immune response induction. *Journal of Surgical Research* **22:** 621–625

Moylan J A, Alexander L G 1978 Diagnosis and treatment of inhalation injury. *World Journal of Surgery* **2:** 185–189

Moylan J A, Wilmore D W, Mouton D E, Pruitt B A 1972 Early diagnosis of inhalational injury using 133 Xe lung scan. *Annals of Surgery* **176:** 477–484

Munster A M 1980 The early management of thermal burns. *Surgery* **87:** 29–40

Nieman G F, Clark W R, Wax S D, Webb W R 1980 The effect of smoke inhalation on pulmonary surfactant. *Annals of Surgery* **191:** 171–181

Pruitt B A 1978 Fluid and electrolyte replacement in the burned patient. *Surgical Clinics of North America* **58:** 1291–1312

Robinson N B, Hudson L D, Riem M, Miller E 1982 Steroid therapy following isolated smoke inhalation injury. *Journal of Trauma* **22:** 876–879

Robinson N B, Hudson L D, Robertson H T 1981 Ventilation and perfusion alterations during smoke inhalation injury. *Surgery* **90:** 352–363

Scheulen J J, Munster A M 1982 The Parkland formula in patients with burns and inhalation injury. *Journal of Trauma* **22:** 869–871

Tranbaugh R F, Elings V B, Christensen J M, Lewis F R 1983 The effect of inhalational injury on lung water accumulation. *Journal of Trauma* **23:** 597–604

United Kingdom Fire Statistics 1979

Venus B, Matsuda T, Copiozo J B, Mathru M 1981 Prophylactic intubation and continuous positive airway pressure in the management of inhalation injury in burn victims. *Critical Care Medicine* **9:** 519–523

Weisman I M, Rinaldo J E, Rogers R M, Sanders M H 1983 Intermittent mandatory ventilation. *American Review of Respiratory Diseases* **127:** 641–647

Whitener D R, Whitener L M, Robertson K J, Baxter C R, Pierce A K 1980 Pulmonary function measurements in patients with thermal injury and smoke inhalation. *American Review of Respiratory Disease* **122:** 731–739

Zawacki B E, Jung R C, Joyce J *et al* 1977 Smoke, burn and the natural history of inhalation injury in fire victims. *Annals of Surgery* **185:** 100–110

Zikria B A, Weston G C, Chodoff M 1972 Smoke and carbon monoxide poisoning in fire victims. *Journal of Trauma* **12:** 641–645

Resuscitation

There has been a recent renewal of interest in cardiopulmonary resuscitation (CPR). Attempts have been made to make the general public aware of life-saving techniques and there has been a move to transform the ambulance and resuscitation services into mobile intensive care units.

Previously accepted physiological principles of external chest compression (ECC) are being questioned and new techniques of cardiopulmonary resuscitation (new CPR) are being evaluated. Traditional drug armamentarium is being revised and recommended clinical indications and doses of drugs such as calcium, sodium bicarbonate and lignocaine have been modified.

TRAINING IN RESUSCITATION

Two decades have passed since external chest compression was shown to produce an arterial pulse during ventricular fibrillation in dogs (Kouwenhoven *et al* 1960) and in man (Jude *et al* 1961). It had been hoped that these observations would lead to improved training of the public and physicians in basic life support based on the standards and guidelines advocated by the American Heart Association (1974, 1980).

However, the competence of young doctors has been questioned by Webb & Lambrew (1978) who found that only 22% could adequately compress and ventilate a manikin. Lowenstein *et al* (1981) tested 45 house officers and found that none passed the American Heart Association's Basic Life Support (BLS) test. Only a third could use a manikin properly and intubate it in 35 seconds and only 31, 40 and 33% could competently manage ventricular fibrillation, asystole and complete heart block respectively. *The Times* (1984) suggested that ambulance crews could save between 2000 and 5000 patients a year in the UK if their training were improved. Such training should include intubation, intravenous infusions and defibrillation.

Public education schemes have shown that the poor performance of nursing and medical personnel can be improved (Cobb 1983) and survival rates can be tripled from 10% to 30% if professional mobile resuscitation units are supplemented by basic CPR begun by the bystander at the time of the collapse.

In Britain there has been political indifference to educational schemes for resuscitation (*British Medical Journal* 1984), but enthusiastic informed groups such as the Resuscitation Council have published booklets describing the necessary life-saving techniques in simple words (Resuscitation Council, UK 1984) and strong advocacy of educational schemes has been provided by Vincent *et al* (1984) and Zideman (1983).

A survey of English health regions (Jones 1983) revealed a hotch-potch mixture with little attempt at quantifying their benefits. Nevertheless, 8 centres had schemes. Brighton's mobile ambulance is now combined with a public education programme, which was successful 31 out of 128 defibrillations in 1981. The Avon scheme treated 49 cardiac arrests in 1981 and defibrillated 37 patients.

The evolution of the Brighton and Frenchay urban mobile resuscitation ambulances are documented by Chamberlain et al (1973) and Baskett et al (1976).

BASIC LIFE SUPPORT AND THE AIRWAY

Basic life support (BLS) is that phase of emergency cardiac care that either (1) prevents circulatory or respiratory arrest or insufficiency through prompt recognition and intervention, or (2) externally supports the circulation and respiration of the victim of cardiac or respiratory arrest through cardiopulmonary resuscitation.

The Resuscitation Council's ABC of resuscitation emphasises a rational sequence or algorithm which includes the approach to the patient and subsequent priorities:

1. Airway
2. Breathing
3. Circulation

In each system a simple assessment is made and consequent therapy advocated.

Some cardiologists have questioned the ABC order of priorities, recommending CAB for both medical and lay personnel (Crul et al 1981). However, the lay public take some time to confirm the diagnosis of cardiac arrest and many cases of arrest are caused by dysrhythmias due to primary anoxia which may well respond to airway clearance and mouth-to-mouth ventilation. Therefore, the ABC sequence seems the widest choice of education for the lay public, but the CAB has advantages when the arrest occurs in situations such as a coronary care unit (Baskett 1984).

The airway

The airway can usually be cleared of foreign matter such as blood, teeth or vomitus and maintained by a combination of head tilting and jaw support. The use of nasopharyngeal airways may overcome difficulties in maintaining an airway via the mouth in patients with trismus or fits.

In an attempt to find an interim solution for paramedics before tracheal intubation can be accomplished, oesophageal obturators (EOA) and oesophageal gastic tube airways (EGTA) have been widely used in the USA (Don et al 1968, Gordon 1977). It is claimed that it is easier to teach paramedics their use than tracheal intubation. Unfortunately, pulmonary ventilation is less efficient than with tracheal tubes (Merrifield & King 1981) and tracheal intubation, oesophageal rupture and aspiration of gastric contents have all been reported.

Intubation of the trachea remains the method of choice to provide a secure airway during resuscitation. On rare occasions, intubation proves to be impossible even in the hands of those skilled in the technique. Cricothyroidotomy can be life-saving in these cases. Baskett (1984) recommends inserting two 14-gauge (2·0 mm) Medicut intravenous cannulae into the trachea through the cricothyroid membrane.

The indwelling needles are removed leaving the plastic cannulae *in situ*. One cannula is attached to a manual resuscitator using a small tracheal tube connector and ventilation gently commenced taking care not to produce overdistension of the lungs. The second cannula is open to the atmosphere.

Ventilation via this route may also be accomplished by intermittent jets of oxygen or high frequency positive pressure ventilation (Swartzman *et al* 1984) but this technique clearly has many potential hazards. A more secure airway must be established using a tracheostomy or cricothyrotomy. A cricothyrotome incorporating a sharp retractable blade is available through Penlon Ltd, Abingdon, Oxford.

Foreign body airways obstruction
The 'Heimlich manoeuvre' (Heimlich 1974) has been modified from the originally described abdominal thrust to a chest thrust. The efficacy of back blows in clearing foreign bodies is also well known.

The typical pattern of complete airway obstruction is that a subject who is eating or has just finished eating suddenly becomes unable to speak or cough and may clutch at his or her throat. Three manoeuvres in sequence are recommended: back blows, manual thrusts (modified Heimlich) and finger sweeps into the mouth or pharynx (Montgomery 1983).

Breathing
Ventilation of the patient can be performed by mouth-to-mouth, mouth-to-nose or with the help of airway aids such as the Brooke and Safar airways. Purpose-made 'pocket' masks, which are transparent, provide a good face seal and can be used with expired air or 100% oxygen, have recently found favour (Standards and Guidelines, JAMA 1980). Nevertheless, more efficient ventilation can be achieved by the use of ventilatory resuscitators, i.e. small portable ventilators designed to be used in emergencies. Resuscitators may be either manually powered or gas powered. Most manual resuscitators consist of a self-refilling bag fitted with a one-way inspiratory-expiratory valve which connects to a face mask or tracheal tube, and a bag inlet valve which allows the bag to fill with air—with or without supplementary oxygen. An evaluation of the performance of several adult manual resuscitators was undertaken by the DHSS (1983) and reviewed by Eaton (1984). In these studies the following criteria were assessed:

1. Ease of use by one person.
2. Possibility of incorrect assembly of components.
3. Ease of cleaning.
4. The attainment of high inspired oxygen levels without jamming of 'patient' valve.
5. Backward leakage through the patient valve.
6. Tidal volume.
7. Maximum airway pressure.
8. Inspiratory and expiratory resistance.

Many resuscitators did not perform adequately and were not recommended.

Gas-powered resuscitators may be manually or automatically triggered. Automatic resuscitators provide reliable ventilation, and free a rescuer to undertake other tasks. Four gas-powered resuscitators were assessed for ventilatory performance, ease of use, strength (dropped on to concrete and run over by an ambulance wheel!), and reliability (Harber & Lucas 1980). Only the 'Pneupac'* resuscitator satisfied all these criteria. Newer resuscitators

---

*'Pneupac' manufactured by Pneupac Ltd of Dunstable.

are available with features such as adjustable inspired oxygen concentration or working as minute volume dividers and mandatory minute volume devices. These sophisticated resuscitators may have special applications but it is not yet apparent that their robustness and reliability make them suitable for general use.

Pressure cycled resuscitators are likely to be triggered during ECC and therefore cannot be recommended.

ADVANCED LIFE SUPPORT (ALS)

ALS includes BLS plus the use of special equipment and techniques for establishing, maintaining and monitoring ventilation and circulation. It includes the employment of drugs and defribillation.

The circulation

The BLS provides a rapid succession of airway care, artificial ventilation and where appropriate external chest compression (ECC). The rates for ECC currently advocated are if working alone, 15 compressions followed by 2 inflations, or with assistance 5 chest compressions per inflation.

A major problem which has stimulated much academic interest in recent years is the failure of ECC, even with perfect technique, to generate much forward blood flow. This led Rudikoff and his colleagues at John Hopkins University in Baltimore (1980) to question the physiology of ECC, which was already known to produce transmission of pressure equally and simultaneously to both arterial and venous systems (Mackenzie et al 1964). The Hopkins group investigated the effects of simultaneous chest compression and ventilation at high airway pressures (Chandra et al 1980) and proposed that a major improvement in cardiac output could be achieved by simultaneous compression and ventilation. They found that the raised intrathoracic pressures increased arterial pressure with no rise in venous pressure and suggested that the whole chest activity was acting as a 'thoracic pump' in which the heart was emptied by lateral compression of the heart due to lung inflation. The theory was supported by cineangiography in dogs (Niemann et al 1981) and echocardiography in man (Rich et al 1981, Werner et al 1981) and by the reports of 'Cough CPR'. Criley et al (1976) demonstrated that coughing more than doubled mean aortic systolic blood pressure and maintained consciousness if brief periods of bradycardia or ventricular fibrillation occurred during coronary angiography.

Chandra's 'New CPR' consisted of a prolonged chest compression forming 60% of the cycle at rates of 10 to 40 per minute accompanied by simultaneous ventilation at high airway pressures (70–110 cmH$_2$O). When this was compared with periods of standard cardiopulmonary resuscitation in alternating 30 second cycles, the 'New CPR' resulted in elevations of systolic blood pressure by 13 mmHg, carotid blood flow by 252% and the carotid flow was found to be directly proportional to intrathoracic pressure suggesting that elevated intrathoracic pressure was essential in CPR (Chandra et al 1980).

Rogers and his colleagues questioned whether the carotid blood flow increase might be due to redistribution of blood flow between the external and internal carotid arteries and whether there were effects on the verterbal circulation (Rogers et al 1981). Other studies have failed to find any difference in cardiac output between interposed ventilation and simultaneous ventilation at high airway pressures (Babbs et al 1982, Redding et al 1981, Bircher & Safar 1981). Babbs related failure of New CPR to the small size of his dogs—which may have relevance in paediatric resuscitation. Moreover, there has been no animal or human study which has produced an improvement in outcome with New CPR, with or without abdominal binding, which would justify any widespread change in clinical practice.

However, in specialised units, after BLS, defibrillation, drugs and transfusion have failed, New CPR may be worthy of use (Birch & Safar 1981). Baskett (1984) suggests that the teaching today should be to continue ECC without interruption for ventilation and an attempt made to interpose a ventilation to synchronise with every fifth compression. He also suggests modifying the technique of external cardiac compression so that the compression phase occupies at least 50% of the cycle. It is likely that this sophistication in ventilation chest compression can only be achieved with the further development of automatic chest compressor/resuscitator units.

Adjuncts to ALS
Abdominal binding. Abdominal binding was suggested by Harris *et al* in 1967 and its efficacy confirmed by Redding (1971). Chandra (1981) successfully applied this technique with similar effect to 10 human subjects, utilising abdominal binding with a 30 cm bladder around the abdomen which was inflated to $60-110$ cmH_2O. Bircher *et al* (1980) and Lilja *et al* (1981) have confirmed that inflation of Medical Antishock Trousers (MAST) augments systolic blood pressure and upper body perfusion during CPR.

The precordial 'thump' has corrected many cardiac arrests, but is now thought to be rarely of benefit.

Open chest cardiac compression
Despite Safar's claim (1981) that open cardiac compression offers the best method of supporting the circulation in cardiac standstill, most feel it should only be used in hospital and then only by specially trained physicians. The indications for opening the chest fall into three groups (Jacobsen 1983):

1. *Immediate opening.* Major chest trauma or penetrating chest wound developing cardiac arrest. Certain patients who develop arrest while undergoing surgery.
2. *Delayed opening.* i.e. shortly after ECC. Patients in whom there is a possibility of cardiac tamponade, profound hypovolaemia or pulmonary air or thromboembolism.
3. *Delayed opening after failure of external resuscitation.* Hypothermic patients plus those with thromboembolism occurring where facilities for immediate cardiopulmonary bypass are available.

Defibrillation
Early defibrillation has resulted in survival rates of over 60% after ventricular fibrillation whereas the prognosis from asystole and electromechanical dissociation is poor (Sowden *et al* 1984).

Kerber *et al* (1981) measured the transthoracic resistance and found it to be related to chest size and highly variable; hence large defibrillator contacts should be used and firm contact obtained. Weaver *et al* (1982) noted that survival was related to the rhythm achieved after the first shock. There was a 40% survival with supraventricular arrythmias, 30% with persistent ventricular fibrillation, 26% with idioventricular rhythms and 14% with asystole. These authors also found that low energy levels of 175 joules were as good as 320 joules.

The Resuscitation Council's recommendations suggest commencing with 180 joule shocks for the first and second defibrillation attempt and if this fails increasing to 360 joules as outlined in Table 17.1.

Table 17.1 Advanced life support—ventricular fibrillation

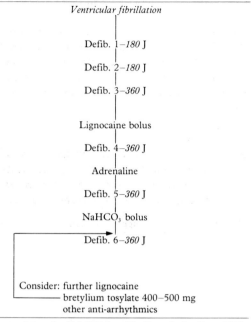

Ventricular fibrillation

Defib. 1—*180* J

Defib. 2—*180* J

Defib. 3—*360* J

Lignocaine bolus

Defib. 4—*360* J

Adrenaline

Defib. 5—*360* J

NaHCO₃ bolus

Defib. 6—*360* J

Consider: further lignocaine
bretylium tosylate 400—500 mg
other anti-arrhythmics

Recommendations for ALS 1984 from The Resuscitation Council UK,
D A Zideman—personal communication.

Automatic external defibrillator pacemakers are now available which work by means of epigastric and tongue terminals and in which safety logic circuits establish ventricular fibrillation and the absence of breathing ($7 \cdot 2$ seconds), charge the capacitator ($4 \cdot 8$ seconds) and deliver 200 joules within 12 seconds (Jugarrao *et al* 1982). Automatic internal defibrillators are also being developed. An implanted defibrillatory device is linked to an e.c.g. monitor and triggers 20–25 joules shock directly through the electrodes (Mirowski *et al* 1981).

Drug therapy

Antiarrhythmic agents
Lignocaine remains the first choice drug for suppressing multiple ectopic ventricular beats and in repeated ventricular fibrillation. It has a rapid onset of action, short duration of effect and relatively few side effects. The action of lignocaine is still controversial. It is known to raise the ventricular fibrillation threshold, suppress automaticity and shorten both the duration of action potentials and effective refractory period. Its efficacy may be due to the creation of temporal homogeneity of action potentials on the distal Purkinge system (Yakaitis 1983).

An initial bolus of 50 to 100 mg should be administered, and this may be followed by a continuous infusion of 4 mg per minute reducing, with the purpose of suppressing ectopic foci but maintaining myocardial contractility.

Bretylium tosylate has been shown to raise the ventricular fibrillation threshold, facilitate electrical defibrillation and has been reported to chemically defibrillate the heart (Badoner

1979, Kock-Weser 1979). Bretylium, unlike other antiarrhythmic agents, causes a decrease in defibrillation threshold and has a positive inotropic effect on the heart. Bretylium should be administered as a 400 mg bolus given early as it takes up to 15 minutes to achieve its maximum effect. Its side effect of hypotension can be managed by appropriate fluid and pressor therapy.

Following lignocaine and bretylium, procainamide and beta-blockers form the first line drugs. The effectiveness of beta-blockers is dependent on the level of sympathetic activity prevailing. Several newer agents are available; disopyramide acts in a quinidine-like way while mexiletine and tocainide which resemble lignocaine. Amiodarone has both coronary vasodilator and antiarrhythmic properties, but may produce an atropine resistant bradycardia and hypotension.

Calcium and calcium antagonists

It is now apparent that calcium should only be administered to treat hypocalcaemia, hyper-kalaemia and massive blood or colloid transfusions. Experimentally, calcium does not increase survival in asystole and hence is not recommended in its treatment (see Table 17.2). Its use after myocardial infarction may accentuate coronary artery spasm (Dembo 1983),

Table 17.2 Advanced life support—asystole

Asystole

|

Atropine

|

Adrenaline

|

$NaHCO_3$ bolus

|

Isoprenaline

Consider: intracardiac adrenaline pacing

Recommendations for ALS 1984 from The Resuscitation Council UK, D A Zideman—personal communication.

increase muscle spasticity and oxygen requirements, lead to an extension of the infarcted area, resulting in failure of resuscitation of digitalised patients. Calcium sometimes improves the performance of a weakly beating heart and is recommended by the Resuscitation Council in the treatment of electrochemical dissociation (see Table 17.3) although Dembo (1983) questions its use in this condition.

Calcium antagonists are protective against ventricular fibrillation and raise the fibrillation threshold. They also improve perfusion to areas around a myocardial infarction and hence reduce the area of cardiac damage. Calcium blockers also antagonise the enhanced adrenergic input to the heart which follows acute coronary occlusion (Rasnekov 1981), reduce systemic vascular resistance and hence cardiac work and slow AV conduction. However, calcium antagonists may induce tachycardia and their place in resuscitation has still to be clarified. They may have a role in cerebral resuscitation (White et al 1983).

Atropine

Atropine is indicated in the treatment of bradycardia and hypotension associated with para-

Table 17.3 Advanced life support—electromechanical dissociation

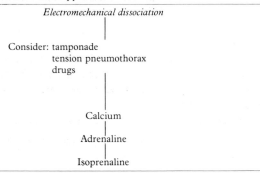

Electromechanical dissociation

Consider: tamponade
tension pneumothorax
drugs

Calcium

Adrenaline

Isoprenaline

Recommendations for ALS 1984 from The Resuscitation Council UK,
D A Zideman—personal communication.

sympathetic stimulation but its recommended use in asystole has been questioned. Nevertheless it can be argued that most salvageable cases of asystole have developed this dysrhythmia due to excessive parasympathetic stimulation and atropine is the appropriate remedy (Laing & Redmond 1982) (see Table 17.2). Atropine produces tachycardia, increased myocardial oxygen consumption and may cause dysrhythmias (Schweitzer & Mark 1980).

Adrenaline and sympathetic stimulants

Adrenaline remains the drug of choice (after atropine) in the treatment of asystole (Table 17.2) and bradycardia with myocardial depression. It should be given as a bolus 2–3 ml of 1/10 000 solution and can be repeated to 10 ml or continued as an infusion. Adrenaline is rapidly and well absorbed after intratracheal administration where 1 mg is diluted to 10 ml of water (Roberts *et al* 1979). The awareness that vasocontrictor drugs are useful and that α receptor stimulation and elevation of diastolic pressure are important has led to new interest in the use of methoxamine because of its lack of inotropic action on the heart and its weak β adrenergic blocking activity.

Once the heart has restarted, maintenance of organ perfusion can be achieved with dopamine. When administered in low dosage it produces dopaminergic and weak β agonist activity whereas α stimulation prevails with higher doses: hence dopamine therapy can be finely tuned to the patient's requirements.

The use of isoprenaline is controversial and should be reserved for patients with severe heart block, refractory asystole (Table 17.2) or electromechanical dissociation (Table 17.3). Treatment may need to be continued until cardiac pacing is established.

Sodium bicarbonate

It is now apparent that the smallest dose of sodium bicarbonate that is required to correct metabolic acidosis should be administered. Excessive bicarbonate therapy causes hyperosmolarity, hypercarbia and brain acidosis, and does not help in correcting arrhythmias (Bishop & Weisfeldt 1976, Yakaitis *et al* 1975).

Sudden cases of cardiac arrest which are promptly treated do not require bicarbonate therapy, which should be reserved for refractory cases or those in whom there is a prolonged period of poor tissue perfusion. Severe acidaemia is commonly seen in drowning victims.

Sodium bicarbonate is generally available as an $8\cdot4\%$ solution; 50 mmol should be administered as a bolus and the need for subsequent doses based on the results of blood gas analysis.

It is essential that hypertonic sodium bicarbonate does not extravasate otherwise extensive tissue damage will ensue. It should not be mixed with calcium as an embolic precipitate will form.

Steroids

It is difficult to prove that steroid therapy is effective, but as it is safe, it is justified in the immediate postarrest situation as a means of combating cerebral oedema.

Route of adminsistration. Adrenaline, lignocaine and atropine are all well absorbed when given by the endotracheal route.

Recommended drug dosages are summarised in Table 17.4.

Table 17.4 Advanced life support—drug dosages (based on 70 kg man)

Atrophine	1–2 mg i.v. or ET
Adrenaline	10 ml 1:10 000 i.v. or ET
Calcium	As glucomate 10 ml of 10% Must not be injected with bicarbonate
Isoprenaline	Bolus 100 μg then infusion 4 μ/min
Lignocaine	Bolus 100 mg i.v. or 200 mg ET then infusion 4 mg/min (reducing)
Sodium Bicarbonate	Not as routine—only refractory cases Bolus of 50 ml 8·4% pH to be measured as soon as possible

Cerebral resuscitation

Treatment of postanoxic cerebral oedema

The important factors are maintenance of satisfactory blood pressure, mild hypocarbia, good arterial oxygenation and normal blood sugar and electrolytes. It is essential that fits are suppressed e.g. using barbiturates. Diuretics also help in the control of intracranial pressure. Steroids may help in limiting cerebral oedema but are without value in head injuries.

In an attempt to supplement these well proven methods, larger doses of barbiturates have been tried but the situation is still that recorded in an editorial in *Anesthesiology* in December 1978, 'To date, there has not been any definitive study clearly proving a specific protective action of barbiturates in global ischaemia' (Rockott & Shapiro 1978). The role of calcium blockers also remains to be determined (White *et al* 1983).

Regimens for ALS

Currently recommended regimens for ALS (1984) from the Resuscitation Council UK are illustrated in Table 17.1 (ventricular fibrillation), Table 17.2 (asystole), Table 17.3 (electromechanical dissociation, i.e. no cardiac output in the presence of e.c.g. complexes), Table 17.4 (summarises drug dosage recommendations).

PHILOSOPHICAL AND ETHICAL PROBLEMS

The development of successful resuscitation has produced problems in the definition of death and anxiety that the privacy and dignity of the deathbed will not be invaded by inappropriate resuscitation attempts.

It is noteworthy that in the two biblical references to resuscitation (Elijah in I Kings, 17:17

and Elisha in II Kings, 4:15) the prophets sought divine guidance before commencing resuscitation.

The essence of resuscitation is to fight for the life of a dying person even into the state of clinical death, but only until it has been established beyond doubt that irreversible brain damage has occurred (Negovsky 1982).

Discontinuing resuscitation or not commencing it are clinical decisions based on medical knowledge of the salvageability of the patient. It is essential that factors which may preserve cerebral function during hypoxia are taken into consideration, such as hypothermia and the presence of sedative drugs. Patients who are housebound are less likely to survive (4%) than those who had pursued activities outside the home (27%). Metabolic or respiratory acidosis existing before cardiac arrest is often associated with diseases in which few patients survive arrest, e.g. pneumonia, renal failure, acute stroke with neurological deficit and hypotension due to myocardial failure or sepsis (Hanson 1984). The age of the patient is less important than the pre-existing disease (Bedall et al 1983). Finally, the response of the patient to resuscitation will greatly influence the likelihood of a successful outcome.

REFERENCES

Babbs C F, Fitzgerald K R, Voorhess W D, Murphy R J 1982 *Critical Care Medicine* **10**: 505–508
Badoner M B 1979 Treatment of ventricular fibrillation and other acute arrhythmias with bretylium tosylate. *American Journal of Cardiology* **21**: 530–544
Baskett P J F, Zorab J S M, Moyer J (eds) 1984 Aspects of cardiopulmonary resuscitation. *WFSA lectures, vol 2.* Blackwell Scientific Publications, London.
Baskett P J F, Diamond A W, Cochrane D F 1976 Urban mobile resuscitation training and service. *British Journal of Anaesthesia* **48**: 377–385
Bedall S E, Delbanco H L, Cook F, Epstein F H 1983 Survival after cardiopulmonary resuscitation in the hospital. *New England Journal of Medicine* **309**: 569–576
Bircher N, Safar P, Stuvert R 1980 A comparison of standard, MAST, augmented and open-chest CPR in dogs. *Critical Care Medicine* **8**: 147
Bircher N, Safar P 1981 Comparison of standard and 'New' closed chest CPR and open chest CPR in dogs. *Critical Care Medicine* **9**: 384–385
Bishop R L, Weisfeldt M L 1976 Sodium bicarbonate administration during cardiac arrest. *Journal of the American Medical Association* **235**: 506–509
Chamberlain D A, White N M, Binning R, Parker W S, Kimber E R 1973 Mobile coronary care provided by ambulance personnel. *British Heart Journal* **35**: 550
Chandra N, Rudikoff M T, Weisfeldt M L 1980 Simultaneous chest compression and ventilation at high airway pressure during cardiopulmonary resuscitation *Lancet* **i**: 175–178
Chandra N, Snyder L D, Weisfeldt M L 1981 Abdominal binding during cardiopulmonary resuscitation in man. *Journal of the American Medical Association* **246**: 351–353
Cobb L A 1983 The benefits of public education in a city wide resuscitation scheme. Abstract from proceedings of the International Conference on cardiopulmonary resuscitation, Rotterdam, p 12
Criley J H, Beaufuss A H, Kissel G L 1976 Cough induced cardiac compression. *Journal of the American Medical Association* **236**: 1246–1250
Crul J F, Bart T J, Meurseng B T J, Ariasin H E, Zimmerman K 1981 The ABC of CPR. Abstract of the 2nd world congress on emergency and disaster medicine, Pittsburgh USA, p 199
Dembo D H 1981 Calcium in advanced life support. *Critical Care Medicine* **9**: 358–359
Don M T A, Lambert E H, Mehran A 1968 Mouth-to-lung airway for cardiac resuscitation. *Lancet* **ii**: 1329
Eaton J M 1984 Adult manual resuscitators. *British Journal of Hospital Medicine* **31** 67–70
Gordon A S 1977 An improved esophageal obturator airway. In: Safar P, Elam J O (eds) Advances in cardio-pulmonary resuscitation. Springer-Verlag, New York
Hanson G C 1984 Cardiopulmonary resuscitation: chances of success (ed). *British Medical Journal* **288**: 1324–1325
Harber T, Lucas B G B 1980 An evaluation of some mechanical resuscitators. *Annals of the Royal College of Surgeons* **62**: 291–293
Harris L Kirimili B, Safar P 1967 Augmentation of artificial circulation during cardiopulmonary resuscitation. *Anesthesiology* **28**: 730
Health Equipment Information 1983 Evaluation issue. DHSS 1983 HE1, 111. DHSS, London
Heimlich H J 1974 Pop goes the café coronary. *Emergency Medicine* **6**: 154

Jacobson S 1983. In: Jacobsen S (ed) Current status of open chest procedures. Resuscitation.
  Clinics in emergency medicine, vol 2. Churchill Livingstone, New York, p 121–128
Jones R H 1983 Management of cardiac arrest in the community: a survey of resuscitation services. British
  Medical Journal 287: 968–971
Jude J R, Kouwenhoven W B, Knickerbocker C G 1961 Cardiac arrest: Report of application of external
  massage in 118 patients. Journal of The American Medical Association 178: 1063–1070
Jugarrao N S, Heber M, Grainger R, Vincent R, Chamberlain D A 1982 Use of an automated external
  defibrillator-pacemaker by ambulance staff. Lancet ii: 73–75
Kerber R E, Graygel J, Hoyt R, Marcus M, Kennedy J 1981 Transthoracic resistance in human
  defibrillation. Circulation 63: 676–682
Koch-Weser J 1979 Medical intelligence—bretylium. New England Journal of Medicine 300: 473–478
Kouwenhoven W B, Jude J R, Knickerbocker C G 1960 Closed-chest cardiac massage. Journal of the
  American Medical Association 173: 1064–1067
Laing G, Redmond A 1982. In: D H Wilson and A K Marsden (eds) Cardiac arrest—a new concept in the care
  of the acutely ill and injured. John Wiley and Son Ltd, Chichester, p 157–159
Lilja G P, Long R S, Ruiz E 1981 Augmentation of systolic blood pressure during external cardiac
  compression by use of the MAST suit. Annals of Emergency Medicine 10: 182
Lowenstein S R, Hansbrough J F, Libby L S, Hill D M, Mountain R D, Scroggin C G 1981
  Cardiopulmonary resuscitation by medical and surgical house officers. Lancet ii: 679–81
MacKenzie G J, Taylor S H, MacDonald A H, Donald K W 1964 Haemodynamic effects of external
  cardiac compression. Lancet i: 1342
Merrifield A J, King S J 1981 The oesophageal obturator airway. A study of cadaver lung ventilation
  through obturator airways and tracheal tubes. Anaesthesia 36: 672–695
Mirowski M, Redi P R, Watkins L, Weisfeldt M L, Mower M M 1981 Clinical treatment of life-threatening
  ventricular tachyarrhythmias with automatic implanted defibrillator. American Heart Journal 102:
  265–270
Montgomery W H 1983 Basic life support directions in the 1980s and an update on airway management. In:
  Jacobsen S (ed) Resuscitation. Clinics in emergency medicine, vol 2. Churchill Livingstone, New York,
  p 39–54
Negovsky V 1982 Reanimatology today. Some scientific and philosophical considerations. Critical Care
  Medicine 10: 130–136
Niemann J I, Rosborough J P, Hausknecht M, Garner D, Cridley J M 1981 Pressure synchronised
  cineangiography in resuscitation 64: 985–991
Redding J S, Haynes R R, Thomas J D 1981 'Old' and 'New' resuscitation manually performed. Critical
  Care Medicine 19: 165
Resnekov L 1981 Calcium antagonist drugs—myocardial preservation and reduced vulnerability to
  ventricular fibrillation during CPR. Critical Care Medicine 9: 360–361
The Resuscitation Council (United Kingdom) 1984 Resuscitation for the citizen. The Resuscitation Council
  (UK), Department of Anaesthetics, The Royal Postgraduate Medical School, Hammersmith Hospital, Du
  Cane Road, London W12 0HS
Rich S, Wix H L, Shapiro E P 1981 Clinical assessment of heart chamber size and valve motion during
  cardiopulmonary resuscitation by two dimensional echocardiography. American Heart Journal
  102: 373–376
Roberts J R, Greenberg M I, Baskin S I 1979 Endotracheal epinephrine in cardiopulmonary collapse.
  Journal of the American College of Experimental Pathology 8: 515–519
Rockoff M A, Shapiro H M 1978 Barbiturates following cardiac arrest: possible benefit of Pandora's box
  (editorial) 49: 385–387
Rogers M C, Weisfeldt M L, Trayston R S 1981 Cerebral blood flow during cardiopulmonary resuscitation
  (editorial). Anesthesia and Analgesia 60: 73–75
Rudikoff M T, Maughan W L, Effran M, Freund P, Weisfeldt M L 1980 Mechanisms of blood flow during
  cardiopulmonary resuscitation. Circulation 61: 345–352
Schweitzer P, Mark H 1980 The effect of atrophine on cardiac arrhythmias and conduction. American Heart
  Journal 100: 255–261
Smith T 1984 Death in the street. British Medical Journal 288: 738–739
Sowden G R, Baskett P J F, Robins D W 1984 Factors associated with survival and eventual cerebral status
  following cardiac arrest. Anaesthesia, in press
Standards for Cardiopulmonary Resuscitation (CPR) and Emergency Cardiac Care (ECC) 1974 Journal of
  the American Medical Association 227 (supplement): 833–868
Standards and Guidelines for Cardiopulmonary Resuscitation (CPR) and Emergency Cardiac Care (ECC)
  1980 Journal of the American Medical Association 244 (supplement): 453–509
Swartzman S, Wilson M A, Hoff B H, Bunegin L, Smith R B, Sjöstrand U 1984 Percutaneous transtracheal
  jet ventilation for cardiopulmonary resuscitation: evaluation of a new jet ventilator. Critical Care Medicine
  12: 8–13

The Times 1984 March 5. Training could save 2000 lives a year. (Nicholas Timmins, Social Services correspondent)

Vincent R, Martin B, Williams G, Quinn E, Robertson G, Chamberlain D A 1984 A community training scheme in cardiopulmonary resuscitation. *British Medical Journal* **288:** 617–20

Weaver W D, Cobb L A, Copass M K, Hallstrom A P 1982 Ventricular fibrillation—a comparative trial using 175 joule and 320 joule shocks. *New England Journal of Medicine* **307:** 1101–1106

Webb D D, Lambrew C T 1978 Evaluation of physician skills in cardiopulmonary resuscitation. *Journal of the American College of Emergency Physicians* **7:** 387–389

White B C, Winegar C D, Wilson R F, Hoehner P J, Trombley J H 1983 Possible role of calcium blockers in cerebral resuscitation: a review of the literature and synethesis for future studies. *Critical Care Medicine* **11:** 202–207

Yakaitis R W 1983 The pharmacology of cardiopulmonary resuscitation. In: Jacobsen S (ed) Resuscitation. *Clinics in emergency medicine, vol 2.* Churchill Livingstone, New York, p 69–82

Yakaitis R W, Thomas J D, Mahaffey J E 1975 Influence of pH and hypoxia on the success of defibrillation. *Critical Care Medicine* **3:** 139–42

Zideman D A 1983 Cardiopulmonary resuscitation: new methods or improved training? *Anaesthesia* **38:** 837–838

Appendix

L. Kaufman

Update from *Anaesthesia Review 2*

APPARATUS

Dinamap

The Dinamap 845 has recently been assessed by Hutton *et al* (1984). They compared the Dinamap, an apparatus designed to measure blood pressure by non-invasive means using oscillometry, with intra-arterial recordings. In the majority of cases they found that the Dinamap gave reasonable trends but at high pressures it under-reads the systolic and mean blood pressure and over-reads at low intra-arterial pressure. The diastolic blood pressure was consistently higher than that obtained by direct measurement. The apparatus also displays the heart rate which is consistent with that obtained from the e.c.g.

The authors felt that the changes in blood pressure using the Dinamap were too slow to be of value in monitoring patients when rapidly acting drugs such as sodium nitroprusside were used. The model tested was an earlier Dinamap but more recently improved models have been introduced.

Green *et al* (1984), in a similar study, compared the results obtained using a similar non-invasive blood pressure monitor (Sentron) with direct intra-arterial measurements. The correlation of the two techniques was better for systolic and mean pressures for adults compared with those of children. The diastolic pressures faired less well and the non-invasive diastolic pressure is higher in the adult compared with the invasive. In children the non-invasive measure was lower. The non-invasive mean blood pressure is nearly always lower than invasive whereas the non-invasive systolic pressure is always higher.

Volume meter

A volume meter for clinical use has been evaluated by Chakrabarti & Loh (1984). They found that the volume meter was simple and accurate to use in intensive care units but the initial outlay and replacement of the disposable sensors made it an expensive item. It was unaffected by oxygen concentration, humidity and temperature but its performance was influenced by high concentrations of nitrous oxide and when the diathermy was used.

Endotracheal tubes

In a recent study of the use of large volume, low pressure endotracheal tube cuffs, it was found that only the balloon of the Lanz tube could not be inflated beyond 27 cmH$_2$O. The cuffs of the other well-known makes of tubes could be inflated beyond 100 cmH$_2$O (Seegobin & Van Hasselelt 1984). A continuous lateral wall pressure above 30 cmH$_2$O reduces the capillary blood flow in the tracheal mucosa and it was recommended that a pressure gauge should be used to measure cuff pressure. However, it has been suggested that high volume, low pressure cuffs may not produce effective seals.*

Oxygen mask

Large reservoir venturi masks (vent mask) have been studied by Jones *et al* (1984). The masks with inspired oxygen concentrations of 24%, 28%, 35% and 40% were reasonably accurate but the 60% mask delivered 10% less than expected. They also advocated that the oxygen flow should be increased by 50% above the recommended flow rate when used with patients whose respiratory rate was greater than 30 per minute.

REFERENCES

Chakrabarti M K, Loh L 1984 Evaluation of Spirolog I volume meter. *Anaesthesia* **39:** 268–271
Green M, Paulus D A, Roan V P, Aa J V D 1984 Comparison between oscillometric and invasive blood pressure monitoring during cardiac surgery. *International Journal of Clinical Monitoring and Computing* **1:** 21–26
Hutton P, Dye J, Prys-Roberts C 1984 An assessment of the Dinamap 845. *Anaesthesia* **39:** 261–267
Jones H A, Turner S L, Hughes J M B 1984 Performance of the large-reservoir oxygen mask (ventimask). *Lancet* **i:** 1427–1431
Patel R I, Oh T H, Chandra R, Epstein B S 1984 Tracheal tube cuff pressure. *Anaesthesia* **39:** 862–864
Seegobin R D, Van Hasselt G L 1984 Endotracheal cuff pressure and tracheal mucosal blood flow: endoscopic study of effects of four large volume cuffs. *British Medical Journal* **288:** 965–968

*Patel *et al* (1984) advised the use of saline to inflate endotracheal tube cuffs to avoid the increase in cuff pressure and volume that occurs when nitrous oxide is used.

PHAEOCHROMOCYTOMA

Although the criteria for the diagnosis of phaeochromocytoma have been outlined in *Anaesthesia Review 1* and *2*, the tumour may present in novel, unusual and even exciting circumstances. Ducatman *et al* (1983) reported the simultaneous presentation of phaeochromocytoma in the right adrenal gland as well as a renal carcinoma on the same side. In another incident, during laparotomy for removal of a large, possible renal tumour, there was a dramatic fall in blood pressure when the tumour was excised. Although the patient had no symptoms suggestive of phaeochromocytoma and the investigations were negative, save for a slight increase in urinary homovanillic acid levels (HVA), a phaeochromocytoma was suspected when it was ascertained that blood replacement was adequate. There were no marked fluctuations of blood pressure even during manipulation of the tumour and this may be related to the anaesthetic technique, which involved the administration of intrathecal diacetyl morphine prior to surgical stimulation and the choice of atracurium as a muscle relaxant. Noradrenaline infusion (2 mg in 500 ml saline) restored the blood pressure: the patient was weaned off the drug within 3 hours. The tumour weighed 770 g and the diagnosis was confirmed by histology. (Personal series.)

Diagnosis

The diagnosis has often relied upon the excretion of catecholamine metabolites but, in an analysis of 64 patients, Stenstrom *et al* (1983) found the measurement of vanilmandelic acid (VMA) was often unreliable. The measurement of urinary adrenaline and noradrenaline was more helpful, although normal levels were found in patients with few attacks. Allison *et al* (1983) have confirmed that computerised tomography (CT) is the investigation of choice in locating the site of phaeochromocytoma and relegates the role of venous sampling of amines to the situation where the diagnosis is still in doubt or the tumour is ectopic or metastatic. Fiorica et al (1982), commenting on the variability of the absolute levels of catecholamines in the adrenal veins, showed that the adrenaline fraction of the total catecholamines secreted was approximately 60% in the adrenal vein draining a normal adrenal gland, but in the gland having a phaeochromocytoma the fraction fell to approximately 30%. This assumes that the secretion of noradrenaline predominates in phaeochromocytoma in the adrenal gland. Ackery et al (1984) have recently reported on the use of iodine-131-meta-iodobenzyl-guanadine, a guanathidine analogue similar to noradrenaline which is selectively taken up by an adrenergic storage vesicles. No adverse affects were observed and the technique had a clinical accuracy of 90%.

Neuropeptide Y (NPY) is a peptide found in the adrenal medulla and autonomic nerves. Adrian et al (1983) found an increased number of cells capable of producing this peptide in tumour tissue from phaeochromocytoma and ganglionneuroplastoma and that plasma NPY concentrations were raised from the normal of 55 pmol/1 to 460 pmol/1. This test affords an additional method of detecting catecholamine secreting tumours.

Management
The control of blood pressure during operation may be extremely difficult due to large amounts of catecholamine secreted when the tumour is manipulated. See *Review 2*. However, this problem does allow the opportunity for the elucidation of drug action on catecholamines. Prazosin, an α 1 receptor blocking agent, although successful in pre-operative management, proved ineffectual in the operative period, when the tumour was localised in the adrenal gland (Nicholson et al 1983). This effect might have been expected as Cubeddu et al (1982) commented on the value of prazosin when the tumours were predominately secreting noradrenaline.

The administration of a β adrenergic blocking drug, such as propranolol, is still fraught with danger, especially if given intravenously. Pulmonary oedema has been reported in an adrenal tumour presumably due to intense peripheral α mediated vasoconstriction (Sloand & Thompson 1984).

The use of labetalol, an α 1 and non-specific β adrenergic receptor blocking agent, has been reported by Rosei et al (1976) and Kaufman (1979). In a study in normotensive patients, Struthers (1983) showed that oral labetalol for 5 days prevented some of the haeomodynamic and metabolic effects of an infusion of adrenaline. These included preventing the cardiovascular action of the adrenaline as reflected by a rise in systolic pressure and a fall in diastolic blood pressure, preventing T wave flattening and QTC prolongation as well as inhibiting the fall in serum potassium level. In contrast, Lin et al (1983a) showed that intravenous labetalol given to hypertensive patients increased plasma levels of noradrenaline and this was linearly related to reduction in the mean arterial pressure. A similar action was noted with sodium nitroprusside. Labetalol apparently also prevents neuronal uptake of noradrenaline, which may explain why the plasma level of the amine is four times higher than that seen with sodium nitroprusside. In a similar study, Lin et al (1983b) compared the effects of hydralazine and sodium nitroprusside on plasma catecholamines and although the mode of action of these drugs differs there was an increase in heart rate related to the increase in plasma noradrenaline which was greater after hydralazine.

There is an increase in sympathetic activity in tetanus not dissimilar from that seen in phaeochromocytoma with hypertension, tachycardia and increased systemic vascular resistance. Domenighetti *et al* (1984) demonstrated that during the early phase of the disease the cardiovascular changes were related to an increase in plasma catecholamine concentrations and these readily responded to an intravenous infusion of labetalol.

The use of theophylline and related compounds may well be contraindicated in patients with catecholamine-secreting tumours (Vestal *et al* 1983). This study of the cardiovascular and metabolic effects in man showed an increase of 260% in plasma adrenaline levels and 64% in plasma noradrenaline levels.

REFERENCES

Ackery D M, Tippett P A, Condon B R, Sutton H E, Wyeth P 1984 New approach to the localisation of phaeochromocytoma: imaging with iodine-131-metaiodobenzylguanidine. *British Medical Journal* **288:** 1587–1591

Adrian T E, Allen J M et al 1983 Neuropeptide Y in phaeochromocytomas and ganglioneuroblastomas. Lancet **ii:** 540–542

Alison D J, Brown M J et al 1983 Role of venous sampling in locating a phaeochromocytoma. *British Medical Journal* **286:** 1122–1124

Cubeddu L X, Zarate N A et al 1982 Prazosin and propranol in preoperative management of phaeochromocytoma. *Clinical Pharmacology and Therapeutics* **32:** 156–160

Domenighetti G M, Savary B, Stricker H 1984 Hyperadrenergic syndrome in severe tetanus: extreme rise in catecholamines responsive to labetalol. *British Medical Journal* **288:** 1483–1484

Ducatman B S, Scheithauer J A, Van Heerden J A, Sheedy P F 1983 Simultaneous phaeochromocytoma and renal cell carcinoma: report of a case and review of the literature. *British Journal of Surgery* **70:** 415–418

Fiorica V, Galloway D C et al 1982 Epinephrine fraction of adrenal vein blood in phaeochromocytoma. *American Journal of the Medical Sciences* **284:** 9–15

Kaufman L 1979 Use of labetalol during hypotensive anaesthesia and in the management of phaeochromocytoma. *British Journal of Clinical Pharmacology* **8:** 229S–232S

Lin M-S, McNay J L, Shepherd A M M 1983a Response of plasma catecholamines to intravenous labetalol: a comparison with sodium nitroprusside. *Clinical Pharmacology and Therapeutics* **34:** 466–473

Lin M-S, 1983b Effects of hydralazine and sodium nitroprusside in plasma catecholamines and heart rate. *Clinical Pharmacology and Therapeutics* **34:** 474–480

Nicholson J P, Daracott Vaughn E et al 1983 Phaeochromocytoma and prazosin. *Annals of Internal Medicine* **99:** 477–479

Rosei E A, Brown J J et al 1976 Treatment of phaeochromocytoma and of clonidine withdrawal hypertension with labetalol. *British Journal of Clinical Pharmacology* **3:** 809S–818S

Sloand E M, Taylor Thompson B 1984 Propranolol-induced pulmonary edema and shock in a patient with phaeochromocytoma. *Archives of Internal Medicine* **144:** 173–175

Stenstrom G, Sjogren B, Waldenstrom J 1983 Excretion of adrenaline, noradrenaline, vanilmandelic acid and metanephrines in 64 patients with phaeochromocytoma. *Acta Medica Scandinavica* **214:** 145–152

Struthers A D, Whitesmith R, Reid J L 1983 Metabolic and haemodynamic effects of increased circulating adrenaline in man. Effect of labetolol, an α and β blocker. *British Heart Journal* **50:** 277–281

Vestal R E, Charles E et al 1983 Effect of intravenous aminophylline on plasma levels of catecholamines and related cardiovascular and metabolic responses in man. *Circulation* **67:** 162–171

ABDOMINAL ANAESTHESIA

The anaesthetic problems involved in the management of large bowel surgery have recently been reviewed (Kaufman 1983). The integrity of the intestinal anastomosis appears to be related to the blood supply of the mucosal layer of the colon and anaesthetic agents and techniques appear to have less influence than had previously been suggested. Flynn *et al* (1983) found that hypotension caused by multiple trauma following motor car accident or gun shot wounds resulted in necrosis of the right colon. The period of hypotension ranged from 30–200 minutes. The initial trauma did not damage the bowel which only became necrotic 2–4 days later.

The use of glycopyrrolate, which has a more profound and prolonged action than atropine, has been shown by Child (1984) to be less effective than atropine in preventing the increase in intraluminal pressure following injection of neostigmine.

A preliminary retrospective study (Sangwan S, personal communication) had failed to confirm an increase in anastomotic breakdown in patients having colonic surgery for diverticular disease. The use of drugs such as morphine and neostigmine said to have deleterious effect in these patients appears not to influence the fate of the intestinal anastomosis.

However, the use of atracurium, a new muscle relaxant which does not depend on enzyme activity for its destruction, has made the use of neostigmine almost superfluous. In a personal study of 150 patients submitted to large bowel surgery there were no cases of anastomotic breakdown that could be attributed to anaesthesia.

Lehr et al (1982) examined potassium in patients suffering from Crohn's disease. They found that the total body potassium deficit was reflected in the severity of the illness but there was no correlation with serum potassium levels. They recommended that 2 weeks prior to surgery the patients should receive a daily intake of 150–200 mmol of potassium.

The effect of β-adrenergic blocking drugs on the gastrointestinal system has been reviewed by Jacob et al (1983), including the effects of gastrointestinal activity, secretion, absorption and mucosal proliferation. They commented on the proliferative peritonitis seen following the use of practolol and also on the interaction between drugs such as propanolol and H_2 receptor anatagonists such as cimetidine. Cimetidine reduces liver blood flow and inhibits liver enzymes resulting in a reduction of clearance of propranolol. Use of intravenous β-blocking agents during the course of anaesthesia may result in an increase of intestinal activity (personal observation).

In animal studies, Fontaine et al (1984) suggested that there are two mechanisms affecting muscle tone and contractility. Tone could be increased with neurogenic cholinergic activity and local prostaglandin synthesis, which is opposed by non-adrenergic, non-cholinergic activity. The second mechanism involves stimulation of α 2 receptors. Mailman (1984) suggested that morphine may affect blood flow in the gut by an indirect action associated with the balance between acetylcholine and noradrenaline release on the intestinal mucosa.

REFERENCES

Child C 1984 Glycopyrrolate and the bowel. *Anaesthesia* **39:** 495

Flynn T C, Rowlands B J et al 1983 Hypotension-induced post-traumatic necrosis of the right colon. *American Journal of Medicine* **146:** 715–718

Fontaine J, Grivegnee A, Reuse J 1984 Andrenoceptors and regulation of intestinal tone in the isolated colon of the mouse. *British Journal of Pharmacology* **81:** 231–243

Jacob H. Brandt L J et al 1983 Beta-adrenergic blockade and the gastrointestinal system. *American Journal of Medicine* **74:** 1042–1051

Kaufman L 1983 Anaesthesia for large bowel surgery: a review. *Journal of the Royal Society of Medicine* **76:** 693–696

Lehr L, Schober O et al 1982 Total body potassium depletion and the need for preoperative nutritional support in Crohn's disease. *Annals of Surgery* **196:** 709–714

Mailman D 1984 Morphine-neural interactions on canine intestinal absorption and blood flow. *British Journal of Pharmacology* **81:** 263–270

ENFLURANE HEPATOTOXICITY

It has become an almost accepted practice not to repeat halothane anaesthesia within 28 days of a previous exposure to halothane. In some centres it is customary to administer enflurane instead during this period, assuming there would be no cross-sensitivity. However, Lewis et *al* (1983) have reported 24 cases of hepatitis associated with the use of enflurane presenting with a clinical picture not dissimilar to that seen following halothane or methoxyflurane. Postoperative fever and jaundice occurred in some patients who had been previously exposed to enflurane or halothane. Five patients died and the liver showed signs of centrilobular necrosis. The relatively low incidence of reported cases of enflurane hepatitis may be due to the fact that very little is metabolised compared with that of halothane or methoxyflurane. The ideal agent for repeated anaesthesia may be isoflurane, which has not been reported to cause liver damage and is resistant to biotransformation (see Eger 1982).

REFERENCES

Eger II E I 1982 Isoflurane (Aerrane). A compendium and reference. Eirco Inc.
Lewis J H, Hyman J *et al* 1983 Enflurane hepatotoxicity. *Annals of Internal Medicine* **98:** 984–992

ALTHESIN

Glaxo have voluntarily withdrawn the intravenous steroid anaesthetic, althesin. Concern was expressed regarding the solvent polyoxyethylated castor oil which has been associated with adverse reactions such as bronchospasm, hypotension, cardiac arrhythmias and cardiac arrest.

ENDOCRINE RESPONSE TO SURGERY

Studies on the endocrine response to surgery are still being undertaken with the introduction of newer techniques of assessment. Arterial plasma levels of adrenaline and noradrenaline have been measured revealing that enflurane anaesthesia is more effective than fentanyl and droperidol in suppressing the catecholamine response (Hamberger & Jarnberg 1983).

Rutberg *et al* (1984) studied the endocrine response to upper abdominal surgery comparing extradural bupivacaine and morphine with postoperative intravenous morphine. Pain relief was much better with either extradural morphine or bupivacaine but neither blocked the increased concentration of cortisol following the skin incision. Extradural analgesia with a local anaesthetic drug suppressed the increase in plasma catecholamines in the immediate postoperative period in contrast to the opiate, which was ineffectual. In the late postoperative period extradural morphine suppresses the endocrine response, presumably by providing pain relief. In another study, Campbell *et al* (1984) showed that plasma concentrations of cortisol and glucose increased during upper abdominal surgery and the hyperglycaemic response was greater in patients receiving halothane in contrast to those receiving fentanyl. In addition, plasma noradrenaline increased in those receiving halothane but did not increase significantly in patients receiving fentanyl. Plasma cortisol levels increased during intubation, but this could be prevented by the prior application of topical lignocaine (Lehtinen *et al* 1984).

Bovill *et al* (1983), found that sufentanil, an opiod 5–10 times more potent than fentanyl, was ineffectual in supressing the increased catecholamine concentration during cardiopulmonary bypass. Diazepam and fentanyl apparently decrease plasma adrenaline and noradrenaline levels, an effect not seen with fentanyl alone (Tomicheck *et al* 1983).

Walsh *et al* (1983) compared intravenous fluid regimes during surgery and found that there was little difference between Hartmann's solution and 0·9% sodium chloride. However, the use of 5% dextrose was associated with an increased hyperglycaemic response to surgical stimulation. The insulin level also increased demonstrating that intravenous dextrose can overcome the insulin suppression usually seen following surgery. Bent et al (1984) found that high dose fentanyl 50 μg per kg had little effect on the endocrine response to surgery if it were administered after the onset of the surgical stimulus. (Measurements included, blood glucose non-esterified fatty acids and cortisol.)

Blunnie et al (1983) compared fentanyl and spinal anaesthesia and found that the latter only partially suppressed the endocrine response and had no effect on the trauma of intubation. Fentanyl was more effective, but was accompanied by prolonged respiratory depression. In contrast, Asoh et al (1983) were able to demonstrate that epidural analgesia suppressed the endocrine response to major upper abdominal surgery. In a further study of upper abdominal surgery, Tsugi et al (1983) demonstrated that stimulation of the splanchnic nerves is responsible for producing the metabolic responses, even under epidural blockade. Some authorities maintain that suppression of the endocrine response to surgery is beneficial, especially on the negative nitrogen balance. In contrast, suppression of the response may be deleterious in patients with multiple injuries.

Medical disorders may also be responsible for endocrine changes. Plasma antidiuretic hormone (ADH) is raised in acute respiratory failure (Szatalowicz et al 1982). There are also changes in cor pulonale (Semple et al 1983). Caution must be exercised in the interpretation of increased levels of hormones during the course of anaesthesia as positive end-expiratory pressure ventilation may affect adrenal function (Priebe et al 1981) with an increase in plasma aldosterone and urinary ADH (Annat et al 1983).

REFERENCES

Annat G, Viale J P, Xuan B B et al 1983 Effect of PEEP ventilation on renal function, plasma renin, aldosterone, neurophysins and urinary ADH, and prostoglandins. Anesthesiology 58: 136–141

Asoh T, Tsuji H, Shirasaka C, Takeuchi Y 1983 Effect of epidural analgesia on metabolic reponse to major upper abdominal surgery. Acta Anaesthesiology Scandinavica 27: 233–237

Bent J M, Paterson J L, Mashiter K, Hall G M 1984 Effects of high-dose fentanyl anaesthesia on the established metabolic and endocrine response to surgery. Anaesthesia 39: 19–23

Blunnie W P, McIlroy D A, Merrett J C, Dundee J W 1983 Cardiovascular and biochemical evidence of stress during major surgery associated with different techniques of anaesthesia. British Journal of Anaesthesia 55: 611–617

Bovill J G, Sebel P S, Fiolet W T, Touber L, Kok K, Philbin D M 1983 The influence of sufentanil on endocrine responses to cardiac surgery. Anesthesia and Analgesia 62: 391–387

Campbell B C, Parikh K R, Naismith A, Sewnauth D, Reid J L 1984 Comparison of fentanyl and halothane supplementation to general anaesthesia on the stress response in upper abdominal surgery. British Journal of Anaesthesia 56: 257–266

Hamberger B, Jarnberg P O 1983 Plasma catecholamines during surgical stress: differences between neurolept and enflurane anaesthesia. Acta Anaesthesiology Scandinavica 27: 307–310

Lehtinen A M, Hovorka J et al 1984 Effect of intrathecal lignocaine halothane and thiopentone on changes in plasma β-endorphin immunoreactivity in response to tracheal intubation. British Journal of Anaesthesia 56: 247–250

Priebe H, Heiman J C, Hedley-Whyte J 1981 Mechanisms of renal dysfunction during positive end-expiratory pressure ventilation. Journal of Applied Physiology: Respiratory, Environmental and Exercise Physiology 50: 643–649

Rutberg H, Hakanson E et al 1984 Effects of the extradural administration of morphine, or bupivacaine, on the endocrine response to upper abdominal surgery. British Journal of Anaesthesia 56: 233–238

Semple P, Watson W S, Beastall G H, Hume R 1983 Endocrine and metabolic studies in unstable cor pulmonale. Thorax 38: 45–49

Szatalowicz V L, Jan P, Goldberg J, Anderson R J 1982 Plasma antiduretic hormone in acute respiratory failure. American Journal of Medicine 72: 583–587

Tomicheck R C, Rosow C E, Philbin D M, Moss J, Teplick R S, Schneider R C 1983 Diazepam—fentanyl interaction—hemodynamic and hormonal effects in coronary artery surgery. Anesthesia and Analgesia 62: 881–884

Tsugi H, Shirasaka C, Asoh T, Takeuchi Y 1983 Influences of splanchnic nerve blockade on endocrine-metabolic responses to upper abdominal surgery. *British Journal of Surgery* **70**: 437–439

Walsh E S, Traynor C, Paterson J L, Hall G M 1983 Effect of different intraoperative fluid regimens on circulating metabolites and insulin during abdominal surgery. *British Journal of Anaesthesia* **55**: 135–140

Owen H, Spence A A 1984 Etomidate. *British Journal of Anaesthesia* **56**: 556–557.

ETOMIDATE

Infusion of etomidate was reported to result in adrenocorticol insufficiency with profound hypotension, hyponatraemia and hyperkalaemia (Fellows *et al* 1983). Wagner *et al* (1984) reported that a 20-hour infusion of etomidate caused adrenocortical suppression for 4 days after the drug had been stopped. 17-α and 11-β hydroxylase activity is suppressed within the adrenal gland leading to depressed production of cortisol. aldosterone and corticosterone (see Owen & Spence 1984).

There have been conflicting reports on the use of etomidate for intravenous induction. Wagner *et al* (1984) found there was adrenal suppression for 4 hours after surgery, but they administered incremental doses during the operation. Duthie *et al* (1984) concluded that a bolus induction dose of etomidate caused no significant adrenocortical suppression while Yeoman *et al* (1984) found there was a significant reducion in the cortisol response to surgery.

REFERENCES

Duthie D J R, Fraser R, Nimmo W S 1984. The effect of induction of anaesthesia by etomidate on corticosteroid synthesis in man. *British Journal of Anaesthesia* **56**: 1292

Fellows I W, Bastow M D, Byrne A J, Allison S P 1983 Adrenocortical suppression in multiply injured patients: a complication of etomidate treatment. *British Medical Journal* **287**: 1835–1838

Owen H, Spence A A 1984 Etomidate. *British Journal of Anaesthesia* **56**: 556–557

Wagner R L, White P F, Kan P B, Rosenthal M H, Feldman D 1984 Inhibition of adrenal steroidgenesis by the anesthetic etomidate. *New England Journal of Medicine* **310**: 1415–1421

Yeoman P M, Fellows I W, Byrne A J, Selby C 1984 The effect of anaesthetic induction using etomidate upon pituitary-adrenocortical function. *British Journal of Anaesthesia* **56**: 1291

Index